HEALTH OF THE SEVENTH CAVALRY

HEALTH OF THE SEVENTH CAVALRY

A Medical History

Edited by
P. WILLEY and DOUGLAS D. SCOTT

UNIVERSITY OF OKLAHOMA PRESS: NORMAN

Also by P. Willey and Douglas D. Scott
(and Melissa A. Connor) *They Died with Custer: Solders' Bones from the Battle of the Little Bighorn* (Norman, Okla., 1998)

Library of Congress Cataloging-in-Publication Data

Health of the Seventh Cavalry : a medical history / edited by P. Willey and Douglas D. Scott.
p. ; cm.
Includes bibliographical references and index.
ISBN 978-0-8061-4839-7 (hardcover : alk. paper)
I. Willey, Patrick S., editor II. Scott, Douglas D., editor
[DNLM: 1. United States. Army. Cavalry, 7th. 2. Military Personnel—history—United States. 3. Occupational Health—history—United States. 4. History, 19th Century—United States. 5. Military Medicine—history—United States. WA 11 AA1]
RC971
616.9′8023—dc23
2015009037

The paper in this book meets the guidelines for permanence and durability of the Committee on Production Guidelines for Book Longevity of the Council on Library Resources, Inc. ∞

1 2 3 4 5 6 7 8 9 10

In memory of Clyde Collins Snow (1928–2014),
whose pioneering work with the Little Bighorn archaeological
skeletons and Seventh Cavalry documents launched our
study of the illness and health of the men with Custer

Contents

Illustrations

Figures

Maps

Tables

Preface and Acknowledgments

The words "Seventh Cavalry" conjure images in nearly any listener. Depending on the person, the pictures summoned may be diametrically opposed—one involving hero soldiers, the other evoking depredators of traditional American Indians. Whichever image comes to mind, it involves officers and troopers who were healthy, fit, and battle ready. Both concepts view the troopers as illness-free and injury-free—at least until their ultimate moments in battle. As often happens, however, reality is much more complex—and far more interesting—than stereotypes.

In earlier works we assessed other myths based on material evidence, contrasting it with documents and other hearsay interpretations. We employed relics found scattered across the battlefields at the Little Bighorn, Yellowstone, and Washita and studied human skeletons from the Little Bighorn. In some instances, our results diverged from or elaborated upon the historic platitudes and myths. In other cases, they supported written documents. We argued from the materials, indicating how they supported, conflicted with, or elaborated historic documents. In the present work we take the opposite stance. We examine how medical documents expand previous understanding of the Seventh Cavalry.

The Seventh Cavalry serves as a proxy for other regiments serving in the post–Civil War period in many ways, although diverging from the norm in others. So when studying the Seventh Cavalry we present not only a more accurate and realistic perspective for that regiment but a model to which other regiments of the period can be compared.

Doug and P. first met fifty summers ago, working as teenaged archaeologists in Elk City Reservoir, southeast Kansas. It required us an additional twenty-five years to be introduced again and reestablish that earlier meeting. A few more years passed before our first substantive collaboration, involving skeletons from the Little Bighorn.

While conducting that research, Doug found medical documents concerning troopers who died at the Little Bighorn and we cursorily reported them. We realized that those medical records held much more information than we could handle then and vowed to pursue them when time permitted. As starry-eyed, overly confident buffoons, we planned to collect and compare the Seventh Cavalry illnesses with those of the Seventh Infantry, demonstrating the impact of occupational specialties on illnesses and injuries. We anticipated that this work would take one or perhaps two years. Even more optimistically, we imagined assessing the health experience of a black regiment to contrast with the white regiment. Now, fourteen years later, we must leave those intriguing but undone comparisons for others to reconnoiter. The present work deals with the Seventh Cavalry alone and is mostly descriptive and explorative.

One idea that persists from the time when we started this work a decade ago is that the illnesses hold enormous insights into life during the post–Civil War period. Now that we are balding and bent (but not broken), our work dealing with the Seventh Cavalry remains more fun than even two teenagers fifty years ago could have imagined.

Over the years, others have joined us in this pursuit. We introduce these relative newcomers, the contributors to this work, in roughly chronological order.

Gary Plank worked with Doug in Lincoln, Nebraska, for decades. His expertise in behavioral psychology, profiling, and insights into Post–Traumatic Stress Disorder demonstrated possible suffering of nineteenth-century Seventh Cavalry combat survivors.

Katie Cohan matriculated at Chico State in fall 2008, working toward a master's degree in anthropology. For her thesis, she undertook a topic that seems tangential to the Seventh Cavalry—human skin pigmentation adaptation. As part of that labor, however, she elucidated a threat that nagged post–Civil War Seventh Cavalry troopers, especially those stationed on the northern plains: frostbite. Her thesis on Seventh Cavalry frostbite won the title of college-level best thesis for 2012. We still believe that she was robbed when the institution gave the overall Chico State's thesis of the year award to someone else.

Our work with Patrick J. Collison, a physician practicing in Yankton, South Dakota, began in February 2009. He and P. met then at the University of South Dakota. A man of many interests and more than considerable energy, Pat adopted the Seventh Cavalry project with relish. Initially he concentrated on his medical specialty—otolaryngology. He quickly agreed to expand his contributions to other areas, including nineteenth-century medicine, military nosology, lower respiratory ailments, and medical terms. We cannot overstate his many contributions to this work.

Billy Markland of Kansas City, Kansas, came into the fold in 2010 when he and Doug met at Fort Leavenworth. Coincidentally, Seventh Cavalry companies formed there in 1866, many were stationed at Fort Leavenworth, and some of the Seventh Cavalry officers killed at the Little Bighorn lie in the national cemetery there. Billy generously offered his western frontier military death database, painstakingly transcribed from original and microfilm records. It contained information on regulars who died on the western frontier from 1848 through 1891, never before assembled in a usable manner. In the present work we have barely scratched the wealth of information that his treasure trove provides. It contains many potential research avenues, which are sure to be valuable to future researchers, thanks to Billy's tireless efforts in transcribing and proofing.

Colleen Milligan arrived at Chico State in fall 2010 with her PhD diploma in hand to undertake teaching four courses a semester, directing the Certificate in Forensic Identification program, and shouldering the considerable labor of forensic cases that the Human Identification Laboratory receives. In her spare time she conducted research. She graciously agreed to contribute a portion of her dissertation for this effort. It provided a different perspective on nineteenth-century health and illness than the one revealed by the Seventh Cavalry. Her contribution involved illness and deaths of midwestern urban civilians of both sexes and all ages in the post–Civil War years and into the early twentieth century. It provided an interesting contrast to the largely young adult all-male Seventh Cavalry data set that we assembled.

Kristina Zarenko, then a graduate student at Chico State, spent the summer there in 2013—no mean feat considering the thermometer-popping temperatures that the region endures. Rather than addressing high temperatures, however, she targeted another summer scourge, which attacked the Seventh Cavalry: malaria-ridden mosquitoes. As her work progressed, she invited her roommate, graduate student Colleen Cheverko, to participate. Now both Kristina and Colleen have completed their master's degrees and moved to doctoral programs elsewhere. May all graduate cohorts and living arrangements be so productive and fruitful!

We are extremely grateful to all of our contributors as well as the many other people who made this effort possible. We cannot adequately express our appreciation for their guidance while gathering information, researching, and writing this book. This brief note acknowledging them in approximate sequence of contact will have to suffice as gratitude for the invaluable aid that they provided.

David Philour and Tony Dunn, Chico State, offered database insights and sage statistical advice. Chico State's College of Behavioral and Social Sciences awarded P. leaves (spring 2001, academic years 2004–2005, 2008–2009, and 2012–13) that permitted transcribing the Seventh Cavalry's carded medical records at the National Archives and Record Administration (NARA), establishing a list of Seventh Cavalry troopers from the period, analyzing those data, and completing draft manuscripts. Chico State's Anthropology Department supported those leaves, despite the administrative and logistical inconveniences that they caused. Our sincere gratitude goes to the department and college for their conviction that this research was not yet another promise made to escape onerous teaching and committee assignments, with little likelihood or intention of fruition.

George Thompson, then of Chico State's Interlibrary Loan, turned somersaults to locate hard-to-find publications in other libraries. Other interlibrary loan staff members at Merriam Library,

Chico State, and Love Library, University of Nebraska–Lincoln, also immensely aided our research.

Dan Tyree, then a Chico State graduate student, now a faculty member at Monroe Community College, Rochester, New York, carefully extracted and transcribed Seventh Cavalry enlistment information. Supporting his labor, the Family History Center, Latter Day Saints, Chico, lent him a microfilmed version of the Register of Enlistment in the U.S. Army from their Church Library as well as a microfilm reader and desk, which they moved to his apartment.

The graduate-level seminar in physical anthropology in the fall semester of 2002 made P. rethink issues associated with this project and stimulated insights into diseases, especially infectious ones. In addition, the several months spent stationed at a forward operating base in northern Iraq in 2004 afforded firsthand experience in some of the challenges that the Seventh Cavalry faced on the post–Civil War Great Plains. Parallels included unpredictable potential hostile action and how rapidly infections spread in a small outpost. In the twenty-first century, contagions occurred despite immunizations and antibiotics, hand washing before all meals, and twenty-four-hour health care. Woe to the poor nineteenth-century Seventh Cavalry troopers lacking such advantages!

Many thanks are due to staff members at the NARA Research Room for service in delivering archival materials. In addition, NARA archivists Michael Musick (retired) and DeAnne Blanton generously offered information concerning records and directions for their use. And P.'s cohort of NARA Research Room "inmates" provided support and encouragement, especially Harold D. Langley, Thomas and Beverly Lowry, and Charles Ritter.

Paul Sledzik and Lore Barbian, then at the National Museum of Health and Medicine, Washington, D.C., shared information and insights concerning nineteenth-century illnesses and treatments. Brian Spatola of the same institution and an anonymous peer reviewer of the book's manuscript provided suggestions for improvement and much-needed encouragement and support.

Housing for the months-long stays while transcribing records in Washington, D.C., was generously provided by friends Lynn Snyder (summer 2001) and Doug Ubelaker (summer 2004).

John A. Doerner (chief historian, retired), Little Bighorn Battlefield National Monument, noted the intriguing case of Private John Fay's insanity. His observation launched our effort to associate symptoms like those of Post–Traumatic Stress Disorder with members of the Seventh Cavalry.

Richard L. Jantz, University of Tennessee, contributed statistical advice that even dummies could—and did—comprehend. Eric Bartelink, Chico State anthropologist, provided aid concerning chart production. With their vast store of knowledge, Michael Magliari (Chico State historian) and other members of Friends of the Nineteenth Century West (Chico Chapter) and Douglas McChristian, Jerome Greene, and Paul Hedren (all retired from the National Park Service) offered help and understanding of the nineteenth-century Indian Wars army.

Cartographic and graphic artist-in-residence Judy Stolen drew or revised the maps, corrected many of the figures, and produced the Post–Traumatic Stress Disorder time line (fig. 12.1).

Charles Rankin and his staff at the University of Oklahoma Press were a pleasure to work with—as always. In particular, we thank Rowan Faye Steineker, who held our hands early in the production process; Emily Jerman Schuster, who laughed at our second-rate humor; and Kathy Lewis, whose sharp pencil and sharper editorial eye made this work a better creation.

Judy Stolen and Melissa Connor, our respective spouses and consummate professionals in their own fields, gave us much support and advice over the years. We owe them a great deal more than can be said here.

Introduction

Douglas D. Scott and P. Willey

The larger-than-life image of George Armstrong Custer and the Seventh U.S. Cavalry has launched hundreds of published works about the man, his soldiers, and the famed Battle of the Little Bighorn. One outcome is that the Seventh Cavalry is one of the best researched and documented units in U.S. Army history. In the volume *They Died with Custer*, we studied the bones of the men who died at the Little Bighorn on June 25 and 26, 1876, which were recovered during professional archaeological investigations. In the course of that work, the medical records of those troopers who participated in the battle were examined and compared to the physical remains of the dead, placing those men's lives and deaths in the larger context of life in the nineteenth century (Scott et al. 1998). Comparisons with works on the Indian Wars army suggested that the men of the Seventh Cavalry represented a cross section of the men who joined the army as a whole. Consequently, the well-studied story of the Seventh Cavalry and its men makes it an ideal exemplar to delve into the history of medicine and health in the nineteenth-century U.S. Army. In addition, the Seventh Cavalry provides a proxy and a model for the aggregate of men who served in the post–Civil War army.

Building on the work of Scott et al. (1998) and others (including Collison 2011; MacLean 2011; Stevenson 2012; Winkler 2013), this endeavor employs multiple lines of evidence to assess the health of the men of the Seventh not just at the time of the Battle of the Little Bighorn but from 1866, when the unit was organized, to 1884. This period includes the Seventh's first recruiting efforts, its early battles, the range of its stations in the central and southern plains, its role in reconstruction of the post–Civil War South, and its assignments on the northern plains. Intersecting many disciplines and specialties (history, health and illness, medicine, human biology, epidemiology, and human osteology), this work provides insights into the health, disease, and trauma that the men of the Seventh Cavalry experienced during those two decades.

The Civil War constitutes the most pivotal period in U.S. history in terms of casualties, mass mobilization, and economic change. Arms and munitions outstripped tactics, resulting in catastrophic battle losses. Mobilization had even more devastating effects. When men assembled in large aggregates with interpersonal contact and exposure to unhygienic camp conditions, circumstances proved ripe for the spread of infectious diseases, which killed more soldiers than all Civil War battles combined.

After the Civil War, most civilian-soldiers returned to communities, families, and their civilian occupations. Some soldiers and sailors, particularly those in regular units, remained in the military. Others completed their enlistments and were discharged, replaced by new recruits. Just as changes in personnel took place after the Civil War, the army's postwar tasks differed from those of the war itself.

The army's assignments after the Civil War were twofold. Its first task was to attempt to control American Indians on the western frontier, rendering the West safe for railroads, settlement, and economic development. The other assignment involved occupying the South, establishing civil rule, pursuing moonshiners, and limiting the influence of the Ku Klux Klan and other segregation-oriented groups. Consequently, the late-nineteenth-century army has been characterized as more of a large police force than a defensive deterrent (Utley 1973; Coffman 1986; Tate 1999). The Seventh Cavalry served in both regions and undertook both assignments (see chapter 1).

The Seventh Cavalry was selected for this study both for its uniqueness among military units and for its commonalities with them. The Seventh's uniqueness derives from its experience in many battles and its glamorous leader. The battles and skirmishes that the Seventh fought increased the number of deaths in action and members dying of wounds compared to those in other regiments. Nevertheless, the Seventh provides a cross section of a typical regiment in the post–Civil War period. Similarities between the Seventh and other regiments include the demography of the enlisted men, their stations, and their duties (Rickey 1963; Coffman 1986; Agnew 2008; Adams 2009; Johnson 2012).

In addition to offering a specific study of the men of the Seventh Cavalry, this book provides a broad understanding of the medical knowledge and practice of the era. Patrick J. Collison develops the topic of the history of medicine and medical practice in chapter 2, but some background is summarized here for context.

In the mid- to late nineteenth century, medical professionals generally treated patients based on one of two prevailing paradigms: miasmatists thought that invisible airborne poisons caused diseases, while contagionists believed that infectious entities spread by contact or vapors caused diseases (Trostle 1986). The physician's goal was to identify the illness and treat ailments with an appropriate course of action, adhering to the Hippocratic oath to do no harm.

In the second half of the nineteenth century, the health disciplines were in competition with each other: the "eclectics" versus the homeopaths. Eclectics embraced formal scientific training and the use of botanical remedies; they opposed traditionally trained physicians and homeopaths. Homeopaths, in contrast, interpreted disease as being primarily an ailment of the spirit, not the physical body. They employed the "law of similar": diseases were cured by administering drugs that induced symptoms in the sick like those in people who were well. Medicines were generally given in minute doses (Starr 1982:96–97). In addition to these two competing groups, botanic physicians (irregulars) emphasized the use of plants as medicines (Freemon 1998:230). Although all these disciplines relied on nonscientific theoretical bases, they largely eschewed toxic drugs and the bleeding or bloodletting that traditional physicians ("allopathics," as the homeopathists called them) practiced as part of their "heroic" steps (Bollet 2002:57).

Heroic treatments involved bleeding patients (through the use of leeches and venesection) and purging with cathartics and enemas.

While these practices were once mainstream in the antebellum era, heroic treatments became infrequent by the time of the Civil War, at least among major medical sects (Bollet 2002:250–52). Technological developments in medicine increased while the heroic treatments declined.

These technological developments during the 1800s included the evolution of new instruments. The stethoscope was developed in the 1820s, the compound microscope in the 1830s, the ophthalmoscope and laryngoscope in the 1850s, the microtome in the 1860s, and thermometers and tissue staining in the 1870s. These advances provided foundations for better understanding the human body and its internal workings (Trostle 1986:39; Bollet 2002:64–70). At the same time, the growth of knowledge about pathogens as the cause of infection and the development of anesthetics and antiseptics produced new methods and treatments of disease and trauma.

The Civil War caused enormous numbers of casualties from combat and disease. Although some authorities (Dean 1997) dispute the quality and improvement of medical practice that occurred during the Civil War, positive steps did reduce the death rate and advance medical knowledge. For instance, the army's surgeon general created well-organized hospitals and standardized treatment procedures during the war. Ambulances, steamships, and railroads proved critical for moving invalids great distances. A system for handling enormous numbers of casualties—including a hierarchy of hospitals and the use of ambulances and female nurses (building on Florence Nightingale's contributions during the Crimean War)—was well established by the end of the war. Bleeding and cupping were abandoned as treatments early in the war. Surgical procedures were developed and refined (Freemon 1998:202); delicate surgeries like trephanation were carried out with reasonable success. In addition, neurological diseases were beginning to be understood in greater detail. Among other new treatments developed during the war was the administration of quinine, which not only mitigated the symptoms of malaria but prevented it when administered daily (Freemon 1998:202). During the Civil War, Union physicians also began the transition from using Latin names for diseases to using their English names.

William Alexander Hammond, surgeon general of the Union Army, established the Army Medical Museum, a collection of medical disease and trauma specimens, with Major John H. Brinton as the museum's first curator. He cited a familiar adage, noting that "there was something in the notion that 'even dry bones may live'" (Brinton 1896:601).

Following the lead of the British publication *Medical and Surgical History of British Forces in Turkey and Crimea*, Hammond also made efforts to collate and publish the medical reports, records, and statistics that flooded his office. Even the title of the U.S. publication echoed the British title: *Medical and Surgical History of the War of Rebellion*, published in six volumes between 1870 and 1888. J. J. Woodward supervised the medical section and George Otis the surgical section (Freemon 1998:200). John Shaw Billings developed and expanded the surgeon general's library and established *Index Medicus* (Freemon 1998:200). Today that library is the core of the National Institute of Health's immense medical library.

In the decades after the war scientists and physicians identified the importance of microorganisms and thereby reduced deaths. Joseph Lister's discovery of antisepsis for sterile surgical fields was made in the 1870s. But the germ theory of disease was not accepted until after the Battle of the Little Bighorn, and materials for implementation became available only later. Disease agents for afflictions such as leprosy and anthrax were identified in the 1870s. The causes of typhoid, tuberculosis, cholera, and diphtheria were identified in the 1880s, the causes of plague and malaria in the 1890s, and the causes of pertussis, syphilis, and epidemic typhus by 1910. Nutritional deficiencies associated with disease and vitamins were not identified until 1920 (Trostle 1986:48).

In developing the story of the Seventh Cavalry's health, we have taken an anthropological approach to the study of human biology. Many of the data on the human medical condition are drawn from historic documents. Human biologists usually study populations of living humans from an evolutionary perspective. Most often they travel into the field and engage living subjects to gather information. Use of archival materials (written or printed sources about past populations) has a history in itself and is increasing among biological anthropologists (Swedlund and Herring 2003; Mitchell 2011).

Earlier anthropological studies using historic documents incorporate census and vital records to understand population structure, migration, birth and death rates, epidemiology, and genetic components. Groups studied have included indigenous peoples, criminals, military recruits, "old" families, and schoolchildren, as well as those living in almshouses (Higgins 2003) and insane asylums (Phillips 2003). The reasons for this development include the potential to extend our understanding of biological diversity and processes into the historic past.

One organization other than the Census Bureau that established and retained extraordinary records is the military. Military documents associated with nineteenth-century enlistment and medical records provide a perspective on who the average soldier was and what diseases he suffered from in the Indian Wars era. Today, of course, the anthropometry and physiology of recruits have been much studied. Demographic and medical data have been collected and analyzed since World War II and increasingly today. The goal has often been to understand how the body functions under stressful conditions. That research has resulted in better-designed uniforms and equipment and more effective educational and training regimes. But more germane to this study, it provided information to analyze questions related to human biology.

Economic historians use stature as a proxy of general well-being—especially in relation to nutrition and health—in addition to representing economic prosperity. In many cases, stature data come from military records. Such studies include Polish military conscripts born in 1957 (Bielicki and Welon 1982), stature of antebellum West Point cadets (Komlos 1984) as an indicator of class and social status, eighteenth-century Austrian Hapsburg soldiers (Komlos 1989), eighteenth- and early-nineteenth-century Irish and British recruits (Steegman 1985; Mokyr and Grada 1994), eighteenth-century French and Indian War soldiers (Steegman and Haseley 1988), and of course the Seventh U.S. Cavalry at the time of the Little Bighorn (Snow and Fitzpatrick 1989; Scott et al. 1998).

In addition to written documents, skeletons provide information about past soldiers, generally limited to basic information such as age, height, ancestry, injuries, and diseases. Human skeletons from military sources include those found at Fort William Henry, dating to the French and Indian Wars, which offered insights into the trauma suffered by the besieged British soldiers as well as their overall health and diet (Steegman 1986; Baker and Liston 1995; Liston and Baker 1995, 1996). Fort Laurens (1778–79), located about eighty miles south of Cleveland, Ohio, yielded human remains of the Revolutionary War period that revealed much about their lives and deaths, indicating that the deaths resulted from accidents and Indian attacks. The skeletons showed that rations were few and of poor quality. In addition, the effects of traveling through the frontier, building a fort, and surviving the winter were hard on the people who died there (Sciulli and Gramly 1989).

Skeletal remains from nineteenth-century wars have also been studied, including those from the War of 1812 site Snake Hill in Canada (Pfeiffer and Williamson 1991) and of Mexicans killed in 1846 at the Battle of Resaca de la Palma in Brownsville, Texas (Ratliff 1993; Wescott et al. 2012). The American Civil War generated many skeletal series, such as the Confederate dead from Glorieta Pass, New Mexico (Owsley 1994), African American troops buried on Folly Island, South Carolina (Rathbun and Smith 1997), and Union remains from Wilson's Creek, Missouri (Willey, Leach, and Grimstead 1999; Willey, Tyree, et al. 2003). Illegal looting of the Fort Craig, New Mexico, cemetery led to a full-scale professional recovery effort. It resulted in the recovery of remains of soldiers and civilians from the antebellum era and amputated limbs from the Civil War Battle of Val Verde as well soldier and civilian remains from the Indian Wars. The Fort Craig cemetery investigations provided new insights into burial practices and the human condition during a thirty-year period (Hanson and Greenwald 2004; Goff n.d.). In the post–Civil War period, the best-known skeletal study is from the Little Bighorn (Snow and Fitzpatrick 1989; Scott et al. 1998). Military dentition from the late nineteenth century has also been studied (Sledzik and Moore-Jansen 1991). These many studies have enhanced our understanding of the lives and deaths of the soldiers.

A telling statement (Sledzik and Sandberg 2002:189) sums up the findings from a study of soldiers' remains in a succinct and poignant manner: instead of taking youths and building men, as militaries have claimed in more recent times, “In the past, they took young men and built physical wrecks.”

Building on these works and expanding the scope to document both change and continuity of health in the Seventh Cavalry, we employ a variety of archival data, including Enlistment Records, Monthly Regimental Returns, and Carded Medical Records. Each record set was established and maintained for various purposes, none of which included a twenty-first-century investigation of health and illness. But they serve the present study well. In the following chapters, we present the results of this broad-based anthropological and epidemiological approach to the study of health and disease in the Seventh Cavalry.

We provide historical and medical contexts for the Seventh Cavalry in the post–Civil War period by using the regiment’s structure, organization, postings, and actions from 1866 to 1884. A discussion of nineteenth-century medical practice and treatment as well as the theory and nature of disease provides a historic context for the Seventh’s medical history. In addition, we examine the structure of disease categories as defined by the nineteenth-century military to place the medical records in a fundamental context.

The soldiers’ backgrounds and illnesses also must be understood. The methods used here required transcribing and interpreting the Monthly Enlistment Records, Monthly Regimental Returns, and Carded Medical Records. We provide descriptive summaries of the Seventh Cavalry troopers’ birthplaces, enlistment ages, heights, occupations, and final ranks. Diseases are documented by their frequencies, dates, and geographic distributions.

With this foundation established, we offer detailed analyses of specific diseases. These ailments include problems of the ear, nose, and throat, lower respiratory troubles, malaria, sexually transmitted infections, cold and other injuries, and Post–Traumatic Stress Disorder (PTSD, a diagnostic category not established until a hundred years later).

The final section of this book places the Seventh Cavalry’s illnesses and trauma in broader contexts by comparing them with three other sources. One such source is paleopathological analyses of Seventh Cavalry skeletons from the Battle of the Little Bighorn. This comparison shows with some exceptions that few of the documented Seventh Cavalry illnesses appear in the skeletons. Second, historic documents on military frontier deaths are summarized and compared to mortality in the Seventh Cavalry. The goal is to build a model of army lifeways and the effect of disease and to elucidate the frequency of accidental and combat deaths suffered by the men of the U.S. Army during the height of the American Indian Wars and their sojourns on the frontier. Finally, we examine a somewhat later nonmilitary urban group to place the specialized nature of the Seventh Cavalry's illnesses in a broader social and health context.

HEALTH OF THE SEVENTH CAVALRY

CHAPTER 1

Seventh Cavalry Regimental History

Douglas D. Scott

Following the Civil War, many and marked changes were afoot for the military. The U.S. military turned from suppressing the rebellion to implementing Reconstruction of the South. In addition, the military brought change to the frontier and stability along the Mexican border and the Rio Grande. Many of these locations were distant from the East and South, where military attention had focused during the Civil War.

Because there was no longer a need for an enormous military, the army was reduced to a peacetime size. The decrease in the size of the force resulted in many career officers being reduced from their Civil War ranks to lower permanent grades. In some ways this reduction in forces dashed the hopes of numerous wartime officers who pursued promotion through the ranks. But as Robert Utley (1967:342) noted, the post–Civil War army was a peacetime army in name and strength only. There were many skirmishes and battles to be fought. And many commanders turned their attention and forces, which had previously subjugated the Confederacy, to dealing with the hostile Indians of the plains and the West in general.

Despite wide and varied duties, including suppressing hostilities on the plains, the primary responsibility of the post–Civil War military was keeping peace, what Edward Coffman (1986:328) called "the army's frontier constabulary phase." Previous military functions in the West included exploration and mapping. During the Civil War, most of the U.S. military had withdrawn from the frontier for engagement in the East and South. In part as a consequence of their absence, unrest on the frontier increased. The numbers of Indians in the West was telling. Of the 270,000 Indians there at the end of the Civil War, 100,000 were considered hostile (Coffman 1986:254). In the three decades that followed the Civil War, the Seventh was involved in more than forty fights with various Indian tribes, frequently involving the Sioux, Cheyennes, Comanches, Kiowas, and Arapahos (Garlington 1896:252). Most of these engagements were skirmishes, but several were major battles, the best-known being the Battle of the Little Bighorn.

When the Civil War concluded, the army had two new roles: policing the Reconstruction efforts of the Republican administration and restoring order on the frontier. The army, reorganized in 1866 by congressional action, was small relative to its wartime size, but it was a vastly expanded army that moved into the frontier, compared to its prewar strength (Utley 1973). The U.S. Seventh Cavalry was created as part of the 1866 reorganization. In July 1866 George Custer was appointed lieutenant colonel of the newly formed Seventh Cavalry. Although second in command, he was frequently in effective command because the colonel was often absent. In late October Custer joined his regiment at its permanent station, Fort Riley, Kansas (Frost 1964; Utley 1988; Daily 1995), to build the newly formed unit.

The Seventh U.S. Cavalry was one of forty regiments of the army during the span of this study, 1866 to 1881. During most of this period, the army's organization consisted of twenty-five regiments of infantry, ten regiments of cavalry, and five regiments of artillery. Those regiments totaled an authorized enlistment of 26,312 men (Utley 1973; Coffman 1986), although the actual number of men on duty seldom exceeded about 22,000 at any one time.

Administratively, the army during the study era was divided into divisions (each commanded by a lieutenant general), departments (commanded by a major general), and districts (commanded by a brigadier general). During the first five years of its existence (1866 to 1871), the Seventh Cavalry was in the Division of the Missouri (encompassing the entire Great Plains and commanded by

William Tecumseh Sherman until 1869) and in the departments of Missouri (Kansas, Missouri, and Indian and New Mexico Territories) and Texas, which formed the southern half of the Division of the Missouri (Leckie 1963:28). The principal responsibilities of the Division of the Missouri were to protect settlers in, travelers passing through, and railroads being built in the division's geographic area. The means of achieving these goals have been called the "sword and olive branch" (Leckie 1963:28). Negotiations with Indians were attempted and were often successful, at least temporarily or to some degree. When negotiations failed, military action was taken.

Regimental Structure

Each cavalry regiment during the study era was headed by a colonel who had a regimental staff and twelve companies under his command. The regimental staff consisted of the colonel, a lieutenant colonel, three majors, a quartermaster, a chief musician, an adjutant, a contract veterinarian, a sergeant major, a quartermaster's sergeant, a saddler sergeant, a chief trumpeter, surgeons or contract surgeons, and hospital stewards.

COMMISSIONED OFFICERS

Fort life on the frontier meant that not only the officers but their wives, families, and servants were intimately familiar with each other. Life at any post, but frontier posts in particular, was a structured affair. Rank had its privileges: ceremony, military courtesy, and military protocol took precedence.

The commanding officer at a post had an entire house for himself and his family (Coffman 1986). At Fort Abraham Lincoln, the Custers occupied the commanding officer's quarters during their tenure. They often invited other officers and their wives to socialize during the evenings and appeared to be the center of one of the regiment's social circles. Other officers had portions of townhouse-like quarters. The quarters were divided, depending on how many lived there. Junior officers could be bumped from their quarters by a senior officer who wanted to live there. Quarters were not assigned on the basis of size of family or number of people: a bachelor senior officer could have three rooms, while a junior officer with a wife and children might live in one room. Officer's wives had no official status or rights within the army. Should an officer die, his wife and children had to vacate the quarters as soon as possible, as Libbie Custer and the other Little Bighorn widows were required to do (Stewart 1972; Cook 1987).

Officers were responsible for their own meals or mess. If they were married, their wives might do the shopping and cooking, although the social status of an officer usually required a servant or soldier striker to do the menial chores and cooking. Unmarried officers sometimes ate with married officers and often pooled their meager resources and messed with other bachelor officers.

NONCOMMISSIONED OFFICERS AND ENLISTED MEN

The lives of the noncommissioned officers were similar to the lives of the enlisted men. They had authority over the enlisted men, carrying out the orders of their superiors and overseeing day-to-day activities at the post and in the field. During this period of the Indian Wars, with understrength units and officers commonly on detached or other duties, noncommissioned officers became de facto small unit leaders (Arms 1991:25–30).

Noncommissioned officers and enlisted men usually lived in communal barracks and messed with their company. Enlisted men received $13 a month and rations; pay for noncommissioned officers was proportionally higher for the different grades. Each company was given a prescribed food ration per man each day. In garrison, individual rations included 12 ounces of pork or bacon (20 ounces of salt or fresh beef could be substituted) and 22 ounces of flour or bread with 16 ounces of hard bread substituted for field rations. For every 100 men in garrison each day, the commissary rationed 8 pounds of ground coffee, 15 pounds of beans or peas, 10 pounds of rice or hominy, 30 pounds of potatoes (if available), 1 quart of molasses, 15 pounds of sugar, 3 pounds 12 ounces of salt, 4 ounces of pepper, and 1 gallon of vinegar (Billings 1974). Each company was also supposed to raise a garden to provide fresh vegetables, but gardens often failed in the harsh plains climate.

Enlisted personnel were discouraged from marrying and in fact had to receive their commanding officer's permission (Kautz 2001:12). Married enlisted men's wives often worked as laundresses for the company and regiment. Laundresses were provided with rations and quarters; these allowances and the pay were incentives for an enlisted man to marry a laundress (Rickey 1963; Coffman 1986). Married enlisted men, often noncommissioned officers, lived with their wives and children in whatever housing they could find. If married to a laundress or hospital matron, the soldier might live in quarters designated for them. Otherwise he might live in a tent or some building that he constructed. No married enlisted quarters officially existed at this period, although some commanding officers did allow use of otherwise unoccupied or unused post buildings.

The Seventh Cavalry was composed of twelve companies. Most were understrength to some degree. In a sense each company was an independent unit, where men ate, slept, and worked together. Within the company, the members knew each other well. Companies stationed together might be acquainted with a few members of other companies, but generally the company was the enlisted man's world. Good officers and noncommissioned officers would make a man's service go well, while a martinet or disciplinarian could make an enlistment miserable. For many enlisted men, the army was the only place to find a decent meal in tough economic times. For others, it was an opportunity for adventure in the West. Each company had its own personality, usually reflected by its officers and noncommissioned officers.

The Seventh Cavalry from 1866 to 1882 and Beyond

The Seventh, which began in 1866, in many ways epitomized the army as a whole during the study period. The men assigned or recruited to join the unit were typical of the entire army in terms of stature, age, and ancestry (Coffman 1986; Scott et al. 1998; Chun 2004; Hedren 2011).

The structure of the unit and its stations during the study period are presented chronologically here, from its organization in 1866 to 1882 to a summary of the Seventh in the later years of the nineteenth and early twentieth centuries (Adjutant General's Office 1909; Chandler 1960; Daily 1995). The year-by-year chronology provides a broad view of the regiment's status. For details of company dispositions and deployments by year, see table 1.1.

1866

Authorization for establishing the new Seventh Cavalry as well as three other regiments occurred in July 1866. By the end of August troops were being organized at Fort Riley, Kansas. The organization of the Seventh was completed late that year (map 1.1). Then the Seventh's companies were dispersed from Fort Riley. By year's end only Regimental Headquarters and three companies remained there, the other companies having been deployed to other forts on the central plains.

The Seventh was assigned to Fort Riley and other posts on the central plains because the central and southern plains were areas of rapid change and intense but sporadic fighting. In particular the Cheyennes, Kiowas, and Arapahos fought to maintain their more traditional lifestyle while settlers, travelers, and hunters traversed or homesteaded the area. The Seventh Cavalry remained in Kansas and adjacent parts of the central plains for the next four and a half years (Garlington 1896:251).

1867

The first few years that the Seventh spent on the plains were particularly well chronicled by Albert Barnitz, an officer who had previously served under Custer during the Civil War. He was newly remarried in early 1867, his first wife and daughter having died in childbirth. He and his new bride (Jennie) headed to the frontier to join the Seventh. Barnitz trudged across the central and southern plains with the Seventh, only to be critically wounded in 1868 during the Battle of the Washita and awarded a disability retirement. His experiences, detailed descriptions, and astute insights on the Seventh's experiences during these formative years provide a humanistic perspective on the events and places and are used in this summary (Utley 1977).

TABLE 1.1. Seventh Cavalry company assignments by year

Year	*HQ*	*A*	*B*	*C*	*D*	*E*	*F*
1866	Ft Riley	Ft Riley	Ft Riley, 11 Ft Lyon	Ft Riley, 11 Ft Lyon	Ft Riley	Ft Riley, 11 Ft Hays	Ft Riley, 11 Ft Harker
1867		3–7 with Custer's scouts, 11 Ft Leavenworth. [Marched] 1,877 miles	1 deserters chased, 4 Ft Dodge. 315 miles	Ft Lyon whole year. After deserters & stolen horses. 515 miles	3–9 with Custer's command. 11 Ft Leavenworth. 2,046 miles	3–9 with Custer's command. 11 Ft Leavenworth. 2105 miles	3 with Custer, 7–11 Monument Station, 11 Ft Leavenworth. 2,000 miles
1868		4 Ft Hays–Ft Larned, 8–9 Bluff Creek, 10 scout, 10 Camp Forsyth. 1,619 miles	7 near Ft Larned, 8 Ft Dodge, 8–9 Bluff Creek, 10 scout, 10 Camp Forsyth. 1,193 miles	8–9 Bluff Creek, 10 scout, 10 Camp Forsyth. 1,133 miles	8–9 Bluff Creek, 10 scout, 10 Camp Forsyth. 1,619 miles	8–9 Bluff Creek, 10 scout, 10 Camp Forsyth. 1,558 miles	8 Ft Harker, 8–9 Bluff Creek, 10 scout, 10 Camp Forsyth. 1,161 miles
1869		1 Ft Cobb, Medicine Bluff Creek, 3 scout, Camp Supply, Ft Dodge,	1 Ft Cobb, Medicine Bluff Creek, 3 scout, Camp Supply, Ft Dodge,	1 Ft Cobb, Medicine Bluff Creek, 3 scout, Camp Supply, Ft Dodge,	1 Ft Cobb, Medicine Bluff Creek, 3 scout, Camp Supply, Ft Dodge,	1 Ft Cobb, Medicine Bluff Creek, 3 scout, Camp Supply, Ft Dodge,	1 Ft Cobb, Medicine Bluff Creek, 3 scout, Camp Supply, Ft Dodge, Ft Hays, 6 Ft Wallace,

(continued)

TABLE 1.1. *(continued)*

Year	*HQ*	*A*	*B*	*C*	*D*	*E*	*F*
		Ft Hays, 8 Camp Supply, Ft Hays, 10 Limestone Creek near Girard. 1,299 miles	Ft Hays, 7 Ft Wallace, Denver, 8 Monument Wells, 9 Redman Station, 10 Ft Lyon. 1,210 miles	10 Ft Leavenworth. 874 miles	Ft Hays, 5 scout, 6 escort captives turned over to tribe (at Ft Harker end of year). 1,061 miles	Ft Hays, 5 Ft Wallace, 6 Reeds Springs, 7 Ft Wallace, 9 march, 10 Smoky Hill camp, 11 Ft Wallace. 1,852 miles	7 escort, Denver, 8 Monument Creek, 10 Sheridan, KS, Ft Leavenworth. 1,244 miles
1870		9 long march, returning to Limestone Creek. 416 miles	5–6 scout, Ft Wallace, 7–10 various scouts, 11 Ft Leavenworth. 1,259 miles	4 Ft Wallace, 5 & 6 scouts, returning to Ft Wallace, 9 Fitz Meadows, CT, 10 Ft Harker. 1,236 miles	2 Lake Sibley, 4 Scandinavia, KS, 6 Ft Hays, 11 Ft Leavenworth. At least 471 miles	~5 Cheyenne Wells & Cedar Pt, 6 scout, 7 River Bend, CT, 8–9 Hugo Station, 10 Ft Leavenworth. 2,965 miles	5 Ft Hays, scouts, 11 Ft Leavenworth. 1,037 miles.
1871		3 Ft Leavenworth, Louisville, 4 Elizabethtown	3 Louisville, Unionville, SC, 7 some	3 Ft Leavenworth, Louisville,	3 Taylor Barracks, Mt Vernon, ? Chester	3 Spartanburg, rest of the year various escorts &	3 Taylor Barracks, 7 Meridian,

		temp duty Spartanburg, SC, 11 Spartanburg	Chester, 6 Rutherfordton		scouts, 12 Unionville, SC.	MS, 11 Taylor Barracks
1872			3 Lincolnton, NC, 10 Charlotte	3 Opelika, AL, 11 Montgomery		
1873	3 Louisville, 4 Cairo, IL, Yankton, 6 Ft Rice, 7–9 NPRR Survey, 9 Ft Lincoln. 1,500 miles	3 Memphis, 4 Cairo, IL, Yankton, 6 Ft Rice, 7–9 NPRR Survey, 9 Ft Lincoln. 1,500 miles.	3 Memphis, 4 Cairo, IL, Yankton, 6 Ft Rice, 7–9 NPRR Survey, 9 Ft Lincoln. 1,500 miles.	3 Memphis, 4 Cairo, IL, Sioux City, Ft Snelling, 6–10 Northern Boundary Survey, 10 Ft Totten.	3 Memphis, 4 Cairo, IL, Yankton, 6 Ft Rice, 7–9 NPRR Survey, 9 Ft Lincoln. 1,500 miles.	3 Louisville, 4 Cairo, IL, Yankton, 6 Ft Rice, 7–9 NPRR Survey, 9 Ft Lincoln. 1,500 miles.
1874	7–8 Black Hills Expedition, 9 Ft Lincoln, 9 Dept of Gulf	7–8 Black Hills Expedition, 9 Ft Lincoln, 9 Dept of Gulf	[Ft Rice] 6 Ft Lincoln, 7–8 Black Hills Exped, 9 Ft Lincoln, 12 some Standing Rock, 12 Ft Lincoln	4 Fts Stevenson & Buford, 6 Lime Creek, 7–8 Sweet Grass Hills, 9 Ft Totten	7–8 Black Hills Expedition, 9 Ft Lincoln, 9 Dept of Gulf	7–8 Black Hills Exped, 9 Ft Lincoln

(continued)

TABLE 1.1. *(continued)*

Year	*HQ*	*A*	*B*	*C*	*D*	*E*	*F*
1875		[Livingston, AL,] 5 Ft Randall, 6–9 scouts, 9 Ft Randall, Ft Rice, 10 Ft Lincoln, Ft Stevenson, Ft Lincoln	Shreveport, LA	(Ft Rice), 3–8 pursuing thieves, 10 Ft Lincoln	4 Ft Lincoln	(Opelika, AL), 5 Ft Randall	Ft Lincoln
1876		5 Expedition (Reno), 9 Ft Lincoln	5 Ft Lincoln, Expedition (pack escort), 9 Ft Lincoln	5 Expedition (Custer), 9 Ft Lincoln, 11 Ft Totten	5 Expedition (Benteen), 9 Ft Lincoln	[Ft Totten] 4 Ft Lincoln, 5 Expedition (Custer), 9 Ft Lincoln	5 Expedition (Custer), 9 Ft Lincoln, 11 Ft Abercrombie
1877		[Ft Rice] 4 Ft Lincoln, 5–9 scout, 9–10 Snake Creek, 10–12 guard Nez Perces, 12 Ft Lincoln	5–10 field, Tongue R Cantonment, escort	8–12 Ft Lincoln, 10–12 guard Nez Perces, 12 Ft Totten?	[Ft Rice] 4 Ft Lincoln, 9–10 Snake Creek, 10–12 guard Nez Perces	6 Tongue R Cantonment, 7–8 scout, 9–12 march	8–9 march, 10–12 guard Nez Perces

1878		7 Camp Sturgis, 10 Red Cloud Agency, 11 Camp Ruhlen, Ft Lincoln	? Ft Yates	? Ft Lincoln, 7 Camp Sturgis, 10 Red Cloud Agency, 11 Camp Ruhlen, Ft Lincoln	? Ft Lincoln, 7 Camp Sturgis, 8 escort, 9 Camp Sturgis, 10 Red Cloud Agency, 11 Camp Ruhlen, Ft Yates	? Ft Lincoln, 7 Camp Sturgis, 8 Camp Ruhlen, 10 Red Cloud Agency, 11 Camp Ruhlen	1 Ft Totten, ? Ft Lincoln, 7 Camp Sturgis, 10 Red Cloud Agency
1879	6 Ft Meade	6 Ft Meade	Ft Yates	6 Ft Meade			
1880		6 scout, 6 Ft Meade	6 scout	8 scout, 9 Ft Meade			
1881				(Ft Pierre) 7–8 guard		(Ft Meade) 6 scout, 10 Ft Meade	(Ft Buford),1 capture Sioux, 8–10 guard NPRR Survey
1882		4–8 Ft Sisseton, 8 Ft Meade		4–8 Ft Sisseton, 8 Ft Meade			(Ft Buford), 7–11 Billings, 11 Ft Buford

(continued)

TABLE 1.1. *(continued)*

Year	*G*	*H*	*I*	*K*	*L*	*M*
1866	Ft Riley, 11 Ft Harker	Ft Riley	Ft Riley, 11 Ft Wallace	Ft Riley, 11 Ft Dodge	Ft Riley, 11 Ft Morgan	Ft Riley
1867	3–4 with Custer, 4–6 Ft Hays, 6–7 Ft Wallace, 6 flood, 7–11? on march, 11 Ft Leavenworth. 1,691 miles	–9 with Custer, 11 Ft Harker. 1,518 miles	Ft Wallace entire year. Indian attacks. [No miles given]	–9 with Custer, 11 Ft Leavenworth. 2,000 miles.	1–7 Ft Morgan, 7–12 Ft Reynolds; 75 men deserted; 1/14 3 NCOs & 21 privates deserted at instigation of 1st sgt. [No miles given]	–9 with Custer, 11 Ft Harker. 1,500 miles
1868	8–9 Bluff Creek, 10 scout, 10 Camp Forsyth. 1,561 miles	8–9 Bluff Creek, 10 scout, 10 Camp Forsyth. 976 miles	6 near Ellis Station, 8–9 Bluff Creek, 10 scout, 10 Camp Forsyth. 1,371 miles	8–9 body guard Sully, 10 Bluff Creek, 10 scout, 10 Camp Forsyth. 1,241 miles	8 Ft Reynolds, 8 Ft Lyon, 11–12 scout, 12 Ft Lyon. 12 to Skull Creek, TX. 469 miles	8–9 Bluff Creek, 10 scout, 10 Camp Forsyth. 976 miles
1869	1 Ft Cobb, Medicine Bluff Creek, 3 scout, Camp Supply,	1 Ft Cobb, Medicine Bluff Creek, 3 scout, Camp Supply,	1 Ft Cobb, Medicine Bluff Creek, 3 scout, Camp Supply,	1 Ft Cobb, Medicine Bluff Creek, 3 scout, Camp Supply,	San Francisco Creek, 2 Ft Lyon, 3 Ft Leavenworth,	1 Ft Cobb, Medicine Bluff Creek, 3 scout, Camp Supply,

	Ft Dodge, Ft Hays, 5–11 Asher Creek, 11 Ft Hays. 714 miles	Ft Dodge, Ft Hays, 4 Ft Dodge. 547 miles	Ft Dodge, Ft Hays, 6 escort, 10 Ft Leavenworth. 1,154 miles	Ft Dodge, Ft Hays, 5 Camp Beecher, scout, 6 Ft Harker, 7 scout, S Fork Solomon R, 11 Ft Harker. 1,067 miles	6 Ft Harker, Saline R, 8 Lake Sibley, 11 New Scandinavia, KS, Ft Leavenworth. 603 miles	Ft Dodge, Ft Hays, 6 scout, 7 Ft Dodge, 8 Ft Hays, 10 Ft Leavenworth. 1,096 miles
1870	2 Solomon R Forks, 6 some at Camp Sturgis, Co scattered, 10 Ft Lyon. 720 miles	(1 at Ft Hays) 4 Saline R, 5 Hays, 6 River Bend, 10 Ft Hays. 820 miles	5 Ft Hays, 7 scouts, 10 Ft Hays. 480 miles	2 Wolf Creek, 4 chase thieves, 5 Ft Harker, Wolf Creek, 6 Ft Harker, 7 scout, 10 Ft Leavenworth. 1,545 miles	5 Ft Hays, Kit Carson, 6 Ft Wallace, 7 Kit Carson, 8 Big Sandy–River Bend, stampede, 9 scouts, 11 Ft Wallace. 1,740 miles	5 Camp Sturgis, 6 various scouts, 10 Solomon R, Ft Hays. 760 miles
1871	4 Ft Hays, 5 Louisville, Columbia, SC, 6 Sumter, 8 McPherson Barracks, 10 Columbia. 295 miles	6 Ash Barracks, 12 Huntsville. 500 miles	3 Ft Leavenworth, Bagdad, 9 Shelbyville	3 Yorkville	5 Louisville, 6 Winnsboro, SC?, 10 Yorkville	3–4 scouts, 5 Louisville, 6 Darlington, SC, 10 Spartanburg, 11 Unionville. 597 miles

(continued)

TABLE 1.1. (*continued*)

Year	*G*	*H*	*I*	*K*	*L*	*M*
1872	8 Laurensville	2 Nashville, 10 Ash Barracks	12 Lebanon, KY		12 Jackson Barracks, New Orleans	12 Oxford, MS
1873	3 Memphis, 4 Cairo, IL, Yankton, 6 Ft Rice, 7–9 NPRR Survey, 9 Ft Lincoln. 1,500 miles	3 Louisville, 4 Cairo, IL, Yankton, 6 Ft Rice, 7–9 NPRR Survey, 9 Ft Lincoln. 1,500 miles	3 Louisville, 4 Cairo, IL, Sioux City, Ft Snelling, 6–10 Northern Boundary Survey, 10 Ft Totten	3 Memphis, 4 Cairo, IL, Yankton, 6 Ft Rice, 7–9 NPRR Survey, 9 Ft Lincoln. 1,500 miles	3 New Orleans, 4 Cairo, IL, Yankton, 6 Ft Rice, 7–9 NPRR Survey, 9 Ft Lincoln. 1,500 miles	3 Memphis, 4 Cairo, IL, Yankton, 6 Ft Rice, 7–9 NPRR Survey, 9 Ft Lincoln. 1,500 miles
1874	7–8 Black Hills Expedition, 9 Ft Lincoln, 9 Dept of Gulf	[Ft Rice] 6 Ft Lincoln, 7–8 Black Hills Expedition, 9 Ft Lincoln, 9 Dept of Gulf	4 Fts Stevenson & Buford, 6 Lime Creek, 7–8 Sweet Grass Hills, 9 Ft Totten	5–6 some scouting, [Ft Rice] 6 Ft Lincoln, 7–8 Black Hills Expedition, 9 Ft Lincoln, 9 Dept of Gulf	7–8 Black Hills Exped, 12 some arrest Rain-in-the-Face	[Ft Rice] 5–6 some scout, 6 Ft Lincoln, 7–8 Black Hills Exped, 11–12 Ft Rice, Standing Rock, 12 Ft Lincoln
1875	Dept of Gulf	5 Ft Randall	4 Ft Lincoln	Dept of Gulf		

1876	5 Ft Lincoln, Expedition (Reno), 9 Ft Lincoln	[Ft Rice], 5 Ft Lincoln, Expedition (Benteen), 9 Ft Lincoln, 11 Ft Rice	5 Expedition (Custer), 9 Ft Lincoln	5 Ft Lincoln, Expedition (Benteen), 9 Ft Lincoln	[Ft Totten] 4 Ft Lincoln, 5 Expedition (Custer), 9 Ft Lincoln	[Ft Rice] 5 Ft Lincoln, Expedition (Reno), 9 Ft Lincoln, 11 Ft Rice
1877	8–9 march, 10–12 guard Nez Perces	4 Ft Lincoln, 8–9 march, 10–12 guard Nez Perces	4–5 march to Cedar Creek, 6–7 Little Bighorn Battlefield exhumation, 8–9 march, 10 guard Nez Perces, 11 Ft Lincoln, 12 stage guard	[9–10 Snake Creek?], 10–12 guard Nez Perces	8–9 march, 10–12 guard Nez Perces	4 Ft Lincoln, 8–9 march, 10–12 guard Nez Perces
1878	? Ft Lincoln, 7 Camp Sturgis, 10 Red Cloud Agency, 11	? Ft Lincoln, 7–8 Cheyenne prisoners, Camp Sturgis,	? Ft Lincoln, 7 Camp Sturgis, 10 Red Cloud Agency, 11	? Ft Lincoln, 7 Camp Sturgis, 8–9 Cheyenne prisoners,	7–8 Cheyenne prisoners, Camp Sturgis, 10 Red Cloud	? Ft Lincoln, 7 Camp Sturgis, 8 escort, Camp Sturgis, 8 Camp

(*continued*)

TABLE 1.1. *(continued)*

Year	*G*	*H*	*I*	*K*	*L*	*M*
	Camp Ruhlen, Ft Lincoln	10 Red Cloud Agency, 11 Camp Ruhlen, Ft Lincoln	Camp Ruhlen, Ft Lincoln	Sidney Barracks, 10 Red Cloud Agency, 11 Camp Ruhlen, 12 Ft Yates	Agency, 11 Camp Ruhlen, Ft Lincoln	Ruhlen, 10 Red Cloud Agency, 11 Camp Ruhlen
1879	6 Ft Meade	6 Ft Meade				
1880						
1881						(Ft Pierre) 7–8 guard
1882		5–9 guard NPRR Survey	(Ft Totten) 8 Turtle Mtn, 9 Ft Totten	(Ft Totten), 11 Ft Meade	6–10 scout, 10 Ft Buford. 1,131 miles	(Ft Meade) 6–10 escort USGS. 1,246 miles

Note: Numbers represent months (1 = January, 2 = February, and so forth).

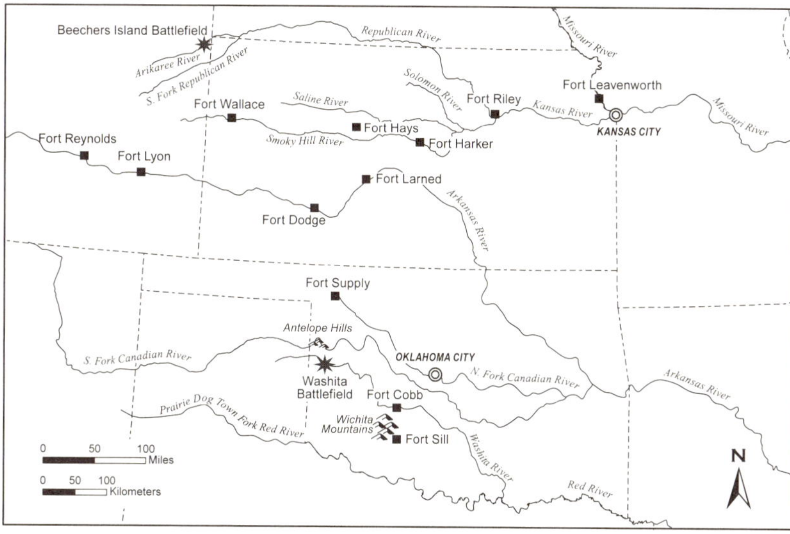

Map 1.1. The central plains, showing principal postings and engagements of the Seventh Cavalry and major cities. Drawn by Judy Stolen. Copyright © 2015, University of Oklahoma Press.

After spending months in winter quarters, the Seventh joined General Winfield Hancock's spring expedition against the Indians on the central and southern plains. In late March Headquarters (HQ), Companies A, D, H, and M, moved from Fort Riley, despite bad weather, to Fort Harker, Kansas, where they joined Companies F and G (Barnitz's company). Barnitz was pleased with the facilities at Fort Harker and how well his troops and horses were housed and cared for. This lull was a time for reequipping and refitting both man and mount (Utley 1977:21).

In early April the combined companies traveled from Fort Harker to Fort Larned, Kansas, joined there by the Seventh Cavalry's Companies E and K. Even that late in the spring they were struck by snowstorms and freezing temperatures (Barnitz in Utley 1977:27). Hancock's expedition against the Kiowas and Cheyennes was off to a slow, cold, and wet start.

They joined Hancock's expedition and chased hostile Cheyennes and Sioux for 300 miles in April, although Barnitz (in Utley 1977) and his company spent most of that time in camp on Big Creek near Fort Hays, Kansas. Desertions were rampant: eighty-five men deserted from the Seventh Cavalry during April 1867 alone (Utley 1977:44). Barnitz attributed the desertions to the capricious and uncaring decisions of his immediate commander, George Custer.

That May scurvy swept through camp (Barnitz in Utley 1977:51), reportedly striking seventy-five men (although our medical record data show only thirty-one for the entire study period and twelve in 1867). Troops were ravenous for canned fruits and vegetables. In June HQ and six companies were encamped near Fort Hays when a flood occurred, drowning five men (Barnitz in Utley 1977:57). After the flood they moved near Fort McPherson, Nebraska, on the Platte River then to the Republican River and remained in that region for the next month. Later they transferred to the vicinity of Fort Wallace, Kansas. Barnitz was at Fort Wallace when he and his Company G were engaged in a skirmish with Sioux or Cheyennes, the first major encounter involving the recently established Seventh. This encounter resulted in the loss of Sergeant Frederick Wyllyams (Company G), whose mutilated corpse was photographed (fig. 1.1).

Cholera appeared in July (Garlington 1896:251). Company G was not immune. The company completed a march from Fort Hays (or Fort Wallace: Utley 1977:85) to Fort Lyon, Colorado, accompanying an engineering party (Chandler 1960:3–4). It was struck by cholera while en route (Barnitz in Utley 1977:85). The company returned to Fort Wallace, where cholera was also present: as many as seven soldiers died each day (none are reported in the Fort Wallace medical records). Among the dead was the surgeon's wife, "Mrs Dr Sternberg," with whom Jennie Barnitz had been particularly close (Barnitz in Utley 1977:85–86; Jennie Barnitz in Utley 1977:91). Barnitz wrote to his wife that "strictest sanatary [*sic*] regulations" in camp prevented or at least minimized the spread of the disease. These regulations included "taking a nice bath every evening, and having nice clean sheets, and white pillow cases" (Barnitz in Utley 1977:89), at least for an officer. Late in the month the epidemic abated, with only one or two soldiers dying each day (Barnitz in Utley 1977:90). Disease was not the only problem of epidemic proportions occurring that month in the regiment.

In July desertions became rampant. During one three-day period, thirty-four men deserted. Officers discovered plans for

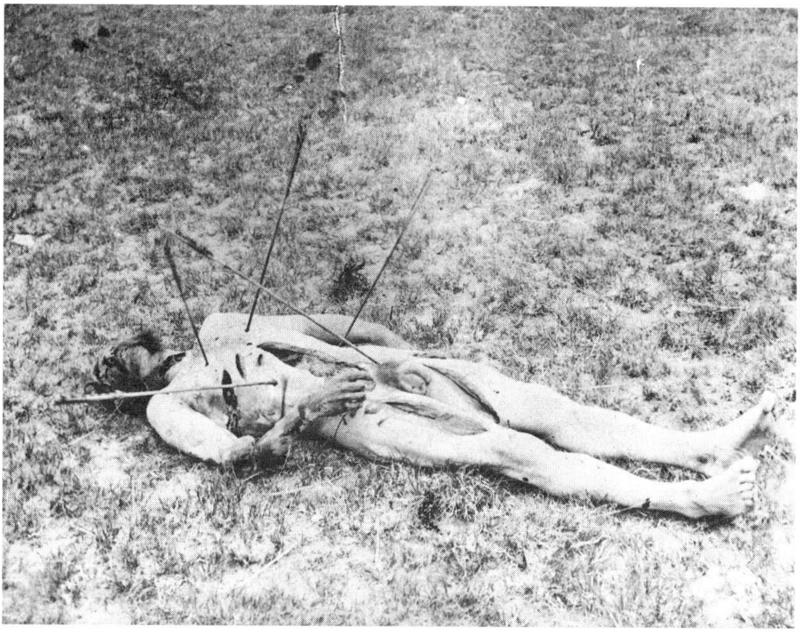

1.1. Victorious warriors sometimes stripped, scalped, and mutilated their vanquished foe, as they did Sergeant Frederick Wyllyams of Company G near Fort Wallace in 1867. Courtesy Kansas State Historical Society.

desertion of another one-third of the command (Utley 1977:86). Custer ordered thirteen broad-daylight deserters hunted down and killed. Although some escaped and others were captured, some of them were killed or wounded. Custer initially refused aid to the wounded prisoners, only later rescinding the order and permitting the surgeon to attend to the wounded.

By August, as Barnitz (in Utley 1977:91–92) worded it, George Custer had the "measels [*sic*]": he was under arrest. Custer had to stand charges that he drove the men and animals so hard during the expedition that men deserted and that he ordered those who did desert shot dead. His recklessness, it was claimed, damaged the animals. In addition to these charges, some of which might possibly be considered in the realm of duty, he faced charges outside the military realm. It is claimed that Custer went absent-without-leave from his command to visit his wife and failed to come to the aid of some members of his escort when they became separated and attacked by Indians. Custer was found guilty and suspended from rank and pay for one year (Chandler 1960:4–5). One man alone does not run a unit, however, and the regiment remained active during Custer's absence.

Major Joel Elliot was in command during Custer's absence. In August parts of the Seventh scouted the Saline River, ending their tour at Fort Hays. During that month, Hancock was transferred from the Department of the Missouri to the East. Major General Philip H. Sheridan received command of the Department and took active command the following year (Leckie 1963:63). In September all Seventh Cavalry companies actively served as escorts and were involved in troop movements, thus spending little time in camp.

During October, portions of the Seventh escorted the Peace Commission to Medicine Lodge Creek, seventy miles south of Fort Larned (Utley 1977:107), among other duties protecting the almost one hundred wagons containing gifts and supplies (Leckie 1963:60). The Medicine Lodge council was part of the grand olive branch, attempting to negotiate a resolution instead of implementing a military solution. The Peace Commission had attempted previously to meet with the northern plains tribes. The absence of the Northern Cheyennes from the council made the meeting pointless, however, and it was postponed (Leckie 1963:58). Consequently the commission members turned their efforts to the southern tribes, attempting to confer with the Arapahos, Cheyennes, Comanches, and Kiowas. This southern council was much more successful than the aborted council with the northern plains tribes.

The Medicine Lodge treaty established more than 7 million acres of reservations north of the Red River, supplied provisions of food, equipment, and clothing, stipulated that tribes retained hunting rights south of the Arkansas River, and staffed the reservations' agencies. In return the tribes agreed to void claims for a larger area, avoid both existing roads and railroads and those being built, and maintain peaceful relations with other Indians and whites alike (Leckie 1963:61–62). The Seventh Cavalry escort then traveled from Medicine Lodge to Fort Harker (Chandler 1960:3–4) and then to winter quarters. The Peace Commission, the tribes, and the military were all happy, although their contentedness was short-lived. The next year their hopes for the olive-branch solution were dashed: the sword was brought to bear.

1868

Early in the year HQ and the Seventh Cavalry companies remained at posts where they had been stationed the preceding winter. During that winter, they were mostly involved in scouting and escorting responsibilities. Sheridan's active assumption of command of the Department of the Missouri occurred at that time. Hopes for a quick ratification of the Medicine Lodge treaty dimmed. The treaty's financial provisions led to loggerheads between the Senate and the House, which finally approved financial support in July (Leckie 1963:67). But by summer many Indians were on the move, which resulted in problems.

Seventh Cavalry companies were in the field in early spring under Major Elliott. They moved to Fort Ellis then Fort Larned to be closer to the Cheyennes, Comanches, Arapahos, and Kiowas in order to be able to thwart hostile acts (Chandler 1960). Indian raids on the Saline and Solomon Rivers occurred in July. Captain Frederick Benteen and portions of the Seventh freed two white captives (Leckie 1963:71).

By fall direct conflict between troops and off-reservation Indians became inevitable. General Alfred Sully was in overall command of the Upper Arkansas district, where most of the activity occurred. Between August and November 1868 in Colorado and Kansas 117 citizens were murdered (32 of these scalped), 16 wounded, 14 women "outraged," 14 women and 2 children captured, 619 mules and horses stolen, and 958 cattle stolen (Chandler 1960:10). Kansas governor Samuel J. Crawford requested permission to muster troops from his state (the Nineteenth Kansas Volunteer Cavalry) to assist the regulars. Organization of the volunteers was too slow to join the Seventh Cavalry in the field for the Battle of the Washita. The volunteers only became a factor late in the campaign. General Sheridan, who had taken over active command of the Department of Missouri, headquartered at Fort Leavenworth, ordered troops to Fort Larned and later to Fort Dodge, where eight of the Seventh Cavalry companies joined Sully's command. In September this combined command crossed the Arkansas River, incessantly harassed by Indians. Indian resistance increased as the troops marched along Beaver Creek, where their villages were believed to be located. An encounter between the troops and Indians was largely inconsequential. The Seventh Cavalry returned to Fort Dodge and from there into camp on Bluff Creek (Chandler 1960).

Early in October 1868 Custer, back on active duty, rejoined the Seventh Cavalry in the field at Bluff Creek. With winter coming nomadic Indians were in a vulnerable position. After an extensive scout the Seventh went into camp at Fort Dodge in preparation for a winter campaign. One of the changes that Custer implemented was improved marksmanship, with the regiment's best shots placed in an elite group under the command of Lieutenant W. W. Cooke (Leckie 1963:94).

In mid-November eleven companies of the Seventh Cavalry left Fort Dodge with Sully's command and headed south. They were joined by infantry and established Camp Supply, now in Oklahoma, on Beaver Creek, where the infantry settled for the duration.

After an early winter blizzard the cavalry under Custer scouted south from Camp Supply, spending the first night on Wolf Creek, then headed southwest up Wolf Creek and from there south toward the Canadian River and Antelope Hills. They found a recent trail of perhaps a hundred warriors on the south side of the Canadian River and followed the tracks through the day and well into the night, reaching a large village in the Washita River bottoms.

At dawn the following day, November 27, the Seventh Cavalry attacked the Cheyennes' village, headed by Black Kettle (Hoig 1979; Kraft 1995; Greene 2008). In the initial action 800–900 ponies were isolated from the village, the village was overrun, and then battle spread and extended to all sides. Part of the pack train with ammunition arrived about an hour into the battle.

As it turned out, Black Kettle's village was the westernmost of a series of camps lower on the Washita River. The shooting and activity at his village brought attention and additional warriors there. Late in the day the Seventh feigned a movement toward the lower villages. After dark they reversed course, traveling back over the destroyed village and retracing the previous day's path to Camp Supply (Chandler 1960:8–25).

Barnitz was seriously wounded during the Battle of the Washita. His wounds were so severe that he was not expected to survive evacuation. The gunshot was fired so close that, according to Barnitz, the blaze singed his overcoat. The ball glanced off a rib and then coursed inferiorly, breaking the rib below it and glancing off the next rib down. From there the bullet passed through his torso, exiting near the spine and continuing through his winter clothing (Barnitz in Utley 1977:226–27). His wound was treated by the two surgeons accompanying the column, who were partially snow blind. They believed that his wound would be fatal. He survived, however, and was moved from the battlefield to Camp Supply, arriving there December 1 in a military ambulance (Utley 1977:235). By Christmas Barnitz was able to sit all day and walk about in his tent. Following an extended convalescence leave of absence and light duty the following year he was awarded a disability retirement in 1870. He lived another forty-two years, dying in 1912 from a growth associated with his Washita wound (Utley 1977:247).

The results of the Battle of the Washita were 800–900 Indian horses captured, the village and its contents destroyed, 103 warriors killed (140 warriors in Garlington 1896:253), 53 women and children taken prisoner, and 2 captive white women freed. The Seventh Cavalry's losses were 2 officers and 19 enlisted men killed, most of them with Elliott's command (25 men killed in Garlington 1896:253), 3 officers (among them Captain Barnitz) and 11 enlisted men (12 in Garlington 1896:253) wounded. Some of the men and officers suffered temporary snow blindness, and many suffered from cold and exposure (Chandler 1960:20–25).

After returning to Camp Supply, the Seventh Cavalry under Sheridan's command left in early December and marched toward Fort Cobb, the location where the tribes were instructed to go for rations and to indicate peaceful intentions. The Seventh was joined by the Nineteenth Kansas (Garlington 1896:254). On that journey the column passed the site of the Battle of the Washita and stopped to recover the bodies of Major Elliott and his sixteen men, which had been abandoned on the field the previous month. The bodies of a white woman and child were also found in one of the lower villages, apparently captives who had been killed during the battle (Chandler 1960:25).

1869

Most of this year the Seventh Cavalry negotiated and rounded up hostiles across the southern plains. In January the regiment (all but Company L) left Fort Cobb, moved to the Wichita Mountains, and from there went to Medicine Bluff Creek, where they stayed until March. Then they returned via Camp Supply to Fort Dodge and Fort Hays (Greene 2008). This winter march caused terrible trepidation: 128 horses were lost. In addition to the regular army's losses, the Nineteenth Kansas lost 148 horses (Garlington 1896:254), apparently from hunger and exhaustion. During this period, the Kiowas, Cheyennes, and Arapahos were mostly subjugated, at least as far as the Department of the Missouri was concerned. The Department of Texas was another matter: the recalcitrants found attractive booty there and depredations continued (Chandler 1960:28–30).

The summer and fall of 1869 were more routine for the Custers and the Seventh than the earlier part of the year had been (Pohanka 1983). Duty at Fort Leavenworth and a return to Fort Hays were the primary agenda.

1870

During this year, only scattered bands of hostiles were present in the southern and central plains, with no large forces in the Department of the Missouri. As a consequence the Seventh Cavalry engaged mostly in separate company actions, with no large regimental movements. Regimental HQ had an active year, but it was mostly social, not military.

1871

In 1871 the Seventh Cavalry's Department of the Missouri assignment ended, and most of the regiment moved into and scattered across the Department of the South. The hostilities in the Department of the Missouri were for the most part done, although smaller actions continued several more years. Decimation of the southern plains bison herd, changes in governmental policies toward Indians, and several more major military encounters were required before the area became safe for travelers, settlers, and railroaders. In the meanwhile the Seventh Cavalry was otherwise engaged. Starting in 1871 and continuing for the next two years, the regiment spread across seven southern states (Garlington 1896:255; Chandler 1960).

At the end of the Civil War, the conquering Union was on the horns of a political and social dilemma. Some Northerners wanted former rebels declared traitors and former slaves elevated to new positions. But the possibility of such social upheaval seemed unlikely considering the political reality of the situation. Thus Reconstruction sought to balance the new regime with the old, allowing time for values and economies to adjust to the new order. To enforce such adjustments the military deployed across the South to ensure that the transition progressed in a peaceful manner. Their major duties involved controlling the activities of the Ku Klux Klan, ensuring fair and honest elections, enforcing civil authority's rule, and pursuing moonshiners. As if these challenges were not enough, the military found itself in a precarious position, forced to deal with civilians and difficult political situations in the midst of social and economic upheavals.

During the first four years after the end of the Civil War, roughly one-third of the army was located in the South (Coffman 1986:234). This proportion of the army in the South decreased until the mid-1870s, when turmoil associated with the presidential election forced additional troops back into the area.

1872

This was the second year that the Seventh Cavalry spent in the Department of the South (except Company L, which remained on the plains). The major duties of the Seventh, as well as the other occupation troops, were protecting and aiding civil authorities, especially destroying illegal distilleries and disrupting the Ku Klux Klan. Company L finally joined the rest of the Seventh late in the year, moving to Jackson Barracks, Louisiana, Department of the Gulf, in December (map 1.2). Otherwise the Seventh Cavalry's companies remained at the locations of their previous postings and continued duties from the previous year (Chandler 1960:37–38).

In January 1872 Custer was ordered to accompany General Philip Sheridan on a buffalo hunt (Scott et al. 2013). This hunt was special because the government sponsored it to entertain Grand Duke Alexis of Russia. According to the participants, it was a success and was a major social event of the winter for western Nebraska and eastern Colorado.

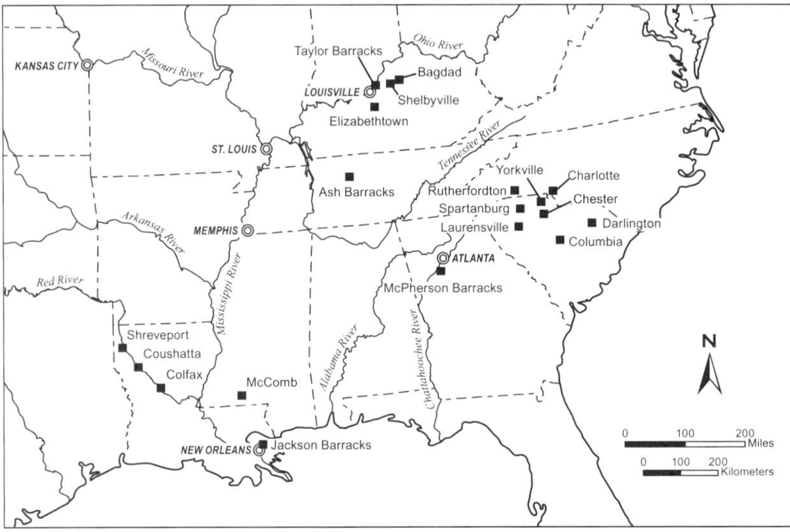

Map 1.2. The South, showing principal postings of the Seventh Cavalry and major cities. Drawn by Judy Stolen. Copyright © 2015, University of Oklahoma Press.

1873

Many changes were afoot for the Seventh Cavalry as well as the nation in this year. During the Economic Panic of 1873, prices fell, unemployment soared, and some prominent banks closed. Government and civil leaders looked for new opportunities and turned to the West for solutions to the problems of the East and South.

After spending two years spread across the South, the Seventh Regiment was ordered to the Department of Dakota, rescinding a previous order to move to Texas. The Seventh not only dodged a posting in Texas but also avoided difficult civil duties, including those involved with the Panic of 1873. After the Seventh Cavalry's occupation of the South, it must have been a relief to be on the plains again.

In March many of the Seventh Cavalry's companies assembled at Louisville, Memphis, and New Orleans then all rejoined at Cairo, Illinois, in early April. From there they moved by railroad to Sioux City, Iowa, where Companies D and I, and HQ separated

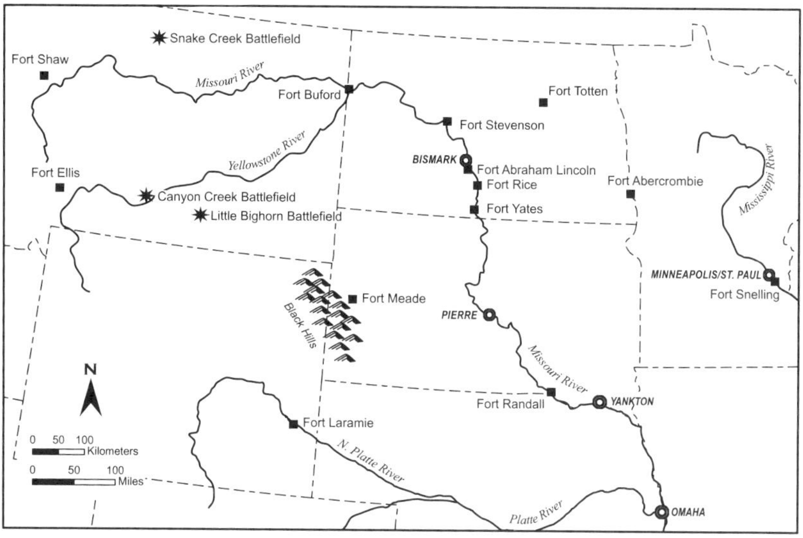

Map 1.3. The northern plains, showing principal postings and engagements of the Seventh Cavalry and major cities. Drawn by Judy Stolen. Copyright © 2015, University of Oklahoma Press.

and traveled to departmental HQ at Fort Snelling, Minnesota. The other companies continued their journey by rail to Yankton, then the territorial capital of Dakota Territory (DT) (Chandler 1960:38; map 1.3).

Just after most of the Seventh arrived at Yankton and was preparing for wagon and steamboat transportation up the Missouri River, a blizzard struck on April 14—"Custer's Blizzard," it was called. Some claimed that this was the worst blizzard that the regiment experienced in its decades on the plains (Garlington 1896:256). Officers stayed in a hotel in Yankton, while some troopers billeted in other hotels and saloons (tough duty for the intemperate among them). Others encamped a few miles downriver from town (Chandler 1960).

Once the ice was off the Missouri River and the grass was green enough to support horses, the Seventh Cavalry left Yankton in early May and headed north. This movement by land was supported by steamship, moving supplies and forage and other important cargo—including invalid soldiers—along the travel route. Six members of command were said to have died while on Snatch Creek near Bon Homme and been buried there, although no regimental record of such deaths apparently exists (Chandler 1960:39).

The Seventh Cavalry completed its movement up the Missouri River, arriving at Fort Rice in mid-June. It escorted the Northern Railroad survey expedition (Eckroth 2013). Approximately 1,500 strong, the troops left Fort Rice later that month, headed west, crossed the Little Missouri River, and reached the Yellowstone River in mid-July. The column marched up the Yellowstone River from there. On August 4 Custer and his detachment were attacked along the Yellowstone River near the future location of Fort Keogh, Montana. After those hostilities one soldier was missing and one wounded. On the same day the veterinarian and a sutler were killed in a separate event (Garlington 1896:256; Chandler 1960:40; Eckroth 2013).

A few days later the trail of a large village was discovered and followed. On August 11 Indians were encountered, first in a stationary fight then in a running battle eight miles long, ending with the Indians escaping across the Yellowstone River (Garlington 1896:256). The results on the U.S. side were one officer and one enlisted man killed and two enlisted men wounded (Chandler 1960:40; Eckroth 2013).

The expedition marched to the Musselshell River, leaving the Yellowstone River. In late August Custer was ordered to Fort Lincoln, DT, via the supply depot on the Yellowstone River. The column arrived at Fort Lincoln in mid-September and dispersed into nearby forts for winter (Eckroth 2013; Chandler 1960:40).

Elsewhere during the summer and fall detached Seventh Cavalry companies under Major Marcus Reno aided the International Northern Boundary Survey. In October their fair-weather work ceased for the year. The companies marched to Fort Totten for the winter (Chandler 1960:40). A presidential proclamation in 1873 provided amnesty for deserters. And "a large number of deserters surrendered to the military authorities" (Chandler 1960:41).

1874

Members of the regiment performed the usual garrison duties during the winter, although they must have been much affected by the weather, especially the cold. It was their first full winter on the northern plains. Small patrols performed scouting duties, deployed to make arrests, and protected people and properties on the agencies. In addition to these small-scale movements, they were also active as larger units, especially as the year continued.

In May Companies D and I left Fort Lincoln, as they had the previous year, to escort the International Northern Boundary Survey Commission. Traveling by way of Forts Stevenson and Buford, the companies established a base of operations in the Sweet Grass Hills of northern Montana Territory (MT). They remained deployed in this service until August, when they returned to Fort Totten and then went into winter quarters in mid-September (Chandler 1960:41–42). At the same time the rest of the regiment was also active in the field.

The likelihood of an expedition became certainty in early July. Most of the regiment (ten companies, according to Garlington 1896:257), supplemented by infantry, scouts, journalists, and scientists, left Fort Lincoln for the Black Hills (Chandler 1960:41). The official purpose of the Black Hills Expedition was to find a place for a new post that would provide a better strategic location to control movements of the Sioux and Cheyennes. Another purpose of the expedition was to map the Black Hills. But an additional and possibly driving goal was to search for gold. For years rumors of gold in the Black Hills spread. In that period of economic difficulties the hopes and possibilities evoked by such a rumor were uplifting.

During the two-month expedition, they had little contact with Indians, although frequent signs and trails indicated their presence. The expedition marched southwest from Fort Lincoln, rounding the north and west sides of the Black Hills. The main body of the expedition went upstream through canyons into the Black Hills' relatively flat valleys and prairies, from there spreading out to explore the south and southeastern portion. The presence of gold was confirmed, and a courier ("Lonesome" Charlie Reynolds, who later died at the Little Bighorn) was sent from the command in early August to carry the news to the nearest telegraph at Fort Laramie. In early August the expedition started its return to Fort Lincoln, backtracking over the trail it had taken in the Black Hills then exiting to the northeast. It camped near Bear Butte, the location that Custer considered most attractive as a place for a future post. Fort Meade was established there three years later. The column returned to Fort Lincoln at the end of August, on schedule and with its orders met.

A few health problems arose during the expedition, including two deaths. Private John Cunningham, Company H, developed diarrhea while on the expedition and died in mid-July after an illness of two weeks. According to one enlisted man's account, Cunningham's death was due to the attending surgeons' maladroitness (Carroll and Frost 1976:32–36). Within a day of Cunningham's death, Private George Turner, Company M, also died. He suffered a gunshot wound during an internecine squabble with another trooper. The two bodies were buried during the same ceremony near present-day Sundance, Wyoming (Progulske and Shideler n.d.:7).

Journalists accompanied the expedition and sent their dispatches from the Black Hills, so the entire nation soon knew of the gold discovery. Some of the expedition members even formed a mining corporation and set claim to French Creek (Progulske and Shideler n.d.:6). Following news accounts of gold, the military was ordered to bar invading prospectors and speculators from the Black Hills, but those efforts were largely futile. Prospectors poured in. When the military apprehended them, the trespassers were delivered to civil authorities, who usually released them. The released prospectors often returned to the Black Hills. Late in the year it became the official policy for the military to cease removing trespassers and withdraw from that area (Chandler 1960:46). An expedition into the Black Hills the next year documented hundreds of trespassers.

Recognizing the untenability of keeping prospectors from the Black Hills, the government arranged meetings with the "treaty" Indians to purchase the territory. That transfer occurred in February 1877 for $4.5 million (Progulske and Shideler n.d.:6).

In late September 1874 six of the regiment's companies left Fort Lincoln, returning to their previous station in the Department of the Gulf. It must have been a relief to leave the northern plains in the fall, thus avoiding another Dakota winter (a trip that migrating fowl have made for millennia and wealthy citizens make today). Those troopers were assigned to posts in Louisiana and

Alabama, remaining in the South until the spring of 1876 (Chandler 1960:41).

In December Tom Custer, commanding men from Company L, arrested Rain-in-the-Face, who had reputedly murdered the veterinarian and sutler the year before near the Yellowstone River. Rain-in-the-Face was jailed at Fort Lincoln but later escaped. He is said to have killed Tom Custer during the Battle of the Little Bighorn (Chandler 1960:43).

1875

Most of the companies remained at their winter quarters until spring, continuing to perform the usual post and escort duties. In April Companies D and I moved from Fort Totten to Fort Lincoln. In May Companies A, E, and H returned from the Department of the Gulf and were stationed opposite Fort Randall, DT. Their main duty involved removing trespassers from the Black Hills. Other troops had various duties, but in general it was a slow year that would belie the activities and tragedies of the next several years.

Many of the events of the following years, however, were related to an order issued late in 1875. In December the Indian Bureau, in the Department of the Interior, ordered all Indians living off the reservations to return promptly to their designated reservations or be considered "hostile." The deadline for their return to reservations was the end of January 1876. Complying with this order was difficult even for those groups who received the order and were willing to return. For others, complying with the order was not a viable option. Following failure of compliance, the power for enforcement of the order passed from the Department of the Interior to the War Department and its army (Chandler 1960:43–46).

1876

The Seventh Cavalry is most remembered for a reputation-defining event that happened during this year. In the years following the Civil War, the Western Indian Wars (1865–91) included 1,067 engagements with the Indians. But almost none of them are as well known as the one involving the Seventh Cavalry and the Sioux,

Northern Cheyennes, and their allies at the Little Bighorn River (Chandler 1960:45). The battle was a watershed for all of the cultures involved. Many causes contributed to the conflict, including trespassing prospectors in the Black Hills, other white expansions into Indian lands, especially by railroads and settlers, and destruction of the bison herds.

Another cause of the conflict was the corruption of the Ulysses S. Grant administration, among the most crooked that the nation has ever seen. Relevant to the Indian situation was the dishonesty of the Department of Interior's Indian Bureau and its Indian agents. The agents were often awarded appointments as political plums, which some agents considered an opportunity for personal economic gain rather than a civic duty. As a result, even the more peacefully inclined Indians living on the reservation attempted to survive under inhumane and insufferable conditions. As an example, the Seventh Cavalry learned during the winter of 1874–75 that the Indians at nearby Standing Rock Indian Reservation had no food, although supplies had been delivered to the railroad head not far from the reservation. The agency had no way of moving supplies from the railroad station to the Indians, so Custer requested permission to divide his surplus military rations with the agency Indians until their supplies could be transported. His offer was declined, and as a result many Indians died on Standing Rock that winter. Similar situations were recorded and comparable offers were made at several places across the West. One of the few options that the starving Indians had was to leave the reservations and join the "hostile" groups that were living a more traditional life off the reservations. The Department of Interior's command late in 1875 was directed against these groups: all Indians must be on the reservation by the end of January 1876. The order, as mentioned earlier, was either not received or ignored for a number of reasons. In early 1876 the problem passed from the hands of the Department of Interior to the War Department (Chandler 1960:45–46).

The War Department's grand plan coalesced as the Campaign of 1876. Its purpose was to force hostiles onto the reservations. During the campaign planning, Custer was summoned before a House of Representatives Committee on Expenditures of the War Department. Custer's testimony, among others, implicated several friends and relatives of President Grant in a scandal revolving around the granting of post traderships and the profits made from those lucrative positions. Based on this testimony, Grant had a poor view of Custer. Custer tried to see the president but was unable to obtain an appointment. Believing that he had permission to leave Washington, Custer traveled to Chicago, on his way to rejoin his regiment. The president, angered that Custer had left Washington without his permission, ordered him through General William Sherman to remain in Chicago. Custer was forbidden to accompany the regiment on the campaign. But in May he was allowed to rejoin the regiment and complete preparations for the upcoming campaign. He returned to Fort Lincoln and rode out on May 17, 1876, as commanding officer of the Seventh, to meet his fate at the Little Bighorn.

The army knew that the Indians wintered somewhere in what is now southeastern Montana. Following a near-disastrous late winter campaign, the army planned a three-pronged offensive to begin in May (Stewart 1955; Gray 1976). General Alfred Terry left Fort Abraham Lincoln with Custer and the Seventh Cavalry and marched west. Colonel John Gibbon left Fort Ellis (near present-day Bozeman, Montana) and marched east down the Yellowstone River. From the south General George Crook led over 1,000 men north from Fort Fetterman, Wyoming Territory (present-day Douglas, Wyoming). The columns were to meet along the Yellowstone River, MT.

On June, 17, 1876, Crook's forces met the Indians at the Battle of the Rosebud. Although losing few men, Crook's forces depleted their ammunition and were forced to withdraw. Meanwhile Terry and Gibbon continued movements, unaware of Crook's engagement. Custer's Seventh Cavalry separated from the rest of Terry's forces on June 22 and followed an Indian trail into the valley of the Little Bighorn. Although Custer did not know it, they were following the trail of many of the Indians who had forced Crook's retreat only days before.

On the morning of June 25, after a night ride, Custer let his men stop briefly as they crossed the divide into the Little Bighorn drainage at a place now known as the Crow's Nest. They made coffee and rested a little. Some said that they could see the Indian camp from there. Custer moved his command into the valley of the Little Bighorn. In the afternoon Custer divided his command into three elements. Captain Thomas McDougall and Company B along with seven men from each of the other companies were assigned to guard the pack train. Captain Frederick Benteen led three companies to scout to the south and prevent potential escapes. Custer took the rest of the men toward the Indian encampment.

Before attacking the village, Custer split his troops again. Three companies were assigned to Major Marcus Reno, who was to follow the west side of the Little Bighorn River and attack the village from the south. Custer followed the east side of the river and apparently planned to cross the river and attack the north end of the village with the remaining five companies. With the two battalions they planned to encircle and capture the Indians. In addition, Benteen, to the south and west, could capture any who attempted to flee in those directions. Reno and Custer paralleled each other on the opposite sides of the river until Reno encountered the village and initiated the attack. As Reno's men began the battle, Custer was seen on the bluffs on the opposite side of the river, riding north.

After initial confusion in the attack on the Indian village, Reno's men encountered heavy opposition. They retreated to the timber near the river and then across the river and up the bluffs on the east side. The retreat was disorderly at best. Skirmishers were not deployed to defend the ford as they forded the river, and men crossing the river made easy targets for the Indians. Many did not hear the retreat call or failed to move from their position and were left in the woods in the valley, straggling in to rejoin the command during the next forty-eight hours.

The men who made it to the top of the bluffs quickly assumed a defensive position and returned the Indians' fire. Meanwhile Custer had ridden north to a ravine now known as Medicine Tail Coulee and sent trumpeter John Martin back with a message to Benteen: "Benteen come on Big Village. Be Quick, Bring packs. P.S. Bring packs." Custer was of course referring to the ammunition packs carried by the pack train under McDougall's charge.

Martin reached Benteen with the message. Benteen followed Custer's trail and found Reno in position on the bluff top. The pack train and McDougall's company followed Benteen and joined the command a short time later. Reno's men wondered what had happened to Custer. They speculated that, like themselves, Custer and his men had assumed a defensive position and were pinned down somewhere to the north. At one point Captain Thomas B. Weir led his company to the north in the hopes of finding Custer's men. The rest of the command followed. They moved about a mile north to an area known today as Weir's Point before being driven back by Indian fire. Some said that from Weir's Point they could see dust and smoke to the north and assumed that Custer and his men were fighting there.

The Indian fire slackened at the Reno-Benteen defense site during the night of June 25 but resumed the next morning. Some of the men who had been abandoned in the valley used the cover of darkness to rejoin the command. The weather produced another blistering Montana June day, and water became a critical factor, particularly for the wounded.

Enlisted volunteers went to the river to get water for the wounded. Sharpshooters were sent to suppress Indian fire during the foray of the water carriers. Several successful trips were made to the river. Individual stories of heroism abound. Some of the men who went for water for the wounded and some of the water carriers and the sharpshooters were later awarded Medals of Honor for their gallantry in action. Twice, when the Indians got too close to the line, Captain Benteen formed his men and charged, driving back the Indians. Captain Benteen walked around the line, encouraging the men and raising their flagging spirits. Another foray to the river was made the night of June 26, to recover the body of Lieutenant Benjamin Hodgson, who had been killed crossing the ford the day before.

Reno's men were pinned down the entire day, but late on June 26 they saw a line of Indians leaving the village. That night Indian fire slackened again, and by the morning of June 27 the Indians were gone. Reno's men saw dust in the distance and then slowly made out cavalry troops. Several of Reno's officers met Terry's and Gibbon's combined command in the Indian village, all wondering where Custer was. Soon a scouting party brought back the news. Custer and his men lay dead on the slopes above the Little Bighorn River about three miles north of Reno's position.

Reno's men were detailed to bury the dead on June 28. The heat that made water such a critical factor during the battle had treated the bodies poorly. Individuals were difficult to identify, even for soldiers who had known them well. The regiment had few digging tools and used and spoons and cups from the mess kits to excavate. Meanwhile the dead in Reno's position were also buried and their equipment was gathered into a pile and burned, to prevent it from falling into the hands of the Indians.

Gibbon and Terry's combined command with the surviving members of the Seventh Cavalry, including about fifty wounded, moved to the mouth of the Little Bighorn, where the steamer *Far West* was waiting. The steamer took aboard the wounded and made record time to Bismarck, DT, bearing the wounded and the news of Custer's defeat to Fort Abraham Lincoln.

After a long summer's march, the remnants of the Seventh Cavalry returned to Fort Lincoln and the Seventh Cavalry's other DT posts in September. Enlistments (dubbed "Custer's Avengers") swelled company troop strength, newly authorized to a strength of 100 men from the 60 per company of the preceding spring (Garlington 1896:160). To keep Indians who were on the reservation from joining the hostiles, October was spent disarming and dismounting the Indians on the Standing Rock and Cheyenne River agencies (Chandler 1960:73).

1877

After the activities of the previous year, 1877 got off to a mercifully slow start but ended with a flurry of activity. The troops moved from winter quarters in April, performing the usual summer scouts. This year, however, emphasis on patrolling the international line reflected the concern that Sitting Bull would return from Canada to the United States.

This year the Nez Perce troubles occurred. After fleeing Washington State and crossing Idaho as well as portions of the newly established Yellowstone National Park, the Nez Perces came into contact with the Seventh Cavalry. The Seventh fought the Nez Perces at Canyon Creek in mid-September, about seventy-five miles from the location of the previous year's Battle of the Little Bighorn. The movement was intended to prevent the Nez Perces' northward flight into Canada to join Sitting Bull's band there. Later in September and October three companies of the Seventh again fought the Nez Perces at Snake Creek ("Bear Paw") in north-central MT. The casualties on the Seventh's side were two officers and nineteen enlisted men killed and two officers and twenty-seven enlisted men wounded (Garlington 1896:262). After the Nez Perces' surrender, nearly the entire regiment guarded and escorted them back to their reservation or incarceration.

In addition to issues involving the Nez Perces, concerns about Sitting Bull's movements and his intentions persisted (Garlington 1896:262). As a consequence, many of the Seventh Cavalry's companies remained in the field late that year. They arrived at winter quarters well into winter, most of them going into winter postings in January of the following year.

1878

The Seventh remained at winter posts through March, when most outlying companies moved to Fort Abraham Lincoln, a central location. From there most companies journeyed to Bear Butte, a strategic location to block Indian movements from the reservations in DT to the Yellowstone River area of MT. In addition to preventing movements of potentially hostile Indians, the troops established more permanent camps. Company F, however, remained at Fort Totten (Garlington 1896:263), at least during the early part of the year.

In the summer portions of the Seventh Cavalry escorted Cheyenne prisoners on their journey from the northern plains south to Indian Territory (IT). That destination did not last long. When the Cheyennes fled the reservations in IT in September and headed north, the Seventh Cavalry was involved. A national perception existed that the Cheyennes' return to DT would destabilize the fragile situation. So in the late fall portions of the Seventh Cavalry moved south to Red Cloud Agency, Nebraska, to thwart the Cheyennes' return. They patrolled sensitive areas and ultimately captured and escorted the Cheyennes. During November, after the capture of the Cheyennes, the Seventh Cavalry contingent except two companies returned to former quarters. Those companies went to the location where the future Fort Meade would be established the next year (Garlington 1896:263).

1879

This year was relatively inactive for the Seventh Cavalry, at least in terms of field activities. They went on a few scouts and fought a prairie fire near Deadwood in the Black Hills. The major change was in postings: four companies moved to Fort Meade (Chandler 1960:78).

1880

For much of the year most of the Seventh Cavalry was occupied guarding the Northern Pacific Railroad construction (Chandler 1960:78). During the winter of 1880–81, Company F accepted the surrender of Sitting Bull and Gall's followers, four years after the Battle of the Little Bighorn (Garlington 1896:263).

1881

This year the Seventh went on many short scouts. It was also a year of substantial change in personnel, with many discharges for expiration of service. The five-year hitch of the "Custer Avengers" was over, and the ranks diminished (Chandler 1960:78).

1882

This year also was mostly spent scouting. In addition to the scouts, the Seventh Cavalry spent considerable time protecting the Northern Pacific Railroad construction. A few companies moved in 1882 (Chandler 1960:78–79). This year approaches the end of the period under study, but any history of the Seventh Cavalry would be remiss if it excluded the following events.

YEARS AFTER 1882

After 1882 the Seventh Cavalry's main duties included return of footloose Indians to their reservations, small-scale scouts, garrison duty, chasing "road agents," patrolling the Canadian-U.S. border, and pursuing cattle rustlers. A general consolidation of companies occurred, moving from more isolated garrisons to larger ones, especially to Fort Meade and Fort Yates (Chandler 1960:79–80).

The final gasps of the wild West occurred in the 1890s. By that time most of the Seventh Cavalry had moved from the northern plains to Fort Riley, Kansas, and Fort Sill, IT, in the central and southern plains, respectively (Garlington 1896:164). Railroads made troop movements more rapid and dependable than marches by horse, which were usually supported by horse-drawn wagons. With the rise of the Ghost Dance movement, some Indians believed that revitalization would occur, that whites would be driven from Indian lands, that the buffalo would return, and that the dead would rise from the grave (Garlington 1896:264). Associated with this revitalization movement was a ceremony called the Ghost Dance. In its wake Sitting Bull was killed on Standing Rock Reservation and the massacre at Wounded Knee occurred (Greene 2014).

In late December 1890 the regiment again engaged the Sioux when it participated in the massacre at Wounded Knee, South Dakota (Utley 1963; Jensen et al. 1991; Greene 2014). That one-sided fight effectively ended the era of the American Indian Wars. The Seventh lost three more Little Bighorn veterans at Wounded Knee: Captain George Wallace, Corporal George Loyd, and Private Gustave Korn, best known as the keeper of Comanche, Keogh's mount from the Little Bighorn. The Seventh Cavalry continued its service to the country during the labor unrest at the end of the century, the Spanish-American War, World War I, World War II, and Korea. The lineal descendent of the Seventh Cavalry is a part of the modern First Cavalry Division.

Summary

In the end the Seventh Cavalry (and the army more generally) was only a contributing factor in the demise of the traditional lifestyle of the Indians (Coffman 1986:254). These tensions caused DT to be what one historian called "the most violent of American frontiers" (Howard R. Lamar, cited in Etulain 2006:171). Larger factors were in effect and drove the Seventh Cavalry's orders. These broader events sealed the fate of the traditional Plains Indians in ways that the Colt revolver and Springfield carbine could not. The factors included continued westward expansion of Euro-Americans, increasing economic opportunities on the plains (especially in time of economic downturns), more rapid transportation (particularly the railroads), and more rapid relay of information (notably via the telegraph). The destruction of the bison herds brought an end to the lifestyle of the nomadic plains tribes. The Indian question had come to a head, and the result was ugly to behold. By the end of the nineteenth century the Indians of the plains were subdued and on reservations. Disease, famine, and apathy had taken their toll. This period has been described as the nadir of Plains Indians.

CHAPTER 2

Overview of Nineteenth-Century Medical Care

Patrick J. Collison

The theory and practice of medicine underwent significant changes during the nineteenth century. The intellectual roots of these advances developed much earlier, with the French Enlightenment and the growth of rationalism. Progress became possible because of profound changes in the epistemology of medicine, with recognition that disease was not punishment for religious transgressions but resulted from physical earthly causes. In general terms, the basis for medical knowledge shifted from faith and fiction at the dawn of the century, to informed speculation at mid-century, and on to the beginnings of evidence-based medicine in the late 1800s. For the individual practitioner, these changes were time- and space-transgressive; old theories and practices persisted in some areas long after new information had undermined their credibility. Military medical care, as provided during the major conflicts of this period, served as a crucible for the refinement of some of these changes to understand and treat disease.

Three Epochs of Nineteenth-Century American Medicine

The first century of United States medicine can be divided into three epochs. The dominant thought between 1776 and about 1832 has been characterized as "Systems of Medicine," promulgated by leaders such as Benjamin Rush, William Cullen, and John Brown (Warner 1997:23, 40). During this period, conventional practitioners evinced a supreme confidence in the art of medicine and a corresponding distrust in the healing powers of nature. Disease etiology was still interpreted in terms of the four humors of the ancients, and treatment involved restoring the balance of an individual's natural state through aggressive intervention. A physician's identity and prestige were established more by displaying quick judgment, experience, and decisiveness than by accumulated knowledge. Therapeutics generally involved "heroic depletion": lowering overactive humors in sthenic (strong or excited) patients by bloodletting, purging with mercury compounds, or inducing vomiting with tartar emetic. These measures reliably demonstrated to the patient that the doctor controlled the situation and could be credited with the favorable outcome that followed, as it does for most self-limited illnesses. In fact, bloodletting provided at least temporary symptomatic relief for several conditions, including congestive heart failure, hematologic diseases causing an excess of red blood cells, and certain psychiatric states for which lowered blood pressure resulted in fainting, a form of "shock therapy." In the absence of effective anesthetics, surgical procedures during this period were risky and traumatic for patient and physician alike. Only simple operations could be executed successfully and had to be performed with skill and alacrity. The essence of professional legitimacy therefore required practical knowledge, close interaction with patients, and moral character: basically the qualities esteemed in American society of the day.

Although in the first half of the century wealthy medical students sought training in Europe, especially in the lecture halls of Edinburgh and the hospitals of Paris, most neophytes learned their craft as apprentices and from preceptor-directed reading. While valuing a European medical education, American practitioners distrusted experimentally based therapeutics, especially the numerical methods of the French, as inappropriate for American constitutions and diseases. They accused the French of being more interested in making the correct diagnosis and confirming it at autopsy than in curing the patient (Warner 1997:189).

In America during the early 1800s orthodox practitioners tended to align themselves with one of two schools of thought:

rational medicine or empiricism. The first and older position emphasized tradition and rules of practice deduced from general principles, while empiricists stressed observation and practical results unclouded by theory. The two terms actually were often synonyms and antonyms of themselves, hurled as invectives to discredit competitors.

The second epoch, 1832 to 1869, is characterized as a time when the value of empirical observation and nature's healing power came to the fore. Prominent individuals such as Louis Bigelow, Elisha Bartlett, and Oliver Wendell Holmes were influenced by French skeptical empiricism to doubt the efficacy and safety of the mercurials, antimony-based emetics, and other harsh inorganic chemicals that had been the mainstays of regular medical practice. In the annual address to the Massachusetts Medical Society in 1860, Holmes expressed his disdain for the current state of medical therapeutics: "I firmly believe that if most of the pharmacopoeia were sunk to the bottom of the sea, it would be all the better for mankind and all the worse for the fishes" (Holmes 1860:140). Despite Holmes's known penchant for hyperbole, these oft-quoted words fueled the therapeutic nihilism that became prevalent in the mid-1800s.

American doctors, especially those practicing far from the academic meccas of the Northeast, took exception to such pronouncements. This skepticism not only undermined their prestige but also provided ammunition to their competitors: the homeopaths, eclectics, and Thomsonians (herbalists). An excess of practitioners, exacerbated by competition from sectarians, diminished practices and made it difficult to make a living. Homeopaths and other irregulars promoted less aggressive therapies, virtually free of side effects—in fact free of all active ingredients. This approach appealed to the general public, especially the well-to-do. Furthermore, advancing knowledge of anatomy, physiology, and pathology forced the insightful practitioner to acknowledge the futility of bloodletting and purging. This admission required a candid acknowledgment of previous ignorance, even harm. Orthodox medicine sought to explain the decline in bloodletting and blunt criticism by several means. One was the "change-of-type" theory, which postulated that diseases and the patients who endured them had changed over time, mainly due to social and environmental factors. In the view of their doctors, people had become less sthenic. This loss of robustness was attributed to "increased delicacy of living and the introduction of those luxuries that tend to enervate the constitution" (Warner 1997:167). Appropriate treatment required a shift from heroic depletion (lancet, tartar emetic, and calomel) to heroic stimulation (alcohol, iron, and "high" diet), permitting a face-saving response to fluctuating circumstances that physicians could build into their medical theory.

A similar principle that traditionalists used to justify resistance to change was specificity. Adhering to a form of states' rights medicine, physicians from certain regions maintained a faith in local therapeutic distinctiveness that persisted into the 1860s. Insisting that "[o]ur medical literature cannot be manufactured for us abroad" (Warner 1997:76), country doctors thought that they saw regional uniqueness in patients and their response to therapy, especially when urban hospitals were contrasted with rural private practice. Discerning an individual's constitution, an inclusive term encompassing all personal characteristics, was considered essential. Nineteenth-century doctors added a fifth temperament to the four temperaments of Hippocrates: nervous. Thus neurasthenia became a malady to which modern city dwellers and participants in industrialization were particularly prone. Urbanites, the wealthy, and whites required elevating therapy: quinine as an antiperiodic and antipyretic, alcohol as a stimulant, iron compounds for anemia, and cod liver oil to nourish those with pulmonary disease. Some of these agents were and still are considered effective. The diet shifted from abstemious to high. Other groups, especially rural laborers, blacks, and Indians, may still have been treated with antiphlogistic (inflammation-suppressing) or debilitative therapies.

Few if any new pharmaceutical agents were introduced during this period that materially advanced the physician's armamentarium. Drugs in the 1860s were not manufactured based on innovative research but rather based on the comforting reassurance of tradition and precedence. The Civil War, which by sheer numbers of victims and force of necessity led to refinements in surgical technique, did not create new and more effective drugs. It served as a proving ground for therapeutic substances, new and old, and mainly advanced medical care by proving some of the old nostrums to be ineffective or unsafe.

The hypodermic syringe with its hollow needle was introduced by Alexander Wood in 1853 (Williams 1981:125). This device facilitated the intravenous administration of analgesics such as morphine as well as local anesthetics. Unfortunately, drug addiction and dependency became so widespread after the Civil War, mainly as the result of intravenous opiate use, that the condition became known as the "soldier's disease."

The discovery of safe and effective general anesthetics was probably the most important advance in medical care during the mid-1800s. Three inhalant agents (ether, nitrous oxide, and chloroform) were all introduced and began to be administered for surgical procedures in the 1840s. This application followed decades of recreational use in parlor games called "ether frolics." The U.S. Congress offered a $100,000 reward to anyone who was proved to be the first to administer an anesthetic effectively. Lacking evidence and mired in endless controversy, none of the early innovators ever collected the prize. General anesthetics were used no less than 80,000 times during the Civil War: chloroform in 76.2 percent of cases, ether in 14.7 percent, and a combination of the two in 9.1 percent (Barnes 1870:887). Titrating the proper concentration while maintaining adequate oxygenation was the most difficult aspect of using these agents. A "large gum catheter" (hard rubber tube) was sometimes utilized to blow air into the lungs for resuscitation but was not yet used for routine inhalant administration and airway protection. It is surprising that anesthetic death rates were only 0.5 percent for chloroform and 0.3 percent for ether. During the period of the early Plains Indian Wars (1865 to 1876), general anesthetics were used 1,210 times. The average length of anesthesia was twenty-two to twenty-six minutes, so only straightforward procedures such as amputations and excisions could be performed (Barnes 1870:898).

Proprietary medical schools multiplied during the second half of the nineteenth century. Many students were educated in these store-front enterprises, although fully equipped teaching hospitals also began to appear, beginning with the University of Pennsylvania in the 1870s. The stereotypical image of proprietary medical schools, operated by mercenary instructors for profit and prestige and offering guaranteed degrees after trivial exams, is probably exaggerated. Although the curriculum and content were not yet uniform, students took their studies seriously and feared failing their tests. They also learned a lot after graduation from patients and other doctors, just as young practitioners do today (Warner 1997:172).

In the third epoch, beginning about the end of the Civil War, universalism began to replace specificity as the guiding principle in medical care, grounded in experimental science. The new professional identity was defined by allegiance to a body of knowledge generated and affirmed by objective laboratory observations and characterized by universal diagnostic and therapeutic categories. Hospital records from the late nineteenth century provide detailed systematic information about current clinical attitudes and activity. By the 1870s the term "normal" had completely replaced "natural" as a descriptor of the model state of patient well-being. The paradigm of thinking about goals of treatment had shifted to measured, quantified norms of bodily function. Graphic representation of variables such as temperature, pulse, respiratory rate, and chemical composition of urine, compared to measured norms, became standard. Clinical assessment moved toward an increasingly reductionist perspective on patients, with shorter and less idiosyncratic record keeping, more instrumental and chemical analyses, quantified signs and symptoms, and more narrowly targeted remedies. The stethoscope, invented by René Laennec in 1847, became de rigueur for every physical exam (Williams 1981:19). The laryngoscope and opthalmoscope were introduced in the 1860s, and Joseph Toynbee's detailed description of ear diseases and pathology in the same decade made ophthalmological and otolaryngologic specialization possible (Toynbee 1860). These were the earliest recognized specialties in medicine, probably because of the precise instrumentation and skills required.

Medical education improved as the twentieth century approached, with the establishment of large university-based teaching hospitals. Johns Hopkins, with pioneering icons such as William Osler and William S. Halsted, opened in 1889. Widespread reforms and closure of nearly all the proprietary schools accelerated with Abraham Flexner's incisive report on medical education in 1910.

Although the germ theory of disease and Robert Koch's famous postulates were not specifically formulated until 1882, much progress was made in the practical aspects of hygiene and surgical antisepsis during the last third of the century. Joseph Lister was distressed by the high rate of infection in his amputation cases and suspected that current ideas about "miasma" (bad air) as a source of contamination were incorrect. Oliver Wendell Holmes also thought doctors might be the most active carriers of disease and observed that the dreaded "hospital gangrene" rarely developed through unbroken skin. Louis Pasteur conducted experiments that allowed him to declare confidently that minute organisms caused infection and were not spontaneously generated. Beginning in 1865 Lister used Pasteur's findings to develop an antiseptic spray, carbolic acid, which disinfected wounds and prevented postoperative infection. This apparatus was used during the Civil War and later, reducing surgical mortality. These antiseptic methods were adopted by Theodor Billroth and others, enabling them successfully to perform complex procedures such as gastrectomies and laryngectomies (Williams 1981:71).

The delivery of medical care received a major boost with the development of nursing services. Before the Civil War nursing was nonexistent as a distinct field. In fact women employed as nurses were described as "slatternly and disreputable" by some observers (Williams 1981:91). Florence Nightingale's efforts during the Crimean War and her establishment of training schools for nurses were critical for the advancement of nursing as a profession (Williams 1981:95). Nightingale was struck by the high mortality rate among soldiers, not from battle wounds but from illness in the barracks. She noted mortality rates of 2.2/1,000 for the general population compared to 10.04/1,000 for soldiers camped in the same districts and acted on this information to improve hospital care. In the North women participated as nurses through the United States Sanitary Commission, an adjunct to the Army Medical Department that was initially rejected by the military and had to be supported by private contributions. The Sanitary Commission was a precursor to the American Red Cross (Kramer 1948:453–55). Then and throughout the later Plains Indian Wars military nurses answered to the hospital steward, who also oversaw cooks, laundresses, food procurement, and quality for the sick and often served as pharmacists (Flannery 2004:81).

Two of the century's most useful medical discoveries came in the 1890s, too late to assist surgeons serving in the immediate post–Civil War period. Diphtheria antitoxin was the first effective antibacterial agent to be developed and, after smallpox vaccine, the first reliable weapon against any microorganism (Ashburn 1929:156). Roentgen rays were discovered in 1895 by William Conrad Roentgen, an experimental physicist with a rigorous academic background. X-ray technology found immediate medical application, especially for orthopedic and dental work (Williams 1981:207).

Military Medicine in the Nineteenth Century

Periods of armed conflict provided impetus for change in medical and surgical care, as well as some resistance to change. Based on the large number of casualties and scope of the conflict, the Civil War has been the focus of most of medical historians' attention. The Mexican-American War of 1846–48 served as a wake-up call for military medicine. Of the 100,000 regulars and volunteers called to duty, casualties totaled 1,500 killed in action contrasted with about 10,000 from disease and accident. The 94 surgeons available were deemed inadequate to care for this many men, and contract surgeons were often viewed as inept and lacking fundamental medical knowledge. Medical attendants also lacked sufficient training (Tate 1999:177). The huge number of casualties in the Civil War forced the issue and compelled improvements.

The most detailed and extensive record of illnesses and injuries during the Civil War period is presented in *The Medical and Surgical History of the War of the Rebellion (1861–65)*. Surgeon General Joseph K. Barnes directed this work, the largest of its magnitude at that time. Insight into current concepts of disease may be obtained by reviewing the Classification of Disease section in this report. Illnesses and injuries were divided into five classes, following a scheme devised by Dr. William Farr of England. Barnes adapted this classification system to facilitate comparisons with data from other countries, an insightful approach that supported the emerging universalist understanding of disease. The classification enacted by the board, adapted for army use, is as follows:

Class I. Zymotic Diseases
    Order 1. Miasmatic
    2. Enthetic
    3. Dietic
Class II. Constitutional Diseases
    Order 1. Diathetic
    2. Tubercular
Class III. Parasitic
Class IV. Local Diseases
    Order 1. Nervous System
    2. Eye
    3. Ear
    4. Organs of Circulation
    5. Respiratory Organs
    6. Digestive Organs
    7. Urinary and Genital Organs
    8. Bones and Joints
    9. Integumentary System
Class V. Wounds, Accidents, and Injuries
    Order 1. Wounds, Accidents, Injuries
    2. Homicide
    3. Suicide
    4. Execution of Sentence

(Barnes 1870:xviii)

This six-volume set consisted of 6,000 pages and weighed 56 pounds. A product of the philosophy of natural history accepted during the 1800s, it is a systematic statistical compilation of the types of injuries and illnesses that a military doctor could expect to treat, along with analysis, interventions, and results. Barnes made an effort to ascertain the incidence of disease and death by recording the number of cases per population of soldiers in a regiment or facility. Particular attention was paid to the morale and sanitary conditions of the troops, the amount and condition of hospital supplies and ambulances, and the quality of food and water supplies. The precise nature and location of each wound was recorded and sometimes illustrated, as well as degree of exposure to the elements and distance and mode of transportation to the hospital. Barnes and George Otis, who detailed wounds incurred during the early Indian Wars period, ensured that medical officers carefully described all aspects of injury to aid in determining best treatments.

The brief military career of Surgeon General William H. Hammond is emblematic of the hard-fought nature of advances in American medical care in general and army medicine in particular. Young and aggressive, Hammond was appointed in 1862 to revitalize an ossified medical department. In response to widespread overprescribing of calomel and tartar emetic, Hammond ordered these substances removed from the standard supply table in Circular No. 6 on May 4, 1863. The use of mercury had been on the wane for decades, and animal experiments by John Hughes Bennett in Edinburgh showed that calomel did not stimulate biliary secretion as most practitioners supposed. Nevertheless, Hammond was pilloried for his order, which orthodox physicians viewed as a betrayal. His military career came to an unfair end when he was court-martialed on August 22, 1864, on trumped-up charges. Hammond was later exonerated and contributed in other ways. He founded the Army Medical Museum (later the National Museum of Health and Medicine) and co-founded the American Neurological Association.

In the 1860s the United States Pharmacopoeia (Boyle 1991:57) listed 871 different substances, 67 percent of which were botanicals (herbs). For army physicians, this list was pared to the Standard Supply Table, a select portion of which is listed in table 2.1.

This list only samples the Standard Table of 1863 (omitting dosages), but it provides the range of drugs available after the Civil War. Modern analysis suggests that for its day the list reflected "a judicious and thoughtful selection of galenicals (botanicals) as well as good judgment in their quantitative allowances" (Flannery 2004:119–23). Many of these substances appeared in the popular patent medicines of the late 1800s, particularly alcohol, opiates, and multiple herbs. Although controlled clinical trials later caused some of these drugs to be discarded as unsafe or ineffective, only a few new pharmaceuticals were added until well into the twentieth century. These included the bromides and chloral hydrate (soporifics) and the salicylates (analgesics and antipyretics).

Four types of illnesses account for most of the medical issues during the Civil War. This same pattern persists throughout the

TABLE 2.1. Drugs approved for use by the U.S. military during the 1860s

Drug	*Use*
Citric acid	Antiscorbutic
Alcohol fortis	Stimulant, anodyne
Ether	Anesthetic
Silver nitrate	Caustic
Chloroform	Anesthetic
Cinchona, quinine	Antimalarial
Belladonna extract	Antispasmodic
Cantharides (Spanish fly)	Counterirritant
Ipecac	Emetic
Iron chloride	Tonic
Buchu extract	Urinary inflammation
Corrosive sublimate	Biliary stimulant
Magnesium sulfate	Laxative
Cod liver oil	Dietary supplement
Opium	Analgesic, antidiarrheal
Syrup of squills	Expectorant
Mayapple	Cathartic
Strychnine	Antispasmodic

Source: This list is abridged from the Standard Supply Table of 1863.

Indian Wars and Reconstruction South, as seen in the Seventh Cavalry medical records that provide the data for the other chapters in this book:

1. Diarrheal ailments. As many as 900 case studies covering 842 pages are included in *The Medical and Surgical History*. Many of these were caused by contaminated drinking water. While some of the harsh remedies (calomel and opiates) may have caused harm, others (such as subnitrate of bismuth) probably relieved cramping and related symptoms.
2. Febrile illnesses. Malaria, typhus, typhoid, and measles are a few examples of the feverish diseases. Cinchona derivatives

were effective for malaria, although they were often used, probably without effect, for the other febrile illnesses as well.

3. Respiratory diseases. These ailments included primarily catarrh (colds), bronchitis, and pneumonia. They were thought to be caused by climatic changes and exposure to inclement weather. Medications used included syrup of squills (derived from the sea onion), quinine, Dover's Powders (ipecac and opium), and cod liver oil. Cupping, bleeding, tartar emetic, and mercurials employed earlier in the century had been abandoned in favor of tonics, stimulants, and a supportive diet.
4. Digestive disorders. These conditions were attributed to the poor and monotonous diet that the soldiers were required to subsist on. Bicarbonate of soda provided some symptom relief.

By the second half of the nineteenth century many physicians, disillusioned by the lack of efficacy of many of the drugs available to them, saw progress in hygienic management and public health as the best means of improving disease outcomes. Public or state preventative medicine became the profession's primary focus, potentially more productive than individual treatment (Warner 1997:241). These trends are seen in military medicine as well. In an annual review of sanitary conditions among the troops, assistant surgeon John S. Billings addressed a number of these concerns (Billings 1974). One was ventilation, based on two specific parameters: carbon dioxide content of living space air and odor. Manuals distributed to hospital stewards urged daily bathing and fresh vegetables to supplement the soldiers' rations (Woodward 2010:12, 81). Scurvy, while still a problem in mid-century, was better recognized and prevented. Virtually all post–Civil War surgeons tried to enhance water quality and safe waste disposal and did not need to understand the germ theory in detail to see the dramatic effect of clean-up campaigns. They recognized the association between filth and disease: what was offensive to the senses was injurious to health. An 1885 regulation made monthly sanitation reports from each commanding officer mandatory, although good bathing facilities in winter were not available to all troopers until 1888. The 1893 appointment of George M. Sternberg as surgeon general brought a new professionalism and scientific rigor to the Army Medical Corps and presaged the modern era of medicine.

The Army Medical School was authorized that same year, ensuring that the latest scientific methods and information were instilled in military doctors' training.

MILITARY SURGEONS

The military surgeons of the post–Civil War period have been both lionized and vilified. They have been called saviors of the troops, bringers of the most recent medical wisdom to the post–Civil War plains and South, and nothing more than butchers. You do not have to search hard to find more examples of sterling professionals among the military surgeons of the period, treating soldiers and civilians alike, than examples of doctors of lesser quality. Often the best physician in the area—if not the only physician—was the one attached to the post hospital. The army surgeon was often the first formally trained practitioner in a region. Army surgeons were among the most rigorously trained and examined medical professionals in the United States during this period.

At the end of the Civil War the army fell from 1 million wartime volunteers to 54,000 soldiers in 1867 and to 26,000 in the 1870s. Many of these troops deployed into small detachments in the South and along the western frontier, each requiring medical care. In 1868 the Army Medical Department covered 289 garrisons. Then as now, support for the soldiers had to be supplemented with civilian employees. By this time more contract physicians (n = 282) served the army than commissioned medical officers (n = 101). Congress saved money by decreasing the number of physicians hired, preventing promotions, and leaving positions vacant (Gillett 1995:11, 15).

At the simplest and most mundane levels the surgeons kept the troops well and in fighting form. When those efforts failed, they treated the ill and injured (Gillett 1989:17). Most nineteenth-century physicians learned their craft through a preceptorship, followed by a few months of lectures then more controlled practice. Army surgeons had to graduate from medical schools. Many of the medical officers had experience in practicing medicine during the Civil War.

In addition, official military physicians took a rigorous two- or three-day examination before a board, consisting of at least three medical officers. The process had been in effect since 1834 (Olch 1982:34) with some modifications during times of war, including the Civil War, when many physicians were needed immediately. The applicant had to be twenty-one to thirty-five years old, be a graduate of a medical school, be of solid mind and character, and pass an examination (Olch 1982:34). Topics covered on the examination included anatomy, chemistry, pharmacology, physiology, surgery, and toxicology. Surprisingly, obstetric knowledge also applied because laundresses, wives of soldiers, and women citizens surrounded posts and required treatment. In addition to considering academic proficiency, the examining board was to "scrutinize rigidly the moral habits, professional acquirements, and physical qualifications of the candidates" (Olch 1982:34).

An applicant who failed the examination could retake it. Of those 160 who took the test in September 1866, only 48 passed. When a physician passed, he was eligible for commission as assistant surgeon, comparable to first lieutenant in rank and pay in the cavalry (Wier 1980:204). After three to five years of service, he would be examined again by the Army Medical Board and, if successful, would be promoted to full surgeon, a rank equivalent to captain. The applicant had to wait for the next available opening, however, just as regular line officers had to do (Olch 1982:34). Rank equivalents for a full surgeon advanced from major to lieutenant colonel and finally colonel; only the surgeon general had the rank of brigadier general (Wier 1980:204).

Each of the nearly three hundred posts and detachments garrisoned between 1866 and 1884 needed the services of a physician. Exam-certified physicians numbered far fewer than the positions required. Garrisons with more troops needed more physicians (Gillett 1989:18). To fill the physician vacancies, the army hired civilian doctors as contract surgeons, officially designated as acting assistant surgeons.

Acting assistant surgeons also underwent a screening process. They were required to have graduated from a reputable medical school, to produce letters of recommendation attesting to their good character, and to show good health. Many applicants also took the comprehensive army medical exams required of regular military physicians, in hopes of eventually receiving commissions. The exam covered medical and surgical topics as well as required proficiency in the arts and sciences, including Latin and Greek. Well over half of those who took the exam failed, including such well-known personages as physician, surveyor, and Indian agent Dr. Valentine T. McGillicuddy. As McGillicuddy was, those not passing the medical exam and those who took and passed the exam but were awaiting a military commission could be employed by the military.

Contract surgeons received $100 to $120 per month, with no reimbursed time for illness or continuing education. Some assignments terminated abruptly, so few physicians could count on an orderly career trajectory or develop a practice of regular patients. Acting assistant surgeons were regarded with disdain by some regular army officers, who were averse to addressing even commissioned medical officers by rank.

Disparaging nicknames, such as "Pills," were used by some enlisted men, who may have lacked confidence in the therapeutics as much as having a personal animus toward individual physicians (Wengert 1997:69). Resentment went both ways. Major Bennett A. Clements, assigned to Crook's arduous "horse meat" campaign in 1876, complained that line officers did not keep the medical staff informed of their plans, making it difficult to secure adequate provisions (Gillett 1995:78). Lieutenant James H. Bradley accompanied the Montana column's march under Colonel John Gibbon from Fort Ellis to join the Bighorn-Yellowstone Expedition. In his journal he notes that Dr. Hart, the only assigned surgeon, left the command after becoming ill in Helena, Montana. "In the absence of a medical officer, Lieutenant Coolidge was appointed acting surgeon. He had amused himself some years past by employing his leisure in the study of medicine, and is well qualified for the post" (Bradley 1961:16). Later he observed that "Doctor *alias* Lieutenant Coolidge examined his patients and prescribed his remedies with the unction of a professional" (Bradley 1961:16). These sarcastic remarks evince an attitude of casual contempt for the medical staff and their work, which would have caused a relatively well educated and underpaid physician to bristle.

Surgeons were not limited to medical treatment: some received military honors as well. Assistant surgeon Leonard Wood earned the Medal of Honor, carrying dispatches through hostile territory during campaigns against the Apaches in 1886 (Carroll 1979:165).

Wood later achieved renown for his discovery of the cause and treatment of yellow fever (Wier 1980:193).

Another Medal of Honor was bestowed on assistant surgeon Henry Tilton for his service to the wounded of the Fifth Infantry and Seventh Cavalry at the Battle of Bear Paw Mountain (Snake Creek) the year after the Little Bighorn. He "fearlessly risked his life and displayed great gallantry in rescuing and protecting wounded men" (Wier 1980:193; see also Carroll 1979:151). Another surgeon who treated Seventh Cavalrymen was Bernard J. D. Irwin, who received the Medal of Honor for previously taking command of troops after their officer was killed at the 1861 Battle of Apache Pass, Arizona. He did not receive his award until 1894, however (Carroll 1979:87). During the westward expansion period (1860 to 1890), at least eight physicians were killed in conflicts with Indians (Wier 1980:196).

Some surgeons were more renowned for their off-hours hobbies than for their medical practice. A number became accomplished geologists, naturalists, ornithologists, botanists, ethnographers, and historians, including Washington Matthews, Elliott Coues, and James Cooper. Others hunted and fished. Many drank and gambled, while others were temperate and pious. Stanley Vestal (1996) describes physicians as "headhunters" due to their practice of recovering the heads of Indians, macerating them to bone, and shipping the skulls to the Army Medical Museum (now the Armed Forces Institute of Pathology's National Museum of Health and Medicine). This practice was not limited to Indians. Executed criminals' bodies were dissected, and some of those remains were sent to the Army Medical Museum too. Cases of soldiers' wounds and diseases were also sent to the surgeon general for the collection. The collection and museum were established during the Civil War to understand the mechanisms of diseases and injuries so that they could better be treated (Devine 2014).

Despite the low pay, boredom, danger, and lack of appreciation, the Seventh Cavalry's surgeons never lacked applicants for positions. Some applicants were attracted to the adventurous life that the western frontier offered. Others established contacts to aid in acquiring land, career advancement, and other financial opportunities. Some signed from a sense of patriotic duty. Utley (1973:87) asserts that primitive living conditions and low pay would discourage "able doctors" and concludes that most army physicians "lacked the competence of their brethren in civil life." A contemporary, Morris Asch (1883:203–204), however, noted that medical officers' pay was comparable to that of newly trained physicians in civilian life and that they benefited from a steady, if modest, income. He also judged them to be as capable as physicians anywhere.

Army Medical Department

In the reduction of the army after the Civil War, Congress authorized 60 surgeons (ranked as majors), 150 assistant surgeons (ranked as lieutenants in the cavalry), and 264 contract surgeons. Budgetary constraints reduced the number of contract surgeons to 75 in 1874 (Coffman 1986:382). The most challenging episode endured by army doctors was the Bighorn-Yellowstone Expedition of 1876, from the standpoint of both the injuries inflicted by the Sioux and Cheyennes and logistical challenges posed by difficult terrain and distance from hospitals. Major William J. Sloan, medical director of the Department of Dakota, supervised the work of a dozen regular medical officers and twice as many contract surgeons and expressed concern about the number and quality of the physicians available (Gillett 1995:69).

The three medical officers at Little Bighorn were probably typical of regimental staffs of the time. Surgeon George E. Lord, post surgeon from Fort Buford, was killed with Custer. His body was later identified by a colleague who recognized a pair of unbleached socks that Lord had purchased earlier and by a staff-style button worn by nonline staff. Contract surgeon James M. DeWolf was wounded and later killed while retreating up the bluff with Reno's command. A third surgeon, Henry R. Porter, was the only physician to survive. He worked heroically to save the injured at an ad hoc field hospital on Reno Hill (Rickey 1963:71). For a list of surgeons who served with or treated Seventh Cavalry members, see the appendix.

Supporting the surgeons were noncommissioned men designated as hospital stewards. They were ranked and paid as sergeants and appear to have functioned as physicians' assistants. Other stewards could be appointed from the enlisted ranks as needed. Although the 1865 *Customs of Service* handbook stipulated that "[n]one but competent men be recommended" (Kautz 2001:85), few wanted this job. Don Rickey (1963:12) noted that "the most shiftless and compromising were assigned to hospital duty, sometimes with tragic results." A third level of health care provider, the medical cadet, was introduced after the Civil War. These were students of medicine between the ages of eighteen and twenty-three with two years of reading medicine and at least one course of lectures at a medical college. They functioned as nurses, dressing wounds in general hospitals, and as ambulance attendants in the field under the direction of medical officers (Kautz 2001:71).

The quality of care provided by army surgeons has been debated by historians, generally supported only by anecdotal evidence. Utley (1977:87) cites primitive living conditions and low pay as reasons why "able doctors" avoided working for the military, concluding that they "lacked the competence of their brethren in civilian life." An 1883 *New York Medical Journal* article asserted, however, that "Army surgeons were as capable as physicians anywhere in the world" (Asch 1883:203). Furthermore, many contract surgeons had comparable experience and training as career military officers: the older ones had served in the Civil War, and the younger ones had good academic and practical training (Gillett 1995:64).

More direct evidence of these surgeons' professional competence is found in detailed reports of injuries suffered during and after the Civil War. Joseph K. Barnes, surgeon general from 1864 to 1882, provides an exhaustive compendium of case reports, including the circumstances and mechanism of injury, signs and symptoms, interventions, and outcomes (Barnes 1870). George Alexander Otis (1871) left us a similarly thorough analysis of war wounds from 1865 through 1871. It is apparent from these texts that the authors and the surgeons providing the reports focused on developing evidence-based medical care, supported by careful observation and assessment of outcomes. The sheer volume of cases ensured that army surgeons' diagnostic and therapeutic skills were developed to a high degree.

Illustrations of equipment and instrumentation from contemporary surgical texts indicate that complex procedures were possible and had been carried out successfully. Relatively safe and effective inhalant and topical anesthetics had become available by this time (nitrous oxide 1844, chloroform 1847, ether 1842, cocaine 1860), facilitating such procedures.

In regard to the surgeon's capacity to deal with injury and illness in the field, we are fortunate to have Dr. Porter's surgical kit on display at the State Historical Society of North Dakota in Bismarck. Two small trunks contain the equipment that he took on field campaigns, including the battle at Little Bighorn. This set includes a variety of suture material and instruments, bone saws, rongeurs, scalpels, knives, elevators, curettes, catheters, an "eye spatula," and bullet probes. A trunk labeled "US Army Field Surgical Chest No. 2" contains various medications including opiates, ether, and chloroform; antiseptics; a tooth extraction case; catgut ligatures; tourniquets; dressing supplies; and an "Ear and Nose Speculum." A contemporary surgical text, Henry Hollingsworth's *A System of Operative Surgery*, is also included (Walker 2008:196).

Summary

A negative assessment of medical progress in the Civil War and later nineteenth century has been asserted by some, who describe the period as "marked by an almost total absence of significant medical discovery or addition to existing knowledge" (Dean 1997:51). In evaluating medical records from this era, it is important to avoid the fallacy of presentism. This term refers to the anachronistic imposition of present-day ideas and perspectives on depictions or interpretations of the past, especially with a triumphalist or teleological stance. As John Harley Warner (1997:4) points out, nineteenth-century "[p]hysicians were not ordinarily simpleminded, passive, or duplicitous, nor were they unobservant of the results of their therapies." Even stories about drastic heroic depletion should be tempered by their context, as "self-satisfied statements about how much medicine has improved" (Warner 1997:94).

Compared to Civil War medicine, historians understandably have ignored military health and medical care of the late nineteenth century. Fewer men served during the post–Civil War period of

Southern Reconstruction and western expansion, specifically the Indian Wars. Class differences also existed between the farmer/citizen soldier of the Civil War and the recruit of the post–Civil War period.

Progress was made in the delivery of medical and surgical services during and after the Civil War. The Surgeon General's Office became well established and effective. Hospitals and nursing services were expanded and made more efficient. Systems of conveyance (ambulances, steamships, and railroads) for transporting the sick improved. Sanitary measures became standard, and ineffective drugs and interventions were abandoned. Through the disciplined work of men like Barnes and Otis, better collection and documentation of specimens and case histories resulted in meaningful surgical data as well as priceless photographic and anatomic collections at the Army Medical Museum. Delicate and extensive surgical operations, such as hip amputation, limb-sparing procedures, repair of cranial trauma, and vessel ligation, were perfected. Indian War surgeons probably made their most significant contributions by implementing the best available technology and clinical methods under particularly adverse circumstances.

CHAPTER 3

Nineteenth-Century Military Nosology

P. Willey and Patrick J. Collison

Chapter 2 presents background to late-nineteenth-century medicine and its application in the U.S. military. This chapter deals with one aspect of that framework: disease categories and their application to Seventh Cavalry illnesses.

Nosology, contrary to what intuition suggests, is *not* the study of noses. It is how diseases are categorized, the structure of illnesses, organizing them into categories with similar diseases, and separating related categories from dissimilar groups of diseases. Diagnosis and these categories function as a culturally and temporally bound means of dealing with otherwise unfathomable illness. Diagnosis and categorization of ailments serve as the first steps toward understanding, treating, and healing. Here we present nineteenth-century illness categories and how the Seventh Cavalry's diagnoses fit those categories.

In the nineteenth century illnesses were often identified by symptoms, presumed causes, or anatomical locations of the disease, not necessarily by the causative organisms or etiology as we understand them today. For our purposes U.S. Army Regulations (1881) provide a framework to situate diseases during the post–Civil War period. This framework divided diseases into classes, which were subdivided into orders, following Linnaean nomenclature. Unlike the Linnaean system, however, nosology included no higher levels (such as kingdom or phylum) and no lower levels (such as genus or species). Such categories were not limited to the past.

Nosology applications continue into the present. Ailments today, like the specialties of many contemporary doctors who treat them, are organized by anatomical location and etiology. Physicians employ such categories for consistency in clinical applications, epidemiological assessments (for example, death records), and health insurance claims. The Systematized Nomenclature of Medicine (SNOMED) and Medical Subject Heading (MeSH) are examples that have been used in this country for fifty years. An even more widely used system is the International Statistical Classification of Diseases and Related Health Problems (ISCD, 10th Revision, version 2012; http://apps.who.int/classifications/icd10/browse/2010/en) of the World Health Organization (WHO). ISCD is employed later in this chapter, after the presentation of nineteenth-century disease categories.

Mid-Nineteenth Century Military Nosology

The mid-nineteenth century military disease classification had been established before the Civil War (Woodward 1870:xvii–xix) and remained fundamentally the same through our study period (U.S. Army Regulations 1881). The system recognized five disease classes, each with varying numbers of subdivisions called orders. Subsumed by the orders were subsubdivisions, usually listing specific diseases or symptoms. We consider diseases by these classes and orders as a means of grouping and presenting the Seventh Cavalry diagnoses.

For these assessments we employ the Seventh Cavalry's Carded Medical Records' primary diagnosis with occasional secondary recourse to marginal notes for clarification. In some instances the first diagnosis is worded differently than the nineteenth-century nosology categories. But often the name is so similar that those probable attributions are included with the ones that are certain for these tabulations. As examples, cephalgia in the records is identified as headache in the nosology and inflammation of the conjunctiva as conjunctivitis. In other cases the categories apparently change during the decades. As an example, inflammation of tonsils in the earlier nosology is recorded as tonsillitis in the later nosology. And some categories appear in one nosology but not in the other. As an example, debility appears in the earlier nosology but not in the later one. All categories of both nosologies are employed here.

Medical terms appear in the Seventh Cavalry's medical records and in the chapters in this book as complaints, diagnoses, or qualifying terms. Many readers may be unfamiliar with some of those terms. So we have provided a glossary.

The nineteenth-century categories and the tallies of Seventh Cavalry diseases in those categories are presented in table 3.1 and discussed below.

Disease Classes and Orders

CLASS I. ZYMOTIC DISEASES

Zymotic diseases were the first of five class categories. In nineteenth-century medical understanding, zymotic diseases included the miasmas, airborne poisons that behaved as "enzymes," fermenting to cause spoilage. Thus it received the prefix "zym," Greek for fermentation (Bollet 2002:51). Most of the zymotic diseases encompassed what we consider infectious diseases today, especially those included in the first two subdivisions (miasmatic and enthetic orders).

More than one-third of all Seventh Cavalry illness diagnoses fell into this category—the greatest portion of any class. Here are the orders and distribution of the diagnoses among the class's three subdivisions.

Order 1. Miasmatic Diseases. Miasma was attributed to airborne poisons produced by decaying materials and carried on stench created by the decay. It emanated from swamps and other festering bodies. Dysenteries, diarrheas, and the so-called childhood diseases (such as chicken pox, measles, and whooping cough) dominated miasmatic diseases. This order also included intermittent fevers, ailments now considered malaria. In addition, some other severe diseases appeared in this order, such as typhoid, yellow and scarlet fevers, and generally less devastating ailments, such as diarrhea.

TABLE 3.1. Post–Civil War Seventh Cavalry diagnoses by class and order (using a nineteenth-century military disease classification system)

CLASS	*Order*	*Disease*	*Number*	*Percentage within order*
I. ZYMOTIC DISEASES, n = 7342 (35.5% of all diagnoses)				
	1. Miasmatic Diseases		6001	99.8
		Typhoid fever	78	1.3
		Typhus fever	4	0.1
		Typho-malarial fever	17	0.3
		Yellow fever	0	0
		Remittent fever	231	3.8
		Quotidian intermittent fever	959	16.0
		Tertian intermittent fever	693	11.5
		Quartan intermittent fever	8	0.1
		Acute diarrhea	2418	40.3
		Chronic diarrhea	37	0.6
		Acute dysentery	133	2.2
		Chronic dysentery	11	0.2
		Epidemic cholera	31	0.5
		Erysipelas	50	0.8
		Hospital gangrene	0	0
		Pyemia	1	0.0
		Small-pox	1	0.0
		Varioloid	6	0.1
		Chicken-pox	1	0.0
		Measles	18	0.3
		Scarlet fever	0	0
		Mumps	23	0.4

TABLE 3.1. *(continued)*

CLASS	*Order*	*Disease*	*Number*	*Percentage within order*
		Tonsillitis (quinsy; inflammation of tonsils [Woodward])	602	10.0
		Diphtheria	1	0.0
		Epidemic catarrh (influenza)	29	0.5
		Whooping cough	0	0
		Cerebro-spinal meningitis	0	0
		3. Common continued fever (Woodward)	0	0
		9. Congestive intermittent fever (Woodward)	3	0.0
		19. Debility (Woodward)	23	0.4
		Others of this category and those with less exact diagnoses	623	10.4
	2. Enthetic Diseases		982	100.1
		Primary syphilis	269	27.4
		Constitutional syphilis	204	20.8
		Gonorrhea	317	32.3
		Gonorrhea orchitis	58	5.9
		Gonorrhea ophthalmia	1	0.1
		Stricture of urethra (gonorrhea)	13	1.3
		Glanders	0	0
		Hydrophobia	0	0
		Bite of serpents	3	0.3
		Malignant pustule	0	0

(continued)

TABLE 3.1. *(continued)*

CLASS	*Order*	*Disease*	*Number*	*Percentage within order*
		Others of this category and those with less exact diagnoses	117	11.9
	3. Dietic Diseases		359	100.0
		Starvation	2	0.6
		Scurvy	32	8.9
		Purpura	0	0
		Inebriation	221	61.6
		Delirium tremens	23	6.4
		Chronic alcoholism	77	21.4
		Others in this category and those with less exact diagnoses	4	1.1
II. CONSTITUTIONAL DISEASES, n = 1238 (6.0% of all diagnoses)				
	1. Diathetic Diseases		1116	100.0
		Gout	1	0.1
		Acute rheumatism	541	48.5
		Chronic rheumatism	337	30.2
		Anemia	18	1.6
		Dropsy (when not a mere symptom of disease of heart, liver, or kidneys)	8	0.7
		Cancer	0	0
		Epithelioma	0	0
		Tumor	19	1.7
		Dry gangrene	0	0
		Others and those with less exact diagnoses in this category	192	17.2

TABLE 3.1. *(continued)*

CLASS	*Order*	*Disease*	*Number*	*Percentage within order*
	2. Tubercular Diseases		72	100.0
		Consumption	68	94.4
		Scrofula	4	5.6
III. PARASITIC DISEASES, $n = 50$ (0.2 percent of all diagnoses)			50	100.0
		Itch	27	54.0
		Tape worms	23	46.0
		Lumbricoid worms	0	
		Ascarides	0	
		Trichimasis	0	
		40. Worms (Woodward)	0	
IV. LOCAL DISEASES, $n = 7289$ (35.3% of all diagnoses)				
	1. Diseases of the Nervous System		933	99.9
		Apoplexy	0	0
		Convulsions	5	0.5
		Chorea	0	0
		Epilepsy	40	4.3
		Headache	312	33.4
		Insanity	20	2.1
		Inflammation of the brain	5	0.5
		Inflammation of the membranes of the brain	0	0
		Inflammation of the spinal cord	1	0.1
		Nostalgia	3	0.3
		Neuralgia	469	50.3

(continued)

TABLE 3.1. *(continued)*

CLASS	*Order*	*Disease*	*Number*	*Percentage within order*
		Paralysis	12	1.3
		Sunstroke	13	1.4
		Tetanus	0	0
		50. Toothache (Woodward)	42	4.5
		Others and those with less exact diagnoses in this category	11	1.2
	2. Diseases of the Eye		355	99.9
		Conjunctivitis	313	88.2
		Iritis	14	3.9
		Cataract	3	0.8
		Amaurosis	0	0
		Night blindness	10	2.8
		57. Ophthalmia (Woodward)	5	1.4
		Others and those with less exact diagnoses in this category	10	2.8
	3. Diseases of the Ear		128	100.0
		Otorhoea (Otorrhea)	70	54.7
		Inflammation of the internal ear	21	16.4
		Deafness	22	17.2
		59. Earache (Woodward)	9	7.0
		Others and those with less exact diagnoses in this category	6	4.7
	4. Diseases of the Organs of Circulation		129	100.0
		Inflammation of pericardium	11	8.5

TABLE 3.1. *(continued)*

CLASS	*Order*	*Disease*	*Number*	*Percentage within order*
		Dropsy of the pericardium	0	0
		Inflammation of endocardium	1	0.8
		Hypertrophy of heart	5	3.9
		Valvular disease of heart	51	39.5
		Dropsy of heart disease	0	0
		Aneurism	0	0
		Phlebitis (also 68. Inflammation of veins; Woodward)	0	0
		Varicose veins	15	11.6
		65. Inflammation of heart (Woodward)	0	0
		Others and those with less exact diagnoses in this category	46	35.7
	5. Diseases of the Respiratory Organs		2543	100.0
		Asthma	13	0.5
		Catarrh	1379	54.2
		Acute bronchitis	513	20.2
		Chronic bronchitis	40	1.6
		Epistaxis (also 76. Hemorrhage from nose; Woodward)	5	0.2
		Inflammation of larynx	19	0.7
		Inflammation of lungs	104	4.1
		Inflammation of pleura	153	6.0
		Dropsy of chest	1	0.0
		77. Hemorrhage from lungs (Woodward)	7	0.3

(continued)

TABLE 3.1. *(continued)*

CLASS	*Order*	*Disease*	*Number*	*Percentage within order*
		Others and those with less exact diagnoses in this category	309	12.2
	6. Diseases of the Digestive Organs		1197	100.2
		Colic	219	18.3
		Constipation	397	33.1
		Cholera morbus	35	2.9
		Dyspepsia	129	10.8
		Inflammation of stomach	15	1.3
		Inflammation of bowels	7	0.6
		Inflammation of peritoneum	1	0.1
		Ascites	0	0
		Hemorrhage from stomach	3	0.3
		Hemorrhage from bowels	1	0.1
		Fistula in ano	14	1.2
		Piles	221	18.4
		Prolapsus ani	3	0.3
		Femoral hernia	4	0.3
		Inguinal hernia	44	3.7
		Acute inflammation of liver	15	1.3
		Chronic inflammation of liver	0	0
		Cirrhosis of liver	0	0
		Dropsy from hepatic disease	1	0.1

TABLE 3.1. *(continued)*

CLASS	*Order*	*Disease*	*Number*	*Percentage within order*
		Jaundice	21	1.8
		Biliary calculi	0	0
		Inflammation of the spleen	2	0.2
		Enlarged spleen	5	0.4
		Others and those with less exact diagnoses in this category	60	5.0
	7. Diseases of Organs	Urinary and Genital	277	100.1
		Inflammation of kidneys	11	4.0
		Bright's disease	0	0
		Diabetes	3	1.1
		Gravel (114. Gravel and stone; Woodward)	3	1.1
		Calculus	5	1.8
		Inflammation of bladder	16	5.8
		Incontinence of urine	24	8.7
		Retention of urine	0	0
		Inflammation of testicle (not gonorrheal)	118	42.6
		Hydrocele	1	0.4
		Varicocele (Woodward's IV, 4, no. 68)	26	9.4
		106. Difficulty of urination (Woodward)	12	4.3
		109. Sarcocele (Woodward)	0	0

(continued)

TABLE 3.1. *(continued)*

CLASS	*Order*	*Disease*	*Number*	*Percentage within order*
		110. Nonsyphilitic ulcer of penis (Woodward)	0	0
		Others and those with less exact diagnoses in this category	58	20.9
	8. Diseases of the Bones and Joints		65	99.9
		Inflammation of periosteum	2	3.1
		Inflammation of bones	1	1.5
		Caries	1	1.5
		Necrosis	6	9.2
		Inflammation of [j]oints	24	36.9
		Anchylosis	5	7.7
		113. Exostosis (Woodward)	0	0
		114. White swelling (Woodward)	0	0
		Others and those with less exact diagnoses in this category	26	40.0
	9. Diseases of the Integumentary System		1712	100.1
		Abscess	238	13.9
		Boil	973	56.8
		Carbuncle	13	0.8
		Ulcers	164	9.6
		Whitlow	164	9.6
		Skin diseases (not including [illegible] or affections or itch)	87	5.1

TABLE 3.1. *(continued)*

CLASS	*Order*	*Disease*	*Number*	*Percentage within order*
		Others and those with less exact diagnoses in this category	73	4.3
V. VIOLENT DISEASE AND DEATH, n = 4625 (22.4% of all diagnoses)				
	1. Wounds, Injuries, and Accidents		4622	100.1
		Burns and scalds	97	2.1
		Contusion	2004	43.4
		Concussion of the brain	12	0.3
		Drowning	0	0
		Sprains	802	17.4
		Dislocations	51	1.1
		Frostbite	301	6.5
		Simple fractures (not gunshot)	142	3.1
		Compound fractures (not gunshot)	8	0.2
		Gunshot wounds	394	8.5
		Incised wounds	330	7.1
		Lacerated wounds	278	6.0
		Punctured wounds	80	1.7
		Poisoning by . . . [name your poison!]	59	1.3
		125. Compression of brain (Woodward)	0	0
		131. Contused and lacerated wounds	0	0
		Others and those with less exact diagnoses in this category	64	1.4
	2. Homicide		1	

(continued)

TABLE 3.1. *(continued)*

CLASS	*Order*	*Disease*	*Number*	*Percentage within order*
	3. Suicide		2	
	4. Execution of Sentence		0	
		Hanging	0	
		Shooting	0	
DIAGNOSIS BLANK, UNIDENTIFIED, UNINTERPRETABLE OR VAGUE			132	
Total (5 classes plus blank/vague) 20,676 diagnoses, 100.0%				

Source: U.S. Army Regulations 1881; Woodward 1870, indicated by numbered diseases.

Miasmatic diseases constituted the most frequent order in the zymotic class in the Seventh Cavalry ailments. More than one-fourth of all diagnoses occurred in this order. Mostly they consisted of diarrheas, intermittent and remittent fevers, and tonsillitis.

Order 2. Enthetic Diseases. These diseases were believed to be caused by "morbid matters" introduced into the body (Woodward 1870:XIX). Sexually transmitted diseases (such as syphilis and gonorrhea) dominated the order. Other illnesses in this order conjured catastrophic Old Testament images. Those "pestilences" included "bite of serpent," malignant pustule (anthrax), and hydrophobia (rabies).

Approximately one-twentieth of all ailments in the Seventh Cavalry data fell into this order. Most of those diagnoses were sexually transmitted diseases (gonorrhea and syphilis), although a few "bite of serpents" appeared.

Order 3. Dietic Diseases. The final subdivision in the zymotic disease class was dietic diseases. As the name implies, it included ingestion of substances, either underconsumption (for example, starvation and scurvy) or overconsumption (for example, inebriation, delirium tremens, and chronic alcoholism). Also encompassed in this order was purpura, an ailment producing reddish or purplish skin color.

A mere 1.7 percent of the diagnoses in the Seventh Cavalry occurred in this category. Most of these involved overconsumption of alcohol.

CLASS II. CONSTITUTIONAL DISEASES

The second class, constitutional diseases, affected the whole individual, not being restricted to one area or focused on one anatomical region. The class included a variety of neoplastic, infectious, and other diseases, subsumed in two subdivisions. Approximately a paltry one-twentieth of the Seventh Cavalry diagnoses fell into this class.

Order 1. Diathetic Diseases. Individuals expressing these diseases exhibited particular hereditary susceptibility or vulnerability to the ailments and showed a predisposition to contract these diseases. From today's perspective this subdivision included an odd combination of diseases, involving joints and muscles (for example, rheumatism) and neoplastic diseases (such as tumor, cancer, and epithelioma). Dropsy (an abnormal fluid buildup in tissues or a body cavity—not physical ineptitude) and anemia were also filed in this category.

This order was the more frequent of this infrequent class in the Seventh Cavalry diagnoses. Rheumatism contributed most to the subdivision's numbers, with tumors and anemias only weakly contributing to the total.

Order 2. Tubercular Diseases. These diseases manifested persistent infections now associated with *Mycobacterium tuberculosis.* That causative agent was only discovered in the early 1880s, however, so that discovery had little impact on Seventh Cavalry health. Symptoms involved a slow wasting or "consumption." Another form, scrofula, was tubercular disease manifested as inflammation of the neck lymph glands. Although not included formally in the category, pulmonary phthisis most likely should be identified as a manifestation of tubercular disease.

A tiny fraction of a percent of Seventh Cavalry diagnoses represented ailments in this order. This frequency was surprising, especially in the mid-nineteenth century. Tuberculosis was widespread then, a significant ailment and frequent cause of death. Possible explanations for this suspected under-representation include misdiagnosis of early stages of tuberculosis by military surgeons and the military population being limited to a youthful group of relatively healthy males, excluding older adults and the most seriously ill.

CLASS III. PARASITIC DISEASES

Diseases in this class consisted of illnesses caused by organisms. As the term was applied in the mid-nineteenth century, parasitic diseases involved ailments whose causative organisms could be observed without recourse to microscopic examination or histological samples. Diagnosis consisted of identification from simple, direct observations. No subdivisions existed in this class. Each parasitic disease, such as itch and those infirmities caused by macroorganisms, was organized directly below the class heading.

Parasitic diseases constituted less than 1 percent of the Seventh Cavalry diagnoses, the least of any class. Most of the diagnoses in this class involved tapeworm and itch.

CLASS IV. LOCAL DISEASES

Diseases in this class involved specific anatomical systems. Most of these nine subdivisions remain in use today and are familiar to modern students of anatomy. Present-day anatomical systems missing from these nineteenth-century categories were the muscular, lymphatic, and endocrine systems. But the rest were included.

More than one-third of all of the Seventh Cavalry's diagnoses fell into this category, nearly eclipsing the zymotic disease sum. The majority of diagnoses in this class's complaints fell in two of the nine subdivisions.

Order 1. Diseases of the Nervous System. Ailments under this heading involved brain, nerves, and their surrounding tissues. Diseases included problems of organic origins, such as inflammation of membranes of the brain. Other diseases in the order, such as insanity, involved unclear or multiple origins. According to one overview of the topic, insanity in the nineteenth century was divided into three subdivisions: mania (mostly identified by the subject's agitation), melancholia (associated with depression, despondency, and lethargy), and dementia (indicated by impaired and distorted thought processes [Schroeder-Lein 2008:161]). Insanity had various causes, both organic, such as late stage syphilis affecting the nervous system, and inorganic, not due to direct injury or other readily identifiable causes.

For present-day readers, several of the order's diseases seem strange. They included nostalgia and sunstroke. Today nostalgia (literally longing for home; Freemon 1998:232) might be interpreted as severe depression. Sunstroke might be considered comparable to the modern definition (symptoms associated with heatstroke) but might employ a broader Civil War-era definition encompassing ailments related to Post–Traumatic Stress Disorder (PTSD; see Dean 1997:131–32).

Nearly one-twentieth of the Seventh Cavalry diagnoses were in the category diseases of the nervous system. Most diagnoses consisted of headaches and neuralgia, with a few more severe manifestations.

Order 2. Diseases of the Eye. Diseases in this subdivision involved organs related to sight. They included ailments resulting from degeneration (such as cataracts), inflammations (for example, conjunctivitis), and other causes, such as malnutrition (when inadequate Vitamin A caused night blindness). Less than 2 percent of the total Seventh Cavalry diagnoses fell into the category of diseases of the eye. Most of these involved conjunctivitis.

Order 3. Diseases of the Ear. These diseases involved structures related to hearing. They resulted from inflammation (for example, otorrhea) or described an inability to hear without specifying a more specific cause (such as deafness). Approximately 0.5% of all the Seventh Cavalry diagnoses involved ear diseases, most often ear inflammations.

Order 4. Diseases of the Organs of Circulation. These diseases affected the heart, arteries, veins, and tissues surrounding those structures. They included inflammations and infections (such as pericarditis and endocarditis), heart defects (such as valvular heart disease), artery or vein alterations (for example, aneurism and varicose veins), and edema (pericardium dropsy).

About 0.5% of all the Seventh Cavalry medical diagnoses were in this category. Although few, many of these were severe when they occurred. Even relatively benign varicose veins constituted a reason for disability discharge. Perhaps such a low frequency of circulatory illnesses should be expected in a group of relatively healthy young men, who had been screened by medical personnel at the time of enlistment.

Order 5. Diseases of the Respiratory Organs. Diseases in this order affected the lungs and related anatomical structures associated with breathing, such as the larynx, bronchi, and pleura. Respiratory diseases included inflammations (such as bronchitis), spasms (for example, asthma), and edema (for example, dropsy of the chest).

A large proportion (12 percent) of the Seventh Cavalry's overall diagnoses fell in the category of diseases of the respiratory organs. Most of the complaints in this order were fairly minor (such as bronchitis and catarrh), but some more severe ones did occur (for example, lung and pleura inflammations). Many of the problems probably reflected issues associated with living in close quarters and being exposed to transmitted diseases.

Order 6. Diseases of the Digestive Organs. These diseases affected structures of the gastrointestinal tract (mostly the lower gastrointestinal tract), including the stomach, bowels, liver, spleen, and anus. Digestive diseases encompassed inflammations (of the stomach, bowels, and peritoneum), bleeding (such as hemorrhage of the stomach and bowels), and degenerative alterations (for example, piles).

Diseases of the digestive organs composed nearly 6 percent of all Seventh Cavalry diagnoses. Most ailments documented in this order involved colic, constipation, dyspepsia, and piles.

Order 7. Diseases of the Urinary and Genital Organs. Ailments in this order affected the kidneys, ureters, bladders, urethra, gonads, ducts, and external genitalia. Diagnoses included inflammatory diseases (of the kidneys, bladder, and testicle) as well as probably congenital ones (hydrocele and varicocele). In addition, gravel (also known as kidney stones), diabetes, and Bright's disease appeared in this order.

Only about 1% of Seventh Cavalry diagnoses fell in the category of diseases of the urinary and genital organs. Most of these complaints involved inflammation of anatomical structures (such as inflammations of the bladder, kidney, and testicle).

Order 8. Diseases of the Bones and Joints. Diseases in this order included inflammations and defects of the skeletal system and joints. They consisted of inflammatory diseases (such as inflammations of the periosteum, bones, and joints), although some may have resulted from many different causes (for example, necrosis and ankylosis).

Less than 1% of the Seventh Cavalry diagnoses were in the category of diseases of the bones and joints. They consisted mostly of joint inflammations.

Order 9. Diseases of the Integumentary System. These diseases included superficial defects, involving skin, nails, and associated external structures.

About 8% of the Seventh Cavalry diagnoses fell in the category of diseases of the integumentary system. That figure is substantial, indicating significant impact on Seventh Cavalry members. Most of these diagnoses consisted of boils, abscesses, ulcers, and whitlow.

CLASS V. VIOLENT DISEASE AND DEATH

Trauma and injuries composed the last class of diseases. It was divided into four orders. Diagnoses in this class constituted more than one-fifth of all the Seventh Cavalry diagnoses, almost all occurring in the first subdivision.

Order 1. Wounds, Injuries, and Accidents. This order included many different physical insults to the body. The injuries recognized involved burns, blunt force trauma (such as contusions and concussions of the brains), cold, fractures, gunshot wounds, and sharp force trauma (such as incised wounds) as well as poisoning. Poisoning was broadly construed in this context. It encompassed poisoning by *Rhus* (the nineteenth-century genus of plants that includes poison ivy, poison oak, and poison sumac) and narcotics (such as opium).

Most of the diagnoses in this category consisted of contusions, sprains, gunshot wounds, incised wounds, lacerations, and fractures in decreasing frequency. Many of these alterations may have left osteological defects.

Order 2. Homicide. This order involved a person killing another individual with or without official approval or sanction. It excluded deaths by execution or self-homicide (suicide), which constituted other orders in this class. No subdivisions were acknowledged in the order.

Only 1 of the Seventh Cavalry diagnoses fell in the category of homicides. The number was surprisingly small, especially considering the many regimental soldiers who died in action at the battles of the Washita, Little Bighorn, Canyon Creek, and Snake Creek. Most Killed in Action (KIA) in the medical records (n = 13 of a total of 19) occurred at the Washita. These results suggest changing or perhaps variable documentation of the Seventh Cavalry's health records. As chapter 14 shows, sources other than the medical records provide better documentation of deaths.

Order 3. Suicide. Purposefully killing oneself constituted suicide. Only 2 suicides were listed in the Seventh Cavalry medical records. One was a primary diagnosis: John Noonan [*sic*], November 1878, at Fort Abraham Lincoln. Another suicide appeared in a medical record's marginal notes, however, not presented as the primary diagnosis (John Steintker aka Stewker). Such omissions probably represented record-keeping protocols, suggesting that suicides and other mortalities were more accurately documented in Enlistment Records rather than in medical documents. Seventh Cavalry Enlistment Records indicated that at least 6 troopers died from suicide.

Order 4. Execution. Killing another person by military command or through civilian legal sanctions constituted execution. In a period before electrocution or injected lethal drugs were options, two execution subdivisions existed: hanging and shooting. No Seventh Cavalry medical or enlistment records indicate execution.

Considering this daunting list of illnesses and potential sources of harm, it is a wonder that any enlistee survived until expiration of service. Fortunately for the soldiers, most illnesses were infrequent or expressed mild diseases. Thus they impacted few Seventh Cavalry troopers. Other pervasive, persistent, and powerful illnesses prevailed, however, and stalked the ranks.

Disease Categories of the Twenty-First Century Found in the Seventh Cavalry Records

In this section we consider two issues. First, how the Seventh Cavalry medical diagnoses compare with the formal disease structures and categories of the nineteenth century. Were those nosological categories mere suggestions for physicians' consideration or were they obligatory categories into which ailments needed to be placed—or even forced?

The second issue is how nineteenth-century illness categories compare and contrast with twenty-first-century categories. Do they neatly dovetail with one another, remaining largely unchanged for 150 years? Or have there been major alterations, indicating paradigm changes during that period?

SEVENTH CAVALRY DIAGNOSES IN NINETEENTH-CENTURY CATEGORIES

Today's medical practitioners follow contemporary nosology—in most instances very closely. In part this conformity is for the sake of consistent reporting and prompt billing. But were nineteenth-century military surgeons under comparable constraints or did they have more latitude in diagnosis and categorization than contemporary physicians do?

The number of Seventh Cavalry diagnoses that fit the nineteenth-century nosology is a measure of this conformity. More than 99 percent (n = 20,544) of the Seventh Cavalry diagnoses find recognizable homes in that nosology, either directly under a disease or as an apparent inclusion within an order.

So we conclude that Seventh Cavalry medical diagnoses mostly fit well the nineteenth-century military nosological categories.

They conform so closely that they appear to be almost prescriptive in nature. Many Seventh Cavalry medical records documented additional details beyond what the nosology required. In those instances the Cavalry medical records provided richer and more detailed accounts than the nosology demanded. They blessed us with more information than was required by mere conformity to the nosology.

NINETEENTH-CENTURY AND CONTEMPORARY CATEGORY CORRESPONDENCES

The next step in this discussion brings the diagnoses into contemporary categories. It compares Seventh Cavalry diagnoses with contemporary disease categories.

Many modern nosology approaches exist. One that is broadly applicable is the WHO's International Statistical Classification of Diseases and Related Health Problems (ICSD: 10th Revision, version 2012; http://apps.who.int/classifications/icd10/browse/2010/en). We selected this classificatory system because of its ease of use, widespread international adoption, broad-spectrum applicability, and electronic accessibility.

INTERNATIONAL STATISTICAL CLASSIFICATION OF DISEASES AND RELATED HEALTH PROBLEMS

The ISCD disease categories are organized in hierarchical ranks, similar to the nineteenth-century illness classifications already presented. Roman numerals mark ISCD chapters, comparable to the nineteenth-century classes. ISCD chapter subdivisions (blocks) parallel the nineteenth-century's orders.

Current categories apparently build on nineteenth-century models. So Seventh Cavalry diagnoses dovetail well with the ISCD, making an easy conversion.

In addition to hierarchical similarities, similar diseases are correlated. As an example, nineteenth-century "Class I. Zymotic Diseases" includes many of the contemporary ISCD's "Chapter I. Certain Infectious and Parasitic Diseases." The nineteenth-century "Class IV. Local Diseases Involving Anatomical Systems" remains similar more than a century later, even in terms of the same titles and same sequence (table 3.2).

Disease categories in the nineteenth century and twenty-first century do differ, however. Nineteenth-century military disease categories fail to identify infectious microorganisms; unknown etiologies; vitamin deficiencies; endocrine irregularities; diseases unique to children, women, and the elderly; and congenital alterations.

Many contemporary disease identifications rely on laboratory identification of the causative microbes (such as salmonella, *Streptococcus*, and *Escherichia coli*). This reliance is especially notable for the diseases in ISCD's chapter I. Among the nineteenth-century diagnoses, in contrast, microscopic infectious agents were not identified.

Ironically, the nineteenth-century use of class and order and omission of the lower Linnaean levels (genus and species) may have had unintended implications. To employ the lower levels of classification required advances in medical thinking—the identification of causative infectious organisms. Those organisms have now been identified in the Linnaean binomial nomenclature. Development and widespread acceptance of the germ theory of disease were just beginning in the late nineteenth century, with the identification of some of the causative microscopic agents after our period of study.

In addition, some new diseases have been discovered or emerged since the nineteenth-century classifications were in use. Probably the most famous of these diseases is HIV (ISCD I, B 20–24).

Although nineteenth-century categories include some diseases attributed to dietary issues, they ignored vitamins, at least as causative entities. Vitamins and their associations were discovered in the twentieth century.

No hormonal imbalances were recognized as such in those earlier days. As a minor contradiction to this statement, consider the nineteenth-century identification of diabetes. At that time it was considered an ailment associated with the urinary and genital structures. Hormones and their critical roles in physiology were discovered in the twentieth century.

Because females and children were excluded from military surgeons' official medical duties, no conditions unique to those

TABLE 3.2. Comparability of disease categories employed in nineteenth-century military nosology and in the ISCD (twenty-first century)

Nineteenth-century military nosology	*ISCD (twenty-first century)*
Class I, Zymotic Diseases	Chapter I. Certain Infectious and Parasitic Diseases
Class IV, Local Diseases	
Order 1, Diseases of the Nervous System	
Order 2, Diseases of the Eye	Chapter VII. Diseases of the Eye and Adnexa
Order 3, Diseases of the Ear	Chapter VIII. Diseases of the Ear and Mastoid Process
Order 5, Diseases of the Respiratory Organs	Chapter X. Diseases of the Respiratory System
Order 6, Diseases of Digestive Organs	Chapter XI. Diseases of the Digestive Systems
Order 7, Diseases of the Urinary and Genital Organs	Chapter XIV. Diseases of the Genitourinary System
Order 8, Diseases of the Connective Tissue	Chapter XIII. Diseases of the Musculoskeletal System and Bones and Joints
Order 9, Diseases of the Integumentary System	Chapter XII. Diseases of Skin and Subcutaneous Tissue
Class V, Violent Diseases and Deaths	Chapter XIX. Injury, Poisoning, and Certain Other Consequences of External Causes; and Chapter XX. External Causes of Morbidity and Mortality

Source: U.S. Army Regulations 1881; WHO's International Statistical Classification of Diseases and Related Health Problems (ISCD).

groups were noted in the official Seventh Cavalry medical records. Nevertheless, military physicians cared for the posts' women and children as well as other people living nearby. Services to these people were beyond normal duties and went without official documentation of their diseases and health challenges in the military records.

The Seventh Cavalry medical records also omitted most congenital malformations, deformations, and chromosomal abnormalities, which now have their own chapter in ISCD. Few were documented.

One possible example was Frank Green's malformed feet, which must have been a minor problem. After a few weeks of medical attention in September 1866, he returned to service at Fort Riley. Surgeons probably identified the most obvious and debilitating congenital problems and deformations during the enlistment physical examination. Such deformations excluded potential recruits from enlistment.

Although chromosomes had been observed by microscopists, not until the mid-1880s did those structures' association with inheritance become understood.

Summary

Although we often believe that marked improvements in medical understanding and healing capabilities occur through time, it is surprising how little disease nosology has changed in nearly 150 years. Nosology is part of that understanding, identification, and interpretation of disease structures and causes. It also indicates which ailments were considered important at that time and which unimportant.

Diseases and how they are categorized are embedded in their cultural context and time. As culture changes, so do the understanding and interpretation of diseases. Such is the case with nineteenth-century military medicine.

The nineteenth-century military nosology nested disease categories in a hierarchy, paralleling Linnaean taxonomy. The list was daunting when a physician was confronted with the number of potential disease entities. It is amazing that any trooper survived his five-year enlistment period. Fortunately for Seventh Cavalry members, many diseases listed in the nosology were infrequent or absent altogether.

The greatest number of Seventh Cavalry diagnoses involved the zymotic diseases, a class that included diseases believed to derive from fermentative processes. Within the class, miasmatic diseases occurred most frequently, with diarrhea and intermittent (malarial) fevers leading the counts.

The next greatest number of diagnoses in the Seventh Cavalry medical records were in the so-called local diseases. These diseases affected specific anatomical systems, such as the nervous and circulatory systems. Among the class's many orders, the most frequent complaints involved the respiratory system; bronchitis and catarrh led that order.

Violent disease and death followed next in frequency. Within that class, the order wounds, injuries, and accidents predominated overwhelmingly; contusions, sprains, and gunshot wounds populated this order.

These three classes—miasmatic, respiratory, and wounds—contributed the greatest numbers of ailments in the Seventh Cavalry.

Seventh Cavalry medical record diagnoses fit into the nineteenth-century military nosology, generally employing those established categories. Nevertheless, a small proportion of the diagnoses or complaints fell outside the nosology. Medical records frequently included additional details beyond those strictly required by the nosology. As examples, some records documented anatomical locations, causes, and circumstances.

The nosology employed in the nineteenth-century military compares favorably with a present-day one, having few major differences. Differences occurred in details and some categories, however. Contemporary disease categories rely on isolating causative microagents and emphasizing emerging diseases. Discovery of the relations of health, vitamins, and hormones happened in the early twentieth century. In addition to medical discoveries not yet made in the post–Civil War period, the military nosology excluded ailments of entire demographic groups (women, children, and elderly males) and severe conditions that would have excluded enlistment, such as major congenital malformations.

CHAPTER 4

Researching the Seventh Cavalry's Medical Records

P. Willey

Most of the following chapters employ the data set that serves as the core of this work. The Seventh Cavalry records summarized in chapters 3 and 5 commence in that pivotal time after the Civil War in 1866, continuing through the late 1860s and 1870s Indian Wars and southern Reconstruction, and ending twenty years later in the early to mid-1880s. It behooves us to understand the materials employed in these studies to know the strengths and weaknesses of conclusions derived from them.

Materials

Nearly all of the materials employed here occur on forms housed at the National Archives and Records Administration (NARA) or available through the NARA on microfilm. The materials include three sources: Regimental Returns, Enlistment Records, and Medical Record Cards. Each source has a standard form, and each preprinted form is completed in handwriting using ink. Only a few of the most recent forms employed a typewriter to complete the form. Each source of information—Regimental Returns, Enlistment Records, and medical records—provides different information on the troopers for the post–Civil War period. They are described below.

REGIMENTAL RETURNS

The first step in this endeavor establishes a list and the number of men who were in the Seventh Cavalry during this period. The Returns from the Regular Army Cavalry Regiments, 1833–1916, NARA Record Group (RG) 94, Microfilm (M) 744 (hereinafter Regimental Returns) provide a monthly list of officers and tabulations of soldiers by company, rank, and other categories. The Regimental Returns provided timely information on troop strength, as well as changes and activities, to Regimental Headquarters. For our purposes, the Regimental Return summary tables offer the number of individuals in the Seventh Cavalry on a month-by-month basis—a critical count for establishing the number of "susceptible" persons for epidemiological analyses.

The Regimental Returns include columns of "Gains" and "Losses" of enlisted men by name, date, company assignment, and the nature of the change. Gains occurred when recruits arrived at the regiment's posts from the training depot, enlisted directly at posts of the Seventh Cavalry, or transferred from one company or another regiment and when deserters surrendered or were apprehended and returned to their posts.

On the opposite end of the service spectrum, the Regimental Returns list losses of enlisted men. Losses occur from discharge for disability, discharge for expiration of enlistment period, desertion, by order, from court martial, and by death. The advantages of the gain and loss lists are that they provide the name, rank, and company of the person being "gained" or "lost." Thus it is possible to track individuals' entrances and exits from the regiment as well as assignment changes within the regiment.

Officers' comings and goings are also noted in the Regimental Returns. The dates when an officer assumed his assignment and when he was relieved of command are noted on those tables, although that officer information is largely disregarded here for reasons discussed later.

The gain and loss dates in the Regimental Returns, as well as those dates of other forms and records employed in this research, are dates in civilian format, in month-day-year sequence. Dates in military format (day-month-year sequence) are rarely used in the mid- to late nineteenth century and occur only occasionally in the latest portion of the period studied. The earliest military format date noted in the Seventh Cavalry medical records is November 1883. As an exception, however, the military date sequence is used eclectically in records related to troopers en route to the northern plains during the 1870s.

The Regimental Returns are from the microfilm of Returns from Regular Army Cavalry Regiments, 1833–1916 (NARA Microcopy 744, Rolls 71–73). The microfilm is generally of high quality, although the original documents had been folded, which obliterated some entries over the decades (an issue discussed in a later section).

ENLISTMENT RECORDS

The second major data source employs the Register of Enlistment in the United States Army, 1798–1914, NARA, RG 94, M 233 (hereinafter Enlistment Register). It documents enlistments and reenlistments. The Enlistment Register is organized chronologically by month and year of enlistment, then alphabetically by the enlistee's name.

The Enlistment Register includes dates, biological and demographic information, and locations. In addition to the enlistee's first and last names, the Enlistment Register sometimes includes a middle initial. The Enlistment Register identifies where and when the recruit enlisted. This location is generally an eastern city, which recruiting officers frequented.

The period of enlistment is included in the Enlistment Register. During the post–Civil War era, the enlistment period was generally five years. Exceptions to this generalization occurred the first year (1866) after the Civil War, when the Seventh Cavalry was being formed, especially in July and August of that year. The enlistment period then was three years. Two recruits that year (Frank Mellville and Andrew J. Davis) enlisted for four years, however, instead of three. But neither of them spent the full four years in the military. Mellville was discharged after two and a half years, and Davis deserted. After 1866 enlistments lasted five years.

The enlistee's birthplace is indicated by town or county and then state or country. The enlistee's age at commencement of enlistment, height, color of eyes, hair, and complexion, and previous occupation are also listed. In addition to this information, the Enlistment Register indicates the nature of the person's final dismissal from service (such as discharge for expiration of service period, desertion from ranks, court martial, or death) and the date. If the person was discharged, his final rank is also recorded in the Enlistment Register. More complicated service periods occurred, such as desertions followed by capture or surrender. Reenlistments follow a similar format, with the additional notation that it is a reenlistment.

For our studies, the microfilm of the Register of Enlistment in the U.S. Army is abstracted for 1866 through the 1878 to 1884 films. The NARA's Microfilm M233 (Rolls 31–43) encompasses those dates.

MEDICAL RECORDS

Individuals' medical histories are presented in the medical records. These were copied beginning in the 1880s (transcriptions continuing through the early 1900s) from the original Hospital Ledgers, Prescription Books, Abstracts of the Quarterly Report of Wounded in the Field, and Operation Forms. The books and records were originally maintained to track admissions and releases, injuries and illnesses, the daily comings and goings—and "passings" —of troopers into and from medical care. These records are collectively called Carded Medical Records, NARA RG 94.

As an example of these original records, Hospital Ledger books provide a chronological, day-to-day list of admissions and discharges occurring at a specific hospital. The Hospital Ledger books, as well as other original records, have disadvantages. Individual soldiers' health careers are disjointed, distributed over the period of their military services at their various post assignments and listed in those various posts' ledgers and records. To overcome that scattering of an individual's records, the ledgers and other documents are transcribed onto cards, which are collated by regiments and names.

The Carded Medical Records are 3.5-inch by 8-inch (88.9 mm by 203.2 mm) forms printed on stiff paper, which are oriented and filed in a vertical ("portrait") orientation. Most forms are preprinted with spaces for the person's name, rank, and company and are preprinted or stamped with the location of the events. On these preprinted forms, transcribers (the "copyists" as indicated on the nineteenth-century forms) copied details concerning the persons and events.

The purpose of the Carded Medical Records was to track individuals' medical histories (Trevor Plante, personal communication, January 4, 2002). Each entry of the original medical records was transcribed onto a card, then all of the cards for a particular individual (regardless of date or hospital) were filed together. The original purpose of the medical cards was to expedite pension claims (Trevor Plante, personal communication, January 4, 2002). So when an applicant made a pension claim, a clerk could find all of a trooper's medical records in one location, rather than searching the disparate records of all posts where the applicant was stationed. For the purposes of the current study, the Carded Medical Record allow us to examine individuals' health records without having to search the separate original Hospital Ledgers, Prescription Books, Reports of Wounded, and Operation Ledgers.

The amount of information noted for individuals on the Carded Medical Records varies. Some soldiers, such as blacksmith Henry Bailey (fig. 4.1) of Company I, had only a single incident of medical treatment recorded. Bailey was treated for having his left thumb hit with a hammer on June 12, 1875, perhaps related to his military specialty. His death at the Little Bighorn just over a year later terminated his military career.

An antithesis of Bailey's apparent health was Private Gustave Korn (fig. 4.2). He joined the Seventh Cavalry in 1873 and served with it until being killed in action at Wounded Knee on December 29, 1890. Korn had twenty recorded treatments between his 1873 enlistment and 1884, the end of our study period. He showed a penchant for injuries, with three cases of incised wounds, three cases of sprains, one case of an ankle dislocation, and three cases of contusions during this eleven-year period. He acted as a farrier during much of this time, and his wounds seem to be an occupational hazard. As an example, Korn's July 1877 contusion resulted when he was "struck . . . in lower region by horse." He was also treated five times for diarrhea or dysentery (mostly between 1875 and 1879), twice for boils, twice for catarrh, and once for bronchitis.

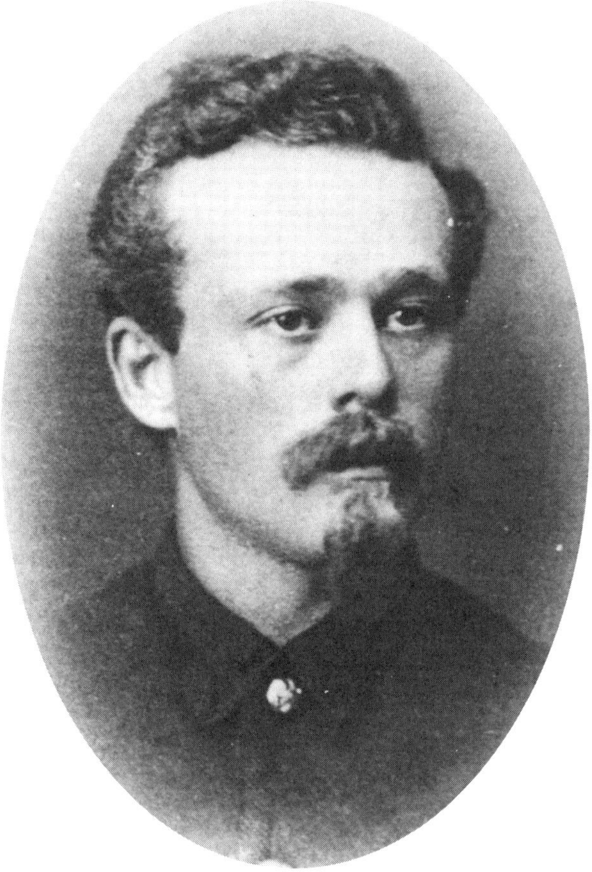

4.1. Blacksmith Henry Bailey of Company I had only one record of medical treatment before dying at the Little Bighorn. Courtesy Little Bighorn Battlefield National Monument, public domain image.

The medical cards are in the NARA's section on Military Service Records. They include those forms in RG 94 Adjunct General's Office, Medical Record Cards, Regular Army, 1821–84, Boxes 396 through 427. The individuals' medical records are arranged alphabetically by last name and are distributed in boxes as indicated in table 4.1. The cards are universally well preserved.

The medical cards are generally completed with first name first and family name last, rather than last name first. Such relative

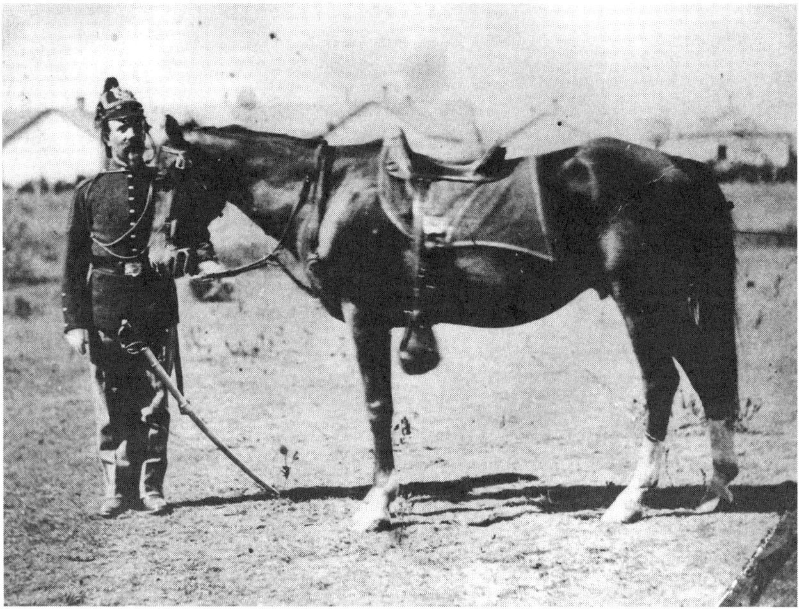

4.2. Private Gustave Korn of Company I had twenty recorded medical treatments between his enlistment in 1873 and the end of the study period in 1884. He was treated for sprains, dislocation, contusions, incised wounds, dysentery, diarrhea, boils, catarrh, and bronchitis, but no combat wounds. Courtesy Little Bighorn Battlefield National Monument, public domain image.

informality is an unusual treatment, at least in present-day bureaucratic situations. The exceptions (last name first, followed by the first name) occur only in some of the latest records inspected, from the early to mid-1880s. But presenting the names in the normal speaking-pattern sequence is the rule through most of the records, not confined to the medical records alone. Although this name sequence might be viewed as a more humane means of addressing a person, it may also represent a time when accounting for persons was easier because of the relatively few individuals involved.

In those thirty-two boxes of transcribed medical records, four kinds of Carded Medical Records appear based on the form formats. They include Medical Record Cards proper, Prescription Book Cards, Quarterly Report of Wounded Cards, and Operation Record Cards.

TABLE 4.1. NARA Record Group box numbers of medical records for the post–Civil War Seventh Cavalry (by soldiers' last names)

Box no.	*Last names*	*Dates examined*	*Dates corrected*
396	Abott–Ball	January 23–26, 2001	January 10–11, 2002
397	Baoline–Blake	January 26–29, 2001	January 11, 2002
398	Blush–Brown, J.	January 29–February 1, 2001	January 11–12, 2002
399	Brown, L.–Cannaran	February 1–2, 2001	January 12, 2002
400	Carey–Cochran	February 3–5, 2001	January 12–14, 2002
401	Coledgs–Crause	February 5–8, 2001	January 14, 2002
402	Creedon–Denny	February 9–12, 2001	January 15, 2002
403	Derr–Dunkerley	February 12–14, 2001	January 15–16, 2002
404	Dunning–Fields	February 14–15, 2001	January 16, 2002
405	Fish–Gaffney	February 16–17, 2001	January 16–17, 2002
406	Gallene–Graham	Feb 17 & June 4–5, 2001	January 17, 2002
407	Grau–Harris	June 6–8, 2001	January 17–18, 2002
408	Harryman–Hoefig	June 9–12, 2001	January 18, 2002
409	Hoffman–Jaimeson	June 12–13, 2001	January 18–19, 2002
410	James–Kennelly	June 13–15, 2001	January 19, 2002
411	Keogh–Lawrence	June 15–19, 2001	January 19, 2002
412	Leary–Lynch	June 19–20, 2001	January 22, 2002
413	Mackey–McCarthy	June 20–21, 2001	January 22, 2002
414	McCarthy, C.–McLead	June 21–25, 2001	June 7–8, 2004
415	McManus–Moore, J.	June 25–27, 2001	June 8, 2004
416	Moore, L.–Neilson	June 27–29, 2001	June 8–9, 2004
417	Nelan–O'Sullivan	June 29–July 2, 2001	June 9–10, 2004
418	Pahl–Quinn	July 2–6, 2001	June 10, 2004
419	Radigando–Roche	July 6–11, 2001	June 10–12, 2004
420	Roeder–Schneider	July 11–13, 2001	June 12, 2004
421	Scholl–Simius	July 13–16, 2001	June 12–14, 2004
422	Skillmano–Staunton	July 16–18, 2001	June 14, 2004
423	Starl–Taylor	July 18–19, 2001	June 14–15, 2004
424	Tempes–Vigny	July 19–24, 2001	June 15, 2004
425	Volkmann–Weller	January 4–7, 2002	June 15–16, 2004
426	Wemster–Winter	January 7–9, 2002	June 16, 2004
427	Wolff–Miscellaneous	January 9–10, 2002	June 16–17, 2004

Note: Dates indicate when the records were examined and transcriptions corrected.

MEDICAL RECORD CARDS

The most frequent forms are the Medical Record Cards, the majority indicating hospitalization in a broad sense. This often meant being restricted to quarters or relieved of specific duties (such as riding or guard duty) and of course, but not necessarily, being housed in the post hospital.

The Medical Record Cards generally follow a standard format (fig. 4.3). Important information begins with the trooper's names, followed by rank, company, and regiment. Next information specific to the illness is presented. Illness-related information starts with date of admission then the location of admission (usually preprinted on the form, although sometimes stamped), "from" status (duty, prison, and so forth), followed by the "complaint" or diagnosis. Details related to wounds (such as missile involved and location where wounded) are emphasized. When and how the trooper was returned to duty or transferred or discharged are presented next. Finally there is a space for remarks, followed by bookkeeping information, such as hospital register and page, and the copyist's signature.

The records concerning complaints are generally consistent, and the category of complaint or diagnosis is completed succinctly. Sometimes a modifier is added to the specific ailment ("acute diarrhea" or "primary syphilis"). Or sometimes a location is indicated under the complaint heading, identifying the anatomical region of the injury or disease. "Contusion, L. instep," for example, indicates a contusion on the left instep of the foot. Comments, such as the cause of an injury, are occasionally added under remarks. In the example above, the form continues, "Rmks: Kicked by horse," indicating that the foot contusion resulted from a horse kick. Remedies, treatments, and medicines are sometimes noted, but these notations are unusual and infrequent. We omitted them from our data collection. Their general absence from the Medical Record Cards presumably represents accurate transcriptions of the original records, which functioned as an inventory of the ill and their recovery, not specifics of their treatment.

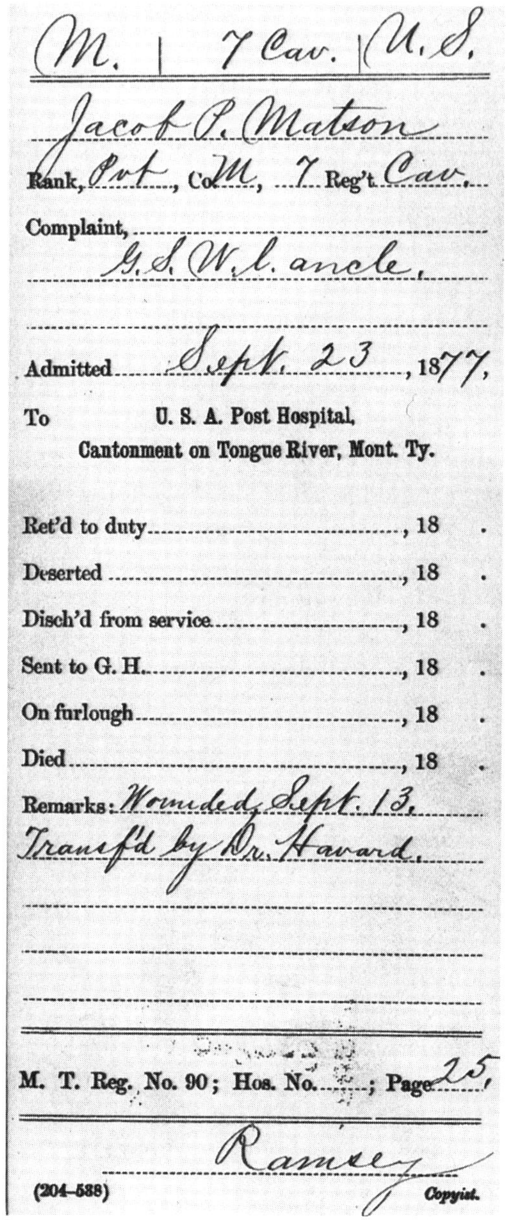

M. | 7 Cav. | U.S.

Jacob P. Matson

Rank, Pvt, Co. M, 7 Reg't. Cav.

Complaint,

G.S.W.l. ancle.

Admitted Sept. 23, 1877.

To U. S. A. Post Hospital,
Cantonment on Tongue River, Mont. Ty.

Ret'd to duty, 18 .

Deserted, 18 .

Disch'd from service, 18 .

Sent to G. H., 18 .

On furlough, 18 .

Died, 18 .

Remarks: Wounded Sept. 13.
Transf'd by Dr. Havard.

M. T. Reg. No. 90; Hos. No. ; Page 25.

Ramsey

(204-588) Copyist.

4.3. Example of typical Seventh Cavalry Medical Record Card. This record shows that Private Jacob P. Matson of Company M was admitted on September 23, 1877, at the Cantonment on the Tongue River, Montana Territory, for a gunshot wound to the left ankle ("G.S.W.1. ancle [*sic*]"). Courtesy National Archives and Records Administration, public domain image.

PRESCRIPTION BOOK CARDS

Included among the Carded Medical Records, although less common than the first group, is a second form: the Prescription Book Cards. Few such records indicate any medicines or treatments being administered. The Prescription Book Cards are the same size as the Medical Record Cards. The information recorded differs, however.

Prescription Book Cards have a standard format (fig. 4.4). Following military affiliations, they begin with the trooper's name, rank, company, and regiment. The location where the illness occurred, which is written on the form (followed by admission date, diagnosis, and return date), is often difficult to determine from the card.

The Prescription Books appear to have been used for minor ailments and frequently employed while in the field, en route between posts, or otherwise outside a post and away from its hospital facility. These are situations in which being hospitalized in the strict sense was not possible.

The Prescription Book Cards often omit important information or present it in a vague fashion. Specifically, dates of admittance and return are often inexact or at least unclear.

QUARTERLY REPORT OF WOUNDED IN THE FIELD CARDS

Third among the Carded Medical Records are abstracts of the Quarterly Report of Wounded in the Field (hereinafter Report of Wounded Cards). Even less frequent than the Prescription Book Cards, the Report of Wounded Cards (fig. 4.5) are the same size and generally in a similar format as the other Carded Medical Records.

The main differences from the Carded Medical Record format are a line for the victim's age and less exact locations of events. The Report of Wounded Cards often contain details concerning injuries or diseases acquired during engagements or while otherwise engaged in the field, as well as the injuries' treatments. In contrast with the other forms, these cards' entries frequently mention treatments.

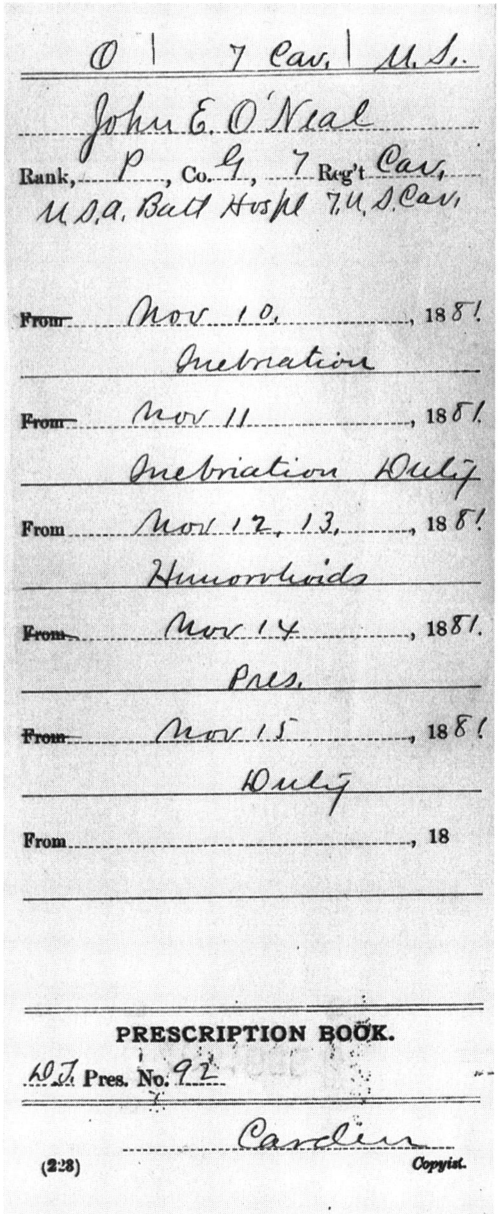

O | 7 Cav. | U.S.

John E. O'Neal

Rank, P, Co. G, 7 Reg't Cav.

U.S.A. Batt Hospl 7 U.S. Cav.

From Nov 10, 1881

Inebriation

From Nov 11, 1881

Inebriation Duty

From Nov 12, 13, 1881

Hemorrhoids

From Nov 14, 1881

Pres.

From Nov 15, 1881

Duty

From ...., 18

PRESCRIPTION BOOK.

W.T. Pres. No. 92

Carden
Copyist.

(228)

4.4. Example of a Seventh Cavalry Prescription Book Card. This record shows that Private John E. O'Neal (elsewhere spelled "O'Neill") of Company G at an unstated location was treated in November 1881 for inebriation and hemorrhoids. Courtesy National Archives and Records Administration, public domain image.

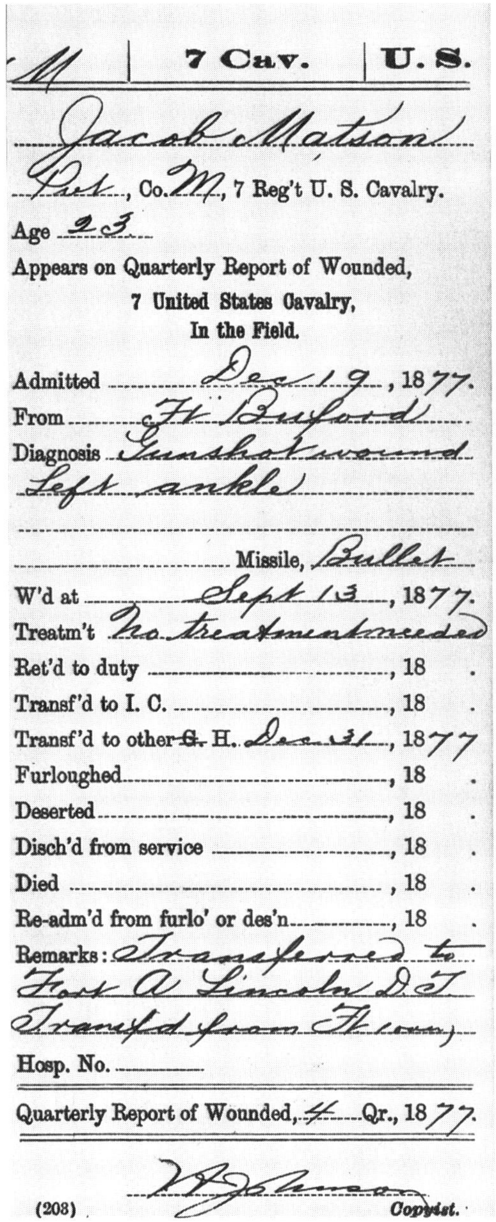

M | 7 Cav. | U. S.

Jacob Matson

Pvt., Co. M, 7 Reg't U. S. Cavalry.

Age 23

Appears on Quarterly Report of Wounded,
7 United States Cavalry,
In the Field.

Admitted Dec 19, 1877.
From Ft Buford
Diagnosis Gunshot wound
Left ankle

Missile, Bullet
W'd at Sept 13, 1877.
Treatm't No treatment needed
Ret'd to duty , 18 .
Transf'd to I. C. , 18 .
Transf'd to other ~~G.~~ H. Dec 31, 1877
Furloughed , 18 .
Deserted , 18 .
Disch'd from service , 18 .
Died , 18 .
Re-adm'd from furlo' or des'n , 18 .
Remarks: Transferred to
Fort A Lincoln D.T.
Transf'd from Ft [illegible]

Hosp. No.

Quarterly Report of Wounded, 4 Qr., 1877.

(208) [illegible] Copyist.

4.5. Example of a Seventh Cavalry Report of Wounded Card. This record shows that Private Jacob Matson of Company M was transferred from Fort Buford on December 19, 1877, to Fort Abraham Lincoln for a gunshot wound to the left ankle. He was transferred again on December 31, 1877. (See fig. 4.3 for an earlier documentation of this wound.) Courtesy National Archives and Records Administration, public domain image.

OPERATION RECORD CARDS

Last and most infrequent of all medical records, Operation Record Cards are filed among the other medical records. Operation Record Cards include the usual information presented on the other forms, as well as details concerning the complaint, a brief presentation of the operation that was performed, and the result of that operation. The categories of results are death, recovered and returned to service, and recuperating.

Accuracy of Records

An issue of vital concern for our study is the accuracy of the records. How well do they describe circumstances, identify ailments, and represent accurate transcriptions? Although it is not possible to determine how accurate the nineteenth-century diagnoses are, other potential errors can be assessed. Errors may occur in the original records, in transcription of the original records, and in deciphering handwritten records.

In a few cases the original records (those in the original ledgers, books, and abstracts) are apparently crossed out. At least some of these "erasures" (using the nineteenth-century term) are noted in the Carded Medical Record. The event is copied to the card then crossed out, with a footnote indicating that the marking occurs in the original records. Our work makes no attempt to transcribe notes concerning these erasures or lining-outs mentioned on the cards. Only the final corrected entries appear in our database.

Proofreaders inspected the copyists' work, making certain that the information was transcribed accurately. If the proofreader's interpretation of the entry differed from the copyist's, a correction was made and noted as being the proofreader's modification. We made no attempt to note copyist's errors indicated by the proofreader or insertions of additional information. The corrected information was recorded without additional notations in our database.

How accurately do the transcribed records reflect the original records? NARA archivist—and national treasure—Michael Musick (now retired) is said to have found only four errors in transcription during his more than thirty years of archival experience (DeAnne Blanton, personal communication, June 10, 2004). If his experience is an accurate indication of error frequency, the transcribed medical records are extraordinarily accurate copies of the original records.

Comparability of Records

Among the various medical record forms (including the Medical Record, Prescription Book, Report of Wounded, and Operation Cards) are occasional duplicate records of the same event. They involve the same person with the same or similar complaints, the same date of admission to hospital, and the same date of return to service. Duplicated records constitute approximately 5 percent of all the medical records; the other 95 percent of the events appear only once in the carded records.

Most duplicate records appear on two different record cards, entered twice in two separate ledgers, and each dutifully copied and collated. Some duplicated records, however, are on different kinds of forms (for instance, on Medical Record and Prescription Book Cards or on Medical Record and Operation Record Cards). These duplications apparently represent transfer of a trooper from one hospital to another (for example, from the post hospital to the general hospital).

As a means of evaluating the consistency of the nineteenth-century records, we compared duplicated records. This evaluation presents methods then results, followed by conclusions.

METHODS

Duplicated record pairs are compared with one another. Both records must include the person's name for inclusion in this assessment, and at least one record must present the trooper's complaint, admittance and return (or transfer) dates, and the location where the illnesses occurred. Paired documents missing important information are excluded from this assessment. As an example, John R.

Lane's gonorrhea complaint during spring 1873 at Taylor Barracks and the other information recorded on one document are thorough, but the paired document is incomplete and thus excluded from this comparison of paired records.

Multiple differences involving one event are counted separately. As an example, if one of the duplicated record pair differs in admittance dates as well as in return dates, then both differences are noted as separate discrepancies. For instance, John N. Alley was admitted on June 12, 1882, in one record but on June 13 in the paired document and was returned to service on June 22, 1882, in one document but on June 28 in the corresponding document. Two discrepancies are noted for Alley in this analysis.

RESULTS

The resulting tally shows similarities and differences among record pairs (table 4.2). Most pairs (61.9 percent of differences) are exactly the same—the same trooper's name, same admittance and

TABLE 4.2. Comparison of duplicated post–Civil War Seventh Cavalry medical records

Differences	*Number*	*Percentage*
No significant or explainable differences	623	61.9
Different trooper's names	90	8.9
Different dates when trooper admitted for treatment	71	7.1
Different dates when trooper returned to duty or transferred	118	11.7
Different locations where illness occurred	5	0.5
Different complaints		
Different complaint modifiers or details	52	5.2
Different diseases or injuries named	41	4.1
Multiple or overlapping diseases	7	0.7
Different complaints subtotal	100	9.9
Total	1007	100.1

Note: Multiple differences between paired records counted separately.

return dates, same location where the illness happened, and same complaint. The high frequency of identical pairs demonstrates precision among the service's surgeons, stewards, clerks, copyists, and proofreaders in identifying, reading, transcribing, and checking medical and related information. Some paired records deviate from this concordance, however, and those discrepancies provide additional insights concerning the accuracy or inaccuracy of records.

Among the differences between record pairs, discrepancies in the person's name occur frequently (8.9 percent of differences). Differences in names usually involve spelling variations of last names. As an example, Samuel Avery's name is spelled Avary in a paired document. Other records omit the trooper's first name, and occasionally the first name of a trooper documented differs between the paired documents. In a few cases, for instance, John and James seem to have been used interchangeably. John aka "James" Costello is an example.

Differences in document-pair admittance and return (or transfer) dates occur more frequently than name differences. As an example of admittance date differences, Frank L. Bunhof [*sic*] was admitted on May 8, 1882, for catarrh, although a paired document indicates admission on May 10. Admittance dates differ less frequently than return date differences. Numbers of return date differences constitute the greatest discrepancy of any recorded category.

Most return date differences involve only a day or two between the paired documents. But others are notable. As an example, Henry Fahler [*sic*] recovered from a headache on February 27, 1874, in one document and March 27, 1874, in another—a month's difference. Some discrepancies in return date pairs may involve ailing troopers being transferred to different posts; the first medical officer may have been unaware of the rest of the illness course and the date when the trooper returned to service. For instance, being transferred from field operations to a post hospital, from one command to another, may cloud the date when the trooper returned to service. As an example, Hugh McGonigle returned to service at Fort Abraham Lincoln on May 5, 1876, but the paired Prescription Book Record shows his return on May 14 while in the field.

Record pair geographic location differences are the least frequent of all categories analyzed. Differences between pairs represent only 0.5 percent. Locations where illnesses happened, especially those at regular posts, are chronicled consistently in the medical records.

Next the complaints written on document pairs are compared to assess their reliability, a critical variable for our purposes. Differences in complaint pairs amount to one of the greatest percentages of all paired document differences. But examining complaint differences by subcategory shows marked variations.

The most frequent complaint differences exist between the record pair's illness by modifiers and details. For example, some paired records include and exclude the severity of the ailment, such as it being acute. As an example, Frederick Tobey suffered from acute diarrhea in one document and "plain" unqualified diarrhea in the paired document. Other differences involve the body part involved, such as hand versus finger. And the medical officer appears to have had latitude as to whether to include or omit details, such as the cause of the event (for example, a fall).

The next most frequent complaint difference occurs in the identification of the ailment. Some different record pairs probably show progression of an ailment. As an example, catarrh may have developed into headache. Other record pairs show more significant differences, such as omission of the ailment name from one record. As example, Herman von Tagan's diagnosis of colic in one document is omitted altogether in its pair. Other paired diagnoses seem to conflict outright. As an example, one of Frank Moulton's complaints is recorded as catarrh, but the paired document indicates quotidian intermittent fever. These discrepancies serve as a warning for the uncritical use of the complaint identifications in our analyses.

Finally, the least frequent differences in complaint record pairs involve multiple and overlapping ailments. In these cases one record shows multiple ailments, while its pair indicates only one. As an example, Robert L. Murphy suffered a simple headache in one record, but the paired document indicates catarrh followed by headache. Such discrepancies might result from a more careful diagnosis while undergoing treatment or represent additional ailments developing while under care.

Based on these duplicated documents, paired records generally display exactly the same information. But paired record differences vary depending on the parameter. Locations where illnesses happen seem consistent, making our analyses of geographic locations and their relationship to ailments reliable. Troopers' names appear less certain. These discrepancies indicate challenges to identifying troopers and suggest caution when analyzing individual health histories and employing individual identities and their associated enlistment information (age, stature, nativity, and so forth). Some identifications may be erroneous (see the next section). Dates of admittance and return to service appear compromised in some of these record pairs. So when we examine the length of an ailment (return date minus admit date = illness length), we must consider that this calculated period is less reliable than some other parameters. Finally, complaint identification demonstrates notable differences between document pairs. As a consequence, subsequent analyses must recognize variability in whether details are included or omitted and that some complaints may be more complex, with multiple, overlapping, or misdiagnoses of diseases present. Most importantly for our analyses, the listing of different ailments in record pairs suggests that diagnosis was—then as now—an imprecise and developing process. This assessment demonstrates that some parameters documented on the medical records can be employed with confidence, while others must be used with caution.

Additional Challenges

As rich and detailed as these medical and enlistment records are, additional challenges to their interpretations and understandings exist, including the identification of individuals, abbreviations and medical terms employed, and faint writing.

INDIVIDUAL IDENTIFICATION

An essential element for much of our research is identifying individuals. This step is required to follow troopers' medical histories and related background information (such as age and birthplace).

Identifying nineteenth-century individuals in the various medical records is a nightmare in the twenty-first century. The nineteenth-century records lack the uniqueness of identification numbers, such as military service, social security, or driver's license numbers. As a consequence, identities are often obscured by the whimsy of orthography, name similarities, and coincidental ranks and enlistment dates.

Most records provide identification information critical to separating one individual from another. That information includes first and last names, company affiliation, dates, and to a lesser extent the location and some chronic complaints. The comparability of post assignments, companies, and period generally serves to separate what appear to be the same individuals. Following the person's name, company assignments and years of enlistment are emphasized to identify individuals. As an example, when several different George Andersons appear in the records, one was assigned to Company H during the 1860s, while an apparently different George Anderson was assigned to a different company, Company K, during the 1870s. Admittedly, errors are likely, with some individuals being represented in our data as two or even several persons, when they are in fact a single person who reenlisted. But without reliable confirmation that we are dealing with a single person, individuals' records have been kept separate.

Middle initials of a single individual often differed in the medical records. As a consequence, we consider middle initials unreliable: they cannot be used either to exclude or to include individuals with the same first and last names as the same or different individuals.

Identifying individuals is often especially challenging early in their military careers. At enlistment, they were recruits, often in transit to their post and usually without company assignments. Because disease dogged recruits as well as the ranks, some of these transients fell ill. If the person's name was unusual and he could be identified easily, those data are included with the individual's health information with relative certainty.

The challenge in identifying specific individuals does not end with their joining companies and metamorphosing from raw recruits into privates. Common last names remain troublesome.

Special problems occur with soldiers whose last names are Smith and Brown. Significant numbers of them had not only the same last name but also the same first name or same initial of the first name.

Another problem identifying specific individuals is name spellings. Considering the high illiteracy rate among troopers, phonetic spellings of names is a perplexing issue, especially with names of French or German origin. But spelling proves difficult even in Irish, English, and some other surnames. It is possible that two or more of those persons may be included as a single person in the database. This lumping is probably more frequent with individuals having common family names and common first names, less frequent with uncommon names.

Occasionally some confusion reigns in the records concerning name sequence, confounding family names (last names or surnames) and first names. For example, take Thomas Allen. Was the name correctly filed for the individual with the family name of Thomas, or did he really have the family name of Allen and thus get misfiled? As another example, August Bockman's record is apparently misfiled among the troopers whose last names began with A as "Bockman August." Regimental Returns are especially troubling in this respect. There are differences within a single month's return as well as discrepancies from company to company's returns.

Our approach includes all medical complaints to assess the regiment's overall health and illness, whether or not the identity of the person can be ascertained. If the person's identity is uncertain, medical data are collected, but no specific individual associated with that illness is noted.

HANDWRITING

The medical forms and enlistment records are nearly all handwritten, with a few rare typewritten forms among the medical records. So entering the transcribed medical records into our database requires interpreting handwriting.

Some nineteenth-century handwriting is esthetically attractive. The most exquisite rivals the beauty of calligraphy. Unfortunately, not all nineteenth-century handwriting is pleasing and easily interpreted by twenty-first-century eyes.

Several nineteenth-century lettering conventions are found. As an example, nearly all of the records' handwriting indicates a letter F by including a serif on the middle line of the letter, a stroke that distinguishes nearly all capital Fs from nearly all capital Ts. As another example, the shapes of some numbers are similar, sometimes making distinguishing one from another difficult. Those numbers include 1 and 7, 4 and 9, and 5 and 6. Depending on the writer's penmanship and the record context, the probability of an erroneous interpretation varies from minuscule to the flip of a coin.

Not all nineteenth-century copyists' penmanship is equally excellent or uniform—or for that matter interpretable. As an example, the Regimental Returns for June–July 1870 in the Gains/Losses table display an idiosyncratic hand. The writer employed small letters and often ran adjacent letters together, frequently making interpretation of names and other information difficult, if not impossible.

Some records or portions of records are illegible or at least indiscernible. Our database, needless to say, omits those records. It is likely that in some cases what appears to be discernible and obvious to contemporary readers is probably not so and is misinterpreted during the data gathering. Assessing how often researcher misinterpretation occurs is beyond the scope of this work but remains a fascinating and important issue.

ABBREVIATIONS

Some of the transcribed records employ abbreviations. Most of these are interpretable based on context. Abbreviations are written for persons' first names, months of the year, military rank, and diseases.

A person's first name is often abbreviated. Some examples follow. "Aug" and "Augt" are interpreted as August or Augustus, "Edw" as Edward, "Geo" as George, "Hy" as Henry, "Jas" and "Ja's" as James, "Jer^{h}" as Jeremiah, "Jos" as Joseph, "J^{no}" and "Jno" as John, "Patr" and "Pk" as Patrick, "Robt" as Robert, "Terr" and

"Ter" as Terrence, "Thos" as Thomas, and "W^{m}" and "Willm" as William.

The months of the year are abbreviated too. When used in the context of a date, "Jany" and similar abbreviations are interpreted as January, "Feby" as February, "Mar" and "Mch" as March, "Apl" as April, and so forth through the rest of the months.

Ranks are almost always abbreviated in the records. A rank of "P" and "Pr" and similar abbreviations are interpreted as private, generally not as prisoner. Some soldiers' ranks, however, are recorded as prisoner, usually indicated by "Pris" or some such abbreviated title. Sometimes the information includes other indications of the soldier's incarceration, such as being admitted to the hospital from the guardhouse. We attempted to record soldiers' status as prisoners based on indications in the medical records, but those attempts are tentative at best. We no doubt missed some prisoners' status. Other rank abbreviations tend to be more obvious, interpretable, and standard.

Abbreviations are also employed for some of the complaints. These too are interpreted and entered in the database. In the context of a diagnosis, as examples, "Ac" or "A" (as in "Diarrhoea A") is interpreted as acute, "C" or "Ch" (as in "C. rheumatism") as chronic, but "C" (as in "C syphilis") as constitutional. "F Int T" is interpreted as tertian intermittent fever. Other complaint abbreviations are similarly interpreted and transcribed.

MEDICAL TERMS AND DIRECTIONS

Sometimes Latin and Greek medical terms are found in the medical records, and for our purposes they are translated into their English equivalents. More Latin and Greek terms seem to be employed in the earlier records, immediately following the Civil War. Later diagnoses employ more English terms, with the fewest non-English terms in the 1880s.

Here are a few examples of the translation of Latinized disease names: "catarrhus" as catarrh, "colica" as colic, "constipatio" as constipation, "febris remittens" as remittent fever, "febris int." as intermittent fever, "ulcero" as ulcer, and "vulnus incision" as incised wound.

We still fight to make illness and health care understandable to laypeople, a battle that probably began with the incantations of the first shaman. Anglicization of illness names by the military of the 1860s was a step in this direction, one that is continuing today. As much as possible, English terms are entered in the database and employed in these analyses.

In addition to the Latin medical terms, some medical records employ antiquated or British spellings for diseases. Examples include "anchylosis," "diarrhoea," "otorrhoea," and "anaemia." The contemporary American spellings are entered in our database.

Although anatomical features and structures are occasionally identified in the nineteenth-century medical records, modern anatomical directions and orientations are limited and usually lacking altogether.

FAINT WRITING

Two additional problems emerge when reading the records. All records are written or printed in ink, almost always black ink. But some of the records' lettering is too light to be legible. This is rarely a problem when the original records are read but becomes an issue more often when records are interpreted from microfilm. As an example, the microfilm Regimental Returns for February 1870 on the page for "Gain—Recruits from Depot" indicate 110 new recruits. But the writing is too light to discern letters and names, although the handwriting appears to be legible. Similar problems probably result from the original documents' fading or poor reproduction quality.

A second problem occasionally occurs. As mentioned earlier, some forms are ripped, with portions of some torn forms missing. This difficulty rarely affects the Carded Medical Records because their paper stock was thick and resisted tearing. But the original Regimental Returns are a different matter, probably due in part to being folded for mailing and storage as well as frequent use over the decades. As an example, the Regimental Returns for portions of the June 1876 column "Gained—Recruits from Depot" and the column "Gained—Enlisted" and all of the reenlistments and losses are torn and missing from the microfilm version.

Summary

The Medical Record, Operation, and Prescription Book Cards and the Regimental Returns and Enlistment Records provide a detailed perspective on health and life, illness and death, in the post–Civil War mounted corps. Although each set of records has issues with completeness, redundancy of the data sets compensates for many of the errors.

As informative as these records are, they are not pristine, interpretation-free, lacking typographical errors, and complete. There are problems in how the troopers' ailments are reported, how medical personnel interpreted those ailments, and how those diagnoses were recorded in the medical records. Further problems involve reporting, transcriptions, and the present interpretations of those documents. All problems confound interpretation, recording, and transcription in the nineteenth century.

Nevertheless, these challenges are relatively few and largely surmountable, at least in contrast with the other records and their interpretations. We hope that interpretation and typographical errors are random and have little influence on the rich, detailed perspective that extant documents provide in understanding the health and illness of soldiers of the mid-nineteenth century.

CHAPTER 5

Regimental Strength and Background of Seventh Cavalry Troopers

P. Willey

Seventh Cavalry troopers did not merely appear unheralded in the regiment, bereft of backgrounds and experiences, to get sick then heal or die. Their illnesses in part reflected their biological heritages and civilian social status. Variables such as age, size, and birthplace affected troopers' likelihood of health or illness. Once they were enlisted, their postings and military activities further exposed them to illnesses, injuries, and other hazards, which built upon their premilitary backgrounds.

This chapter describes those parameters introduced in chapter 4, summarizing and presenting the soldiers' preenlistment backgrounds as well as chronicling military measures. In addition to these preenlistment data, the numbers of troopers serving in the Seventh Cavalry are documented as well as the number of troopers who unilaterally terminated their enlistment through desertion.

Chapter 4 outlines the documents available to examine these dimensions. This chapter summarizes those data by document sources. It begins with information derived from the Regimental Returns then presents data from enlistment records. We consider medical records in the more focused chapters that follow.

Regimental Returns

Our work requires establishing trooper numbers in service—a critical count for establishing the number of potentially susceptible individuals for epidemiological analyses (tables 5.1 and 5.2). The Regimental Returns yield the number of individuals who served in and those who deserted from the Seventh Cavalry each month.

TROOP STRENGTH

Examining the overall monthly numbers of enlisted men (table 5.3), the regiment size swings from a low of 489 (November 1881) to a high of more than double that number (n = 1,244 in September 1876). The average month finds about 813 enlisted men in the regiment.

Differences in numbers of enlisted men occurred by year too (fig. 5.1). Following inception of the Seventh Cavalry in 1866, a general increase in numbers happened annually from the mid-1860s through 1871, then the numbers decreased to a low in 1875. After that year the greatest monthly number of enlisted men during our study period was in 1876, reflecting the increased enlistments during the months following June 1876 and the Battle of the Little Bighorn. After this increased strength in 1876 and 1877, annual declines reoccurred in 1878 and continued through the rest of the period. Those later average monthly numbers by year approached and in some cases exceeded the low number in 1875.

TABLE 5.1. National Archives microfilm rolls employed to assess post–Civil War Seventh Cavalry troop strength and desertion rates

Microfilm roll	*Dates included*
Microcopy 744, Roll 71	September 1866–December 1873
Microcopy 744, Roll 72	January 1874–December 1881
Microcopy 744, Roll 73	January 1882–(transcribed through December 1884)

Source: Regimental Monthly Returns.

TABLE 5.2. Comparison of column titles employed in table 5.3 and the original column titles in Regimental Monthly Returns

Column title	*Original Monthly Return titles and explanations*
Date	Month and year of the return
Enlisted number	Number of enlisted men present (including hospital stewards?)
Aggregate number	Total number of officers and enlisted men present
Officers died	
In action	Number of officers who died that month "in action or of wounds rec'd there"
Of disease	Number of officers who died that month "of disease & c."*
Enlisted men died	
In action	Number of enlisted men who died that month "In action or of wounds rec'd there"
Of disease	Number of enlisted men who died that month "of disease & c."*
Deserted	Number of enlisted men who deserted that month

*Note that "of disease & c." seemed to include all deaths other than those associated with battle-related deaths, whether caused by disease or not. At least some suicides, for instance, were included as "of disease & c."

As well as annual differences, the number of enlisted men showed variation by month within the years (fig. 5.2). Considering all years (1866 to 1884) combined, the greatest average occurred in February, the lowest average in August. Note, however, that the numbers of enlisted men each month varied greatly.

In some ways these monthly differences are more interpretable when considered by season. The greatest average number of enlisted men happened in winter. The lowest average number of enlisted men occurred in summer (June–August). These highs and lows probably reflected the seasonal availability of civilian work, contrasted with the year-round convenience of military employment. Fluctuations in fair-weather work probably influenced individuals' decisions to enlist in the fall, hole up for the winter

TABLE 5.3. Post–Civil War Seventh Cavalry enlisted men and officers present, deaths, and desertions by month and year

			OFFICERS DIED		ENLISTED DIED		
Date	*Enlisted number*	*Aggregate number*	*In action*	*Of disease*	*In action*	*Of disease*	*Deserted*
September **1866**	764	882				13	89 (—)
October	846	849				9	41 (5.4%)
November	851	861			1	2	1 (0.1%)
December	963	977					38 (4.5%)
January **1867**	1001	1022					65 (6.7%)
February	993	1020				2	116 (11.6%)
March	1011	1038					116 (11.7%)
April	1045	1072				1	85 (8.4%)
May	966	996				3	76 (7.3%)
June	897	926			8		80 (8.3%)
July	840	870			1	12	60 (6.7%)
August	796	827			1	7	41 (4.9%)
September	1041	1074				2	31 (3.9%)
October	999	1037			1	1	41 (3.9%)
November	976	1017				3	38 (3.8%)
December	937	979			1		54 (5.5%)
January **1868**	1101	1144					57 (6.1%)
February	1130	1172				1	31 (2.8%)
March	999	1041					155 (13.7%)
April	930	972					64 (6.4%)
May	897	938					38 (4.1%)
June	872	914					27 (3.0%)
July	865	908					12 (1.4%)
August	864	907				2	8 (0.9%)
September	849	892			4	2	16 (1.9%)
October	840	883			1		1 (0.1%)
November	954	995	2		19		2 (0.2%)
December	952	993			1		4 (0.4%)

(continued)

TABLE 5.3. *(continued)*

Date	*Enlisted number*	*Aggregate number*	OFFICERS DIED *In action*	OFFICERS DIED *Of disease*	ENLISTED DIED *In action*	ENLISTED DIED *Of disease*	*Deserted*
January **1869**	925	965		1		1	30 (3.2%)
February	921	961				2	8 (0.9%)
March	920	959					8 (0.9%)
April	863	901		1		2	65 (7.1%)
May	799	836				1	71 (8.2%)
June	775	811					26 (3.3%)
July	702	745				4	37 (4.8%)
August	667	710				1	20 (2.8%)
September	666	709				1	5 (0.7%)
October	666	708					10 (1.5%)
November	674	716					8 (1.2%)
December	745	787					10 (1.5%)
January **1870**	759	801					12 (1.6%)
February	885	927				3	13 (1.7%)
March	879	920					33 (3.7%)
April	863	904				1	30 (3.4%)
May	859	899					28 (3.2%)
June	1034	1074					35 (4.1%)
July	1045	1085				2	73 (7.1%)
August	1089	1131				2	51 (4.9%)
September	1021	1062				3	50 (4.6%)
October	1002	1044				2	16 (1.6%)
November	978	1018				1	33 (3.3%)
December	981	1017				3	12 (1.2%)
January **1871**	981	1022				2	19 (1.9%)
February	987	1028				1	6 (0.6%)
March	965	1006					24 (2.4%)
April	1139	1180					26 (2.7%)
May	1110	1151				2	32 (2.8%)

TABLE 5.3. *(continued)*

Date	Enlisted number	Aggregate number	OFFICERS DIED In action	OFFICERS DIED Of disease	ENLISTED DIED In action	ENLISTED DIED Of disease	Deserted
June	988	1029					49 (4.4%)
July	962	1003		1		1	17 (1.7%)
August	808	849					51 (5.3%)
September	784	825				1	12 (1.5%)
October	770	811				3	10 (1.3%)
November	741	782				3	7 (0.9%)
December	717	758				1	25 (3.4%)
January **1872**	703	744					5 (0.7%)
February	987	1028				2	13 (1.8%)
March	964	1003				1	24 (2.4%)
April	917	956				2	47 (4.9%)
May	905	944					18 (2.0%)
June	851	890					55 (6.1%)
July	795	834				3	32 (3.7%)
August	759	801				1	16 (2.0%)
September	736	778					23 (3.0%)
October	719	761					27 (3.7%)
November	713	755				1	9 (1.3%)
December	922	964				2	18 (2.5%)
January **1873**	909	951				1	22 (2.4%)
February	972	1015				4	31 (3.4%)
March	899	942				1	72 (7.4%)
April	845	888				4	67 (7.5%)
May	796	839					55 (6.5%)
June	813	856				1	17 (2.1%)
July	801	844					10 (1.2%)
August	790	833			1		9 (1.1%)
September	761	804				3	3 (0.4%)
October	961	1004					17 (2.2%)

(continued)

TABLE 5.3. *(continued)*

Date	Enlisted number	Aggregate number	OFFICERS DIED In action	OFFICERS DIED Of disease	ENLISTED DIED In action	ENLISTED DIED Of disease	Deserted
November	958	1001				2	2 (0.2%)
December	957	1000					3 (0.3%)
January **1874**	938	981				2	6 (0.6%)
February	936	979					3 (0.3%)
March	937	980					12 (1.3%)
April	906	949			1	1	25 (2.8%)
May	864	907					42 (4.6%)
June	856	899				1	15 (1.7%)
July	845	887				2	8 (0.9%)
August	839	882				2	3 (0.4%)
September	814	857					14 (1.7%)
October	784	827				2	17 (2.1%)
November	756	799					8 (1.0%)
December	743	786				2	5 (0.7%)
January **1875**	737	780					5 (0.7%)
February	790	832		1			4 (0.5%)
March	769	811					16 (2.0%)
April	759	801				1	6 (0.8%)
May	728	770				1	14 (1.8%)
June	699	742					4 (0.5%)
July	666	709					4 (0.6%)
August	656	699				1	2 (0.3%)
September	648	691				1	2 (0.3%)
October	797	840				1	1 (0.2%)
November	796	839					3 (0.4%)
December	797	837				3	1 (0.1%)
January **1876**	796	836				1	1 (0.1%)
February	784	825				2	2 (0.3%)
March	748	789					3 (0.4%)

TABLE 5.3. (*continued*)

			OFFICERS DIED		ENLISTED DIED		
Date	*Enlisted number*	*Aggregate number*	*In action*	*Of disease*	*In action*	*Of disease*	*Deserted*
April	797	838					0
May	790	831					2 (0.3%)
June	552	580	13		237		0
July	545	588			3	1	1 (0.2%)
August	707	749				1	5 (0.9%)
September	1244	1287			1		8 (1.1%)
October	1237	1279			1	1	7 (0.6%)
November	1218	1260					8 (0.6%)
December	1210	1251		1		1	5 (0.4%)
January **1877**	1162	1203				2	11 (0.9%)
February	1121	1162					17 (1.5%)
March	1097	1138				1	31 (2.8%)
April	1047	1088				1	39 (3.6%)
May	990	1031					42 (4.0%)
June	960	1001					12 (1.2%)
July	934	978				1	14 (1.5%)
August	922	966				1	8 (0.9%)
September	896	938	2		19		7 (0.8%)
October	884	928			1		9 (1.0%)
November	868	912					5 (0.6%)
December	826	870					22 (2.5%)
January **1878**	798	842				2	14 (1.7%)
February	795	839					2 (0.3%)
March	742	786					31 (3.9%)
April	722	766				1	1 (0.1%)
May	694	737					15 (2.1%)
June	676	718					8 (1.2%)
July	662	702					11 (1.6%)
August	650	693				1	11 (1.7%)

(*continued*)

TABLE 5.3. *(continued)*

Date	Enlisted number	Aggregate number	OFFICERS DIED In action	OFFICERS DIED Of disease	ENLISTED DIED In action	ENLISTED DIED Of disease	Deserted
September	635	678					4 (0.6%)
October	732	775			1		0
November	785	828			1		5 (0.7%)
December	784	827				1	2 (0.3%)
January **1879**	786	829					1 (0.1%)
February	775	818			1		1 (0.1%)
March	775	818					2 (0.3%)
April	759	802					15 (1.9%)
May	750	792		1			10 (1.3%)
June	741	783					3 (0.4%)
July	728	771					5 (0.7%)
August	728	771				1	2 (0.3%)
September	721	764					1 (0.1%)
October	721	764					2 (0.3%)
November	714	757				1	3 (0.4%)
December	704	747					1 (0.1%)
January **1880**	702	745				1	2 (0.3%)
February	718	760					2 (0.3%)
March	766	808					3 (0.4%)
April	764	805					4 (0.5%)
May	759	801					2 (0.3%)
June	747	789					10 (1.3%)
July	754	797			1	1	1 (0.1%)
August	734	777					5 (0.7%)
September	711	754					4 (0.5%)
October	718	761					2 (0.3%)
November	791	834					1 (0.1%)
December	786	829					4 (0.5%)
January **1881**	784	827				1	0

TABLE 5.3. *(continued)*

			OFFICERS DIED		ENLISTED DIED		
Date	*Enlisted number*	*Aggregate number*	*In action*	*Of disease*	*In action*	*Of disease*	*Deserted*
February	780	822		1		1	0
March	760	802					1 (0.1%)
April	740	782					4 (0.5%)
May	732	774					3 (0.4%)
June	696	738					8 (1.1%)
July	675	717					13 (1.9%)
August	649	690				1	7 (1.0%)
September	490	533				1	7 (1.1%)
October	495	538					4 (0.8%)
November	489	532					16 (3.2%)
December	610	653				1	8 (1.6%)
January **1882**	687	730					0
February	691	734					4 (0.6%)
March	681	724					8 (1.2%)
April	666	709					7 (1.0%)
May	627	670					41 (6.2%)
June	628	671					11 (1.8%)
July	602	644					22 (3.5%)
August	601	643					8 (1.3%)
September	593	635					12 (2.0%)
October	607	649					8 (1.3%)
November	698	740					8 (1.3%)
December	696	738				1	3 (0.4%)
January **1883**	691	733					6 (0.9%)
February	682	723					4 (0.6%)
March	674	715					2 (0.3%)
April	664	705					12 (1.8%)
May	648	689				1	19 (2.9%)
June	623	664				2	22 (3.4%)

(continued)

TABLE 5.3. *(continued)*

			OFFICERS DIED		ENLISTED DIED		
Date	*Enlisted number*	*Aggregate number*	*In action*	*Of disease*	*In action*	*Of disease*	*Deserted*
July	610	653					4 (0.6%)
August	710	753					12 (2.0%)
September	710	752				1	8 (1.1%)
October	740	782				1	9 (1.3%)
November	736	778				1	18 (2.4%)
December	739	781					8 (1.1%)
January **1884**	755	797				1	2 (0.3%)
February	749	790					4 (0.5%)
March	736	777					14 (1.9%)
April	728	768					7 (1.0%)
May	689	730			2		40 (5.5%)
June	687	728				1	7 (1.0%)
July	698	741				1	21 (3.1%)
August	733	776				2	3 (0.4%)
September	765	808					23 (3.1%)
October	768	810				1	7 (0.9%)
November	772	814					12 (1.6%)
December	764	806					3 (0.4%)
Total			17	7	308	191	4083

Note: Enlisted number column indicates the number of enlisted men present; aggregate number is the total of enlisted men and officers present. Counts abstracted from the Seventh Cavalry's Monthly Returns, Nation Archives and Records Administration microfilms (see tables 5.1 and 5.2 for more details).

months, then jump ship as the grass greened and spring's opportunities knocked.

These differences in enlistee numbers must be considered when assessing frequencies of illnesses. Monthly, seasonal, and annual differences are critical to determining relative illness frequencies.

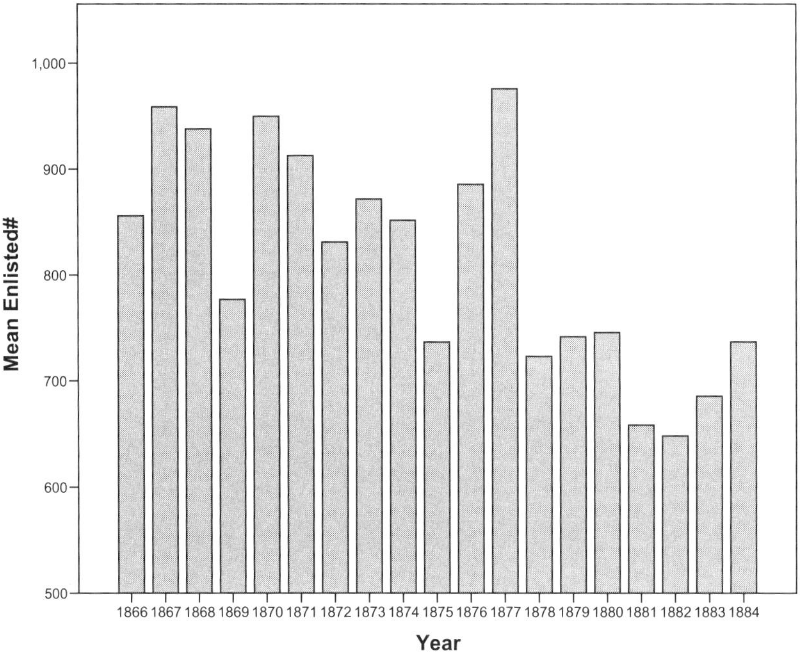

5.1. Average monthly number of post–Civil War Seventh Cavalry enlisted men by year.

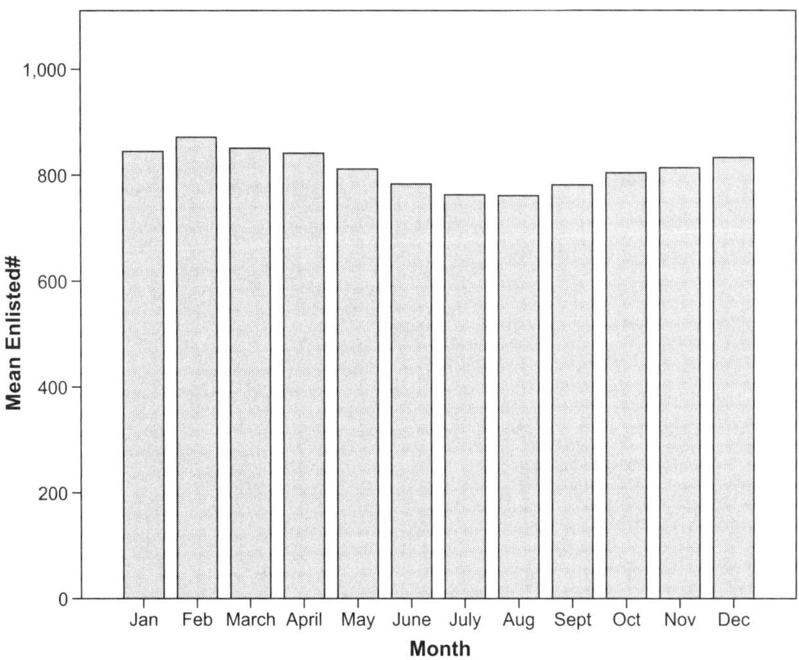

5.2. Average number of post–Civil War Seventh Cavalry enlisted men by month.

DESERTIONS

In addition to troop strength, Regimental Returns record the number of men deserting on a month-by-month basis. Contrasted with present rates, desertion occurred in shockingly high proportions during the post-Civil War period, including the Seventh Cavalry. Some background on desertion during this period is merited before summarizing those Seventh Cavalry figures.

In the nineteenth century desertion was defined as absence from duty for the briefest period. Such an absence even included wandering a short distance from camp without authorization. This nineteenth-century definition of desertion contrasts with the present-day definition, which usually requires thirty days of being absent without official leave (AWOL) before the absent service member is assigned deserter status. Even today this time requirement may be voided if the service member is determined not to return. No formal AWOL category existed in the nineteenth century. You were either in the military or not, however fleeting the absence.

When a deserter was caught, the penalty could be two to five years of imprisonment followed by a dishonorable discharge (Coffman 1986:373). That severe punishment was usually used only as a last resort. Based on Seventh Cavalry desertions, most returning deserters suffered few apparent long-term penalties.

Edward Coffman (1986:371–72) provides a lengthy list of reasons for desertions: "the inordinate demands on soldier labor, poor quarters, poor or inadequate food, lack of recreation, harsh noncoms or officers, low pay and lengthy intervals between paydays, drunkenness, poor quality of recruits, lack of understanding of the difference between the enlistment oath and an ordinary job contract, and the indifference if not outright hostility of society."

Whatever the causes, desertions occurred at an amazingly high rate during the post–Civil War period. Coffman (1986:371) estimated that during a 24-year period (1867 to 1891) 88,475 men deserted from the U.S. Army out of a force that averaged only 22,000 soldiers/year. This rate was so high that General James W. Forsyth was ordered on an inspection tour during the summer of 1868 to identify the reasons for such a high rate of desertion. Similarly, it was claimed, during the first two years of the Seventh Cavalry's existence, 1,200 men deserted (Barnitz in Utley 1977:161).

For the U.S. military as a whole, however, the worst year was yet to come. In 1871 the already-low enlisted man's pay was further reduced. A private's monthly pay fell from $16 to $13 in 1871—nearly a one-fifth decrease (Coffman 1986:346; McDermott 1997:170). With the reduction of pay, as might be expected, came an increase in desertions, which rose to 32.6% that year (Coffman 1986:346).

Looking at overall post–Civil War trends, desertions increased in spring, following a winter's service. These spring deserters constituted the "snowbirds." Those troopers, after dodging winter's teeth in the relative comfort of heated barracks and with regular meals, chose to hit the trail, leaving post and comrades. One adjutant general claimed that two-thirds of the desertions occurred in the spring (Coffman 1986:372).

Inserting some methodological steps for clarification, we turn to desertion frequencies documented by the Seventh Cavalry's Regimental Returns (1866 to 1884). To calculate monthly desertion rates, the number of desertions for a particular month is divided by the number of enlisted men from the previous month. Consider, as an example, the earliest months after establishment of the Seventh Cavalry (table 5.3). The records show 41 desertions for October 1866. That figure (41) is divided by the number of enlisted men (764) at the end of the previous month, September 1866. The resulting relative frequency (41/764) is 5.4%.

Applying those methods, it is clear that Seventh Cavalry monthly desertion rates varied tremendously. Some months there were literally zero desertions in the entire Seventh Cavalry. As might be expected, this occurred most often in the colder months and during the later years of our study. The months with no desertions include October 1878, January and February 1881, and January 1882. As exceptions to these generalizations, no desertions were reported during two warm months (April and June 1876) in the middle of our study period—the spring and month coinciding with the Battle of the Little Bighorn. If judicious men considered desertion, April and June 1876 would be the likely months. Perhaps the lack of desertions in June 1876 was because the Seventh Cavalry marched through territory where desertion made the solitary sojourner vulnerable to being discovered and killed by hostiles.

On the other extreme, some months had huge numbers of desertions. The greatest number and highest relative frequency of desertions occurred in March 1868, when 155 enlisted men, nearly 14% of the available troop strength, deserted. The next greatest months for desertions (a tie in terms of numbers) occurred surprisingly in February and March 1867. In each of those two months 116 men deserted, almost 12% of the enlisted men. As noted earlier, desertion rates usually ebbed during colder months of the year, not rose, as during those bitter winter months of 1867.

Those were the desertion lows and highs by month. What about the average? The average desertion rate for the entire period was 2.25% per month. Such reduction in manpower, whatever the month, must have had a tremendous effect on morale and battle readiness.

We now turn to annual and seasonal differences in desertion rates. To determine seasonal desertion rates, the monthly rates are summed by the four seasons: winter, spring, summer, and fall. The percentages of monthly desertions (calculated above) for the three months of each season for each year are added. As an example, for the winter of 1867, the percentages of desertions in December 1866, January, and February 1867 (4.5, 6.7, and 11.6%, respectively) are summed; the resulting total indicates a 22.8% desertion rate during winter 1867 (table 5.4). Exceptions to this approach include fall 1866 and winter 1885, when incomplete data invalidate this approach. So the initial season of the Seventh Cavalry's existence and the terminal season of our study period are omitted from this consideration.

It is claimed that desertions rose in the spring. To test that assertion using the Seventh Cavalry seasonal desertion rates, statistical assessments employ both ANOVA and Kruskal-Wallis tests in SPSS (2008).

Seasonal desertion rates are compared with broader claims for the military of the time. On average, the Seventh Cavalry data set had 54.85 desertions per season (table 5.5). The fewest desertions occurred during the winters of 1876, 1879, and 1881, with only

TABLE 5.4. Post–Civil War Seventh Cavalry desertion percentages by year and season

Year	Winter	Spring	Summer	Fall	Total
1867	22.8	27.4	19.9	11.6	81.7
1868	14.4	24.2	5.3	2.2	46.1
1869	4.5	16.2	10.9	3.4	35.0
1870	4.8	10.3	16.1	9.5	40.7
1871	3.7	7.9	11.4	3.7	26.7
1872	5.9	9.3	11.8	8.0	35.0
1873	8.3	21.4	4.4	2.8	36.9
1874	1.2	8.7	3.0	4.8	17.7
1875	1.9	4.6	1.4	.9	8.8
1876	.5	.7	1.1	2.3	4.6
1877	2.8	10.4	3.6	2.4	19.2
1878	4.5	6.1	4.5	1.3	16.4
1879	.5	3.5	1.4	.8	6.2
1880	.7	1.2	2.1	.9	4.9
1881	.5	1.0	4.0	5.1	10.6
1882	2.2	8.4	6.6	4.6	21.8
1883	1.9	5.0	6.0	4.8	17.7
1884	1.9	8.4	4.5	5.6	20.4

Note: Percent desertion is number of enlisted men who deserted divided by total number of enlisted men that season.

TABLE 5.5. Post–Civil War Seventh Cavalry desertion percentages by season

	Winter	Spring	Summer	Fall
Average number	41.22	89.28	55.33	33.56
Standard deviation	55.435	81.074	51.857	29.230
Minimum	4	5	6	6
Maximum	219	277	181	110

4 desertions in each of those 3 winters. The greatest number of desertions in a season was in spring 1867, with 277 desertions. This is consistent with what one officer of the day claimed for the post–Civil War period as a whole (Coffman 1986:372).

For all seasons combined, the overall average was 6.26% desertions per season and year. Seasonal desertion averages were lowest in fall (4.15%) with winter a close second (4.61%). The highest average season desertion rate occurred in spring (9.72%). The other warm-weather season, summer, approximated the overall mean for all seasons (6.56%).

The statistical assessment supports what the descriptive statistics suggest and what authority claimed. One-way ANOVA (F = 3.496, df = 3, 68, p = 0.020) and Krushal-Wallis tests (χ^2 = 9.732, df = 3, p = 0.021) are statistically significant. Based on these statistical assessments, desertions were not randomly distributed by season.

To assess the authority's claim that two-thirds of desertions occurred in spring (in Coffman 1986:372), we use the Seventh Cavalry seasonal desertion counts. Dividing the Seventh Cavalry mean desertions for spring (89.28) by the summed means for all seasons (219.39) yields a relative frequency of 40.7% overall during the period, not supporting the two-thirds figure that was claimed. Nonetheless, it is clear that desertion rates differ by season, with spring having the greatest number, and winter and fall the fewest.

Annual desertion rates are based on the average monthly rates. Average monthly desertion rates are summed by calendar year, from January through December. Annual desertion percentage is the number of desertions divided by the total number of enlisted men for that year. For the first year of the Seventh Cavalry's existence, which began in September 1866, the figures are reduced to those last four months of 1866.

Total annual desertion percentage employs the monthly desertion percentage as defined above and sums the desertion percentages for each month for a calendar year. As an example, the total annual desertion percentage of 1867 is the percentage of January 1867 desertion, plus the percentage of February 1867 desertion, plus the percentage of March 1867 desertion, and so forth through the percentage of December 1867 desertion. Other years follow the same procedure, except for the partial year of the Seventh Cavalry's inception (1866). Only September through December 1866 are summed for that year, the first four months of the regiment's existence.

As a cautionary note, the total annual desertion percentage differs from the "annual" total by season. Those two totals consist of slightly different months. When calculating the seasonal desertion rates, the figure for December of the previous year is added to January and February of the subsequent year and the December of that subsequent year is omitted from the sum. The annual desertion rates, in contrast, are those from January through December of a single calendar year.

When examined on an annual basis, the rate of desertion echoes the monthly and seasonal data. Annual desertion rates were often high and differed from one year to the next (table 5.6, total annual desertion frequency column). In this section we first examine the overall annual trends for Seventh Cavalry desertions and then assess some historic claims.

Annual Seventh Cavalry desertion rates vary from a high of 82.7% (803 men) in 1867 to a low of 4.9% (42 men) in 1876. The overall average desertion percentage was 24.1% (214.9 men). Although this is not a high desertion rate by the standards of the day, it is much higher than the desertion rate of modern military forces. In 2004, for example, 2,376 soldiers deserted from the U.S. Army, which had a strength of 483,880, a rate of 0.49% for the entire year (Powers 2005). Even at that rate, the army has major concerns about today's desertions. That modern rate, however, is a mere 2% of the Seventh Cavalry's desertion rate.

We find a general trend in examining the Seventh Cavalry's annual desertion rates. During our study period the annual number of desertions decreased from 1866 through 1884 ($R^2 = 0.45$; df 1, 17, $F = 13.890$, $p = 0.002$; $Y = 41379.368—21.954X$). Although the number of deserters varies considerably and changes in desertion numbers are not uniform from one year to the next, the overall trend is for the number of desertions to decrease from the earlier years to the later ones. Similar changes occur using the annual desertion percentage by year ($R^2 = 0.570$; $F = 24.851$, df = 1, 17, $p = 0.000$). Besides the temporal trend, our annual

TABLE 5.6. Post–Civil War Seventh Cavalry desertions by year

Year	*Total enlisted men*	*Number of desertions*	*Average monthly desertion frequency (%)**	*Total annual desertion frequency***
1866***	3424	169	4.9	11.0
1867	11502	803	7.0	82.7
1868	11253	415	3.7	41.0
1869	9323	298	3.2	36.1
1870	11395	386	3.4	40.4
1871	10952	278	2.5	28.9
1872	9971	287	2.9	34.1
1873	10462	308	2.9	34.7
1874	10218	158	1.5	18.1
1875	8842	62	0.7	8.2
1876	10628	42	0.4	4.9
1877	11707	217	1.9	21.3
1878	8675	104	1.2	14.2
1879	8902	46	0.5	6.0
1880	8950	40	0.4	5.3
1881	7900	71	0.9	11.7
1882	7777	132	1.7	20.6
1883	8227	124	1.5	18.4
1884	8844	143	1.6	19.7

*Average monthly desertion frequency is defined as number of desertions during that year divided by total enlisted men for the same year.

**Total annual desertion frequency is the sum of each month's desertion frequency for that year.

***Note that the Seventh Cavalry was formed in September of 1866, so these counts and percentage reflect a partial year.

desertion figures have a bearing on two claims: the number of Seventh Cavalry deserting in the mid-1860s and high numbers deserting in 1871.

It has been claimed that the Seventh Cavalry had a very high desertion rate in its earliest years. Barnitz asserted in July 1868 that 1,200 men deserted during the first two years of the Seventh Cavalry's existence (in Utley 1977:161). As remarkably high as this figure is, our data from the monthly regimental returns indicate that Barnitz may have understated the number of desertions. From the inception of the Seventh Cavalry (September 1866) through the time of Barnitz's claim (July 1868), 1,356 men deserted, 156 more men than he identified. Note that the entire two years had not elapsed when Barnitz made his claim. Barnitz's figure of 1,200 desertions dates a little over a year and a half after the Seventh Cavalry formed: with 1,215 desertions at the end of March 1868, its nineteenth month. Barnitz, it seems, understated the actual number of desertions during that period.

But perhaps Barnitz was not in error. It is possible that he counted the number of men who deserted and remained on the loose, not those who deserted but for one reason or another (such as being captured or surrendering) were back in service in July 1868. It is also possible that Barnitz was counting deserters by individuals, excluding from the count the second timers—men who deserted, returned to service, then deserted a second time. Our monthly regimental returns tallied each time a man abandoned his post as another desertion. Some men did exactly that. Whatever the specific details, an enormous number of men deserted in the Seventh Cavalry's early years.

Turning to a broader perspective, it has been claimed that desertions hit an all-time high in 1871. That year a private's monthly pay was decreased from $16 to $13 (Coffman 1989:346), a reduction of nearly one-fifth. For the military as a whole, nearly one-third of the men (32.6%) deserted that year alone (Coffman 1986:346). How does that generalization about the military as a whole fit the Seventh Cavalry desertion rate?

According to the Seventh Cavalry's monthly Regimental Returns, 278 desertions happened during the 12 months of 1871 (table 5.6). The Seventh Cavalry's desertion rate in 1871 was as low as it had been since the regiment's inception in 1866 and was not achieved again until 1874. The Seventh Cavalry desertion data for 1871 do not follow the trend claimed for the military as a whole. In fact they show the reverse.

The numbers of troopers and deserters come from the Regimental Returns and provide an overall portrait of the Seventh

Cavalry by month, season, and year for 1866 to 1884. In many ways they also serve as the demographic foundation, permitting comparisons of troop strength. Enlistment Records identify individual soldiers and their military careers and are also employed here to portray the Seventh Cavalry.

Enlistment Records

"A regiment is recruited from all classes and conditions of men," including "the lowest specimens of humanity recruited in the crowded cities" (Libbie Custer quoted in Coffman 1986:305).

The second data source employed here is the Enlistment Register, which documents enlistment and reenlistment information. It includes pivotal military dates on an individual-by-individual basis, biological information related to each enlistee, and locations where events occurred. The Enlistment Records indicate where the trooper enlisted; enlistment period (usually five years); birthplace; age at enlistment; height; color of eyes, hair, and complexion; and civilian occupation. In addition to this information, the Enlistment Register indicates the nature of the person's final dismissal from service (for example, expiration of enlistment period, desertion, or death) and rank at that time. Reenlistment documents follow a similar format, including the additional notation that the trooper is reenlisting.

Of particular importance for our analyses are enlistment location, nativity, civilian occupation, enlistment age, stature, complexion, discharge rank, and nature of discharge. Those variables are considered below after a general consideration of the enlistment process.

Before enlistment became official, a medical officer conducted a physical examination of the recruit, in the presence of the recruiting officer. As Charles Ewing (1894:168) insightfully noted, the surgeon was caught on the horns of dilemma. On one hand, he attempted to obtain the best recruits for the military, while on the other he tried to appease the recruiting officer. Then as now the recruiting officer was more interested in quantity than in quality. The surgeon confirmed the fitness and qualifications of the recruit for military service. As an overriding body superseding the surgeons, Boards of Inspectors at the recruit depots checked the medical officers' assessments (Ewing 1894:168).

NATIVITY

Birth location is assessed next. But first background information relating to nativity and military enlistment is required.

Throughout our period of study U.S. citizens and noncitizens could join the army. Starting in the 1890s, a law required enlistees to be citizens or at least to make declarations of their intentions to become citizens before they could become soldiers (Coffman 1986:331). But no such requirement was in effect during our period of study.

Place of birth is recorded on enlistment records. Some adjustments are made for analytical purposes, including grouping small jurisdictions into larger ones. All questionable birthplaces (for example, "Canada?") are included with the state or country indicated, disregarding the qualifying question mark. For those troopers whose birthplaces are listed as Baden, Bavaria, Hanover, Hesse, Hesse Castle, Prussia, Saxony, Silesia, and Würtemburg, their nativities are included under Germany. Those troopers whose birthplaces are listed as Berne and Suissi are included with those born in Switzerland, and those listed as being born in Bohemia are included under Austria. Troopers born in Canada West, New Brunswick, and Nova Scotia are included in Canada; those listed as born in Loraine are included in France; and those recorded as born in Great Britain, Wales, and South Wales are included in England.

Using Enlistment Records, birthplaces by state and country are summarized for the Seventh Cavalry (table 5.7). Approximately one-third of the troopers claimed foreign births, while half were native-born citizens and the other one-sixth went unrecorded. This ratio is similar to other research concerning nativity of enlistees from the period (Adams 2009:25). The proportion of immigrants, however, is remarkable.

Decisions to move from one country to another result from a combination of push-pull factors (Lee 1966). Some influences push potential migrants from their homelands, encouraging emigration.

TABLE 5.7. Birthplaces of post–Civil War Seventh Cavalry troopers by nation and state

Nation	*State*	*Number*	*Overall*	*1870 Census Adult males**
Africa		2 (0.07)		
Argentina		1 (0.04)		
At sea		3 (0.11)		
Australia		1 (0.04)		
Austria		24 (0.88)		
Barbados		1 (0.04)		
Belgium		9 (0.33)		
Canada		176 (6.49)		
Cuba		2 (0.07)		
Denmark		30 (1.11)		
England		298 (10.65)		
Finland		1 (0.04)		
France		69 (2.54)		
Germany		893 (32.92)		
Greece		1 (0.04)		
Holland		17 (0.63)		
Hungary		12 (0.44)		
Ireland		965 (35.57)		
Italy		11 (0.41)		
Mexico		1 (0.04)		
Norway		17 (0.63)		
Poland		7 (0.26)		
Russia		8 (0.29)		
Scotland		84 (3.10)		
Spain		3 (0.11)		
Sweden		19 (0.70)		
Switzerland		58 (2.14)		
Subtotal		2713 (99.69)	33.45	

TABLE 5.7. *(continued)*

Nation	*State*	*Number*	*Overall*	*1870 Census Adult males**
US	Alabama	4 (0.10)		340,984
US	Arkansas	4 (0.10)		175,194
US	California	5 (0.12)		283,740
US	Connecticut	58 (1.44)		209,123
US	Dakota Territory	1 (0.02)		7,047
US	Washington, DC	31 (0.77)		46,652
US	Delaware	16 (0.40)		46,274
US	Georgia	11 (0.27)		401,547
US	Illinois	188 (4.67)		946,717
US	Indiana	179 (4.44)		612,832
US	Indian Territory	2 (0.05)		—
US	Iowa	47 (1.17)		445,064
US	Kansas	5 (0.12)		148,152
US	Kentucky	149 (3.70)		466,762
US	Louisiana	29 (0.72)		261,170
US	Maine	91 (2.26)		245,704
US	Maryland	171 (4.24)		281,294
US	Massachusetts	313 (7.77)		554,886
US	Michigan	111 (2.75)		460,408
US	Minnesota	6 (0.15)		167,456
US	Mississippi	6 (0.15)		288,185
US	Missouri	85 (2.11)		632,179
US	Nebraska	3 (0.07)		52,588
US	New Hampshire	43 (1.07)		126,353
US	New Jersey	96 (2.38)		335,819
US	New York	847 (21.02)		1,658,504
US	North Carolina	30 (0.74)		365,528
US	Ohio	519 (12.83)		976,588

(continued)

TABLE 5.7. *(continued)*

Nation	*State*	*Number*	*Overall*	*1870 Census Adult males**
US	Pennsylvania	677 (16.80)		1,292,518
US	Rhode Island	36 (0.89)		82,824
US	South Carolina	3 (0.07)		241,492
US	Tennessee	45 (1.12)		436,154
US	Texas	9 (0.22)		297,356
US	Vermont	46 (1.14)		129,248
US	Virginia	67 (1.66)		427,455
US	West Virginia	25 (0.62)		154,234
US	Wisconsin	72 (1.79)		391,603
	Subtotal	4030 (99.94)	49.69	
None	None	1366		
Not recorded	?	1		
	Subtotal	1367	16.86	
	Total	8110	100.00	

Source: From Enlistment Records.

Note: Parentheses indicate percentages by nation and state.

*Male population over age of ten years (U.S. Census Bureau 1872, table 26, 670).

Pull factors encourage migrants to settle at a particular destination. Because push-pulls affect different people unequally, migrants represent a nonrandom subset of the original population that they left. Those migrants who leave their native lands often demonstrate differences from the stay-behinds in sex, age, number of sibs, socioeconomic status, property ownership, and access to work.

Here we were concerned with late-nineteenth-century international migration. Those immigrants consisted predominantly of males, largely fleeing famine or economic issues, mostly from northern and western Europe (Haines 2000:350–57).

Approximately one-third of the foreign-born Seventh Cavalry troopers hailed from Ireland (35.57% of foreign-born) and one-third from Germany (32.92%), again similar to other studies (Adams 2009:26; Wittke 1967:xv). Next came enlistees from England (10.65%) and Canada (6.49%). Most of the remaining foreign-born enlistees reported being born in Europe. Other birthplaces included Africa, Argentina, Australia, Barbados, and Mexico. Note that few troopers came from eastern and southern Europe or Central and South America and none from eastern Asia. In the years to come those other regions produced waves of immigrants to the United States, but they were in few numbers during the mid-1800s.

Consider changes in migration since then from a broader perspective. After the outpouring of immigrants from western and northern Europe to the United States that typified the Civil War period, the homelands of the migrants changed. Late in the nineteenth century eastern and southern European immigration accelerated (Parillo 2003). As a response, stringent immigration laws were established in the early 1900s. More recent immigrants have come predominantly from eastern, southeastern, and southwestern Asia as well as Latin America (Reimers 2005; Portes and Rumbault 2006). Migration surged in the 1970s. Immigration has formed a larger percentage of U.S. population growth (contrasted with birth-death rates in the indigenous population) since then, exceeding even nineteenth-century proportions (Haines 2000:316).

Although we commonly think of immigrants moving internationally from one country to another, movements also happen internally inside a country's boundaries. Military service guaranteed that all soldiers would move within the United States. Many of the native-born troopers were forced for the first time to live in crowded conditions, consume a substandard diet, and be regimented.

Most native-born Seventh Cavalry enlistees hailed from the eastern United States and Great Lakes area. The most frequent birth states were New York (21.02% of native-born troopers), Pennsylvania (16.80%), and Ohio (12.83%). Those three states constituted more than half of the native-born enlistees' birth states. No other state approached 10% of troopers—not even Massachusetts, which one study found contributed many western frontier soldiers in the 1870s (Adams 2009:28). Some states or territories were not represented at all among the enlistees' birth locations: Arizona, Colorado, Florida, Idaho, Nevada, New Mexico, Oregon, Utah, Washington, and Wyoming. For the most part, these states were the relatively underpopulated western states.

The infrequency of reported southern birthplaces is intriguing. Here we compare trooper birthplaces in former Confederate states (Alabama, Arkansas, Florida, Georgia, Louisiana, Mississippi, North Carolina, South Carolina, Tennessee, Texas, and Virginia) with those in the non-Confederate states and territories, standardized by the 1870 census of males ten years and older. The distribution of Confederate versus Union troopers in relation to population is statistically significant ($\chi^2 = 731.5$, df $= 1$, $p < 0.001$). Troopers from the non-Confederate states and territories were over-represented, and troopers from the former Confederate states were under-represented.

This distribution may indicate a bias against Southerners joining the military soon after the Civil War. Or troopers may have declared that they were born in Union states even when their actual birth state was southern. Based on similar results, Kevin Adams (2009:26–27) interprets the lack of white southerners in the military West as indicating perceived Reconstruction excesses or resistance to the effect of the Civil War.

For the rare trooper with two conflicting birthplaces (different enlistment records listing different birthplaces), the birthplace listed for the period when the illness occurred is employed in our health analyses.

OCCUPATION

The military had a conforming effect on dress, behavior, and manners of the soldiers. The uniformity, however, masked the differences in backgrounds and personalities of a disparate group of men. Some of those experiences and abilities included skills and training gained while engaged in previous civilian occupations, also noted in enlistment documents.

The recruits' civilian occupations may have been recorded to identify individuals with skills of particular value to the regiment. For instance, if the enlistee's civilian profession was blacksmith, farrier, musician, or the like, his services might be especially valuable in a comparable military position.

Occupations in the nineteenth century reflected the economic change that the country was experiencing. The Jeffersonian ideal of an agrarian society shifted toward a more industrial foundation, and farming became less frequent as the century progressed. New economic activities and other occupations emerged, such as photographer, steam engineer, and machinist. And young men of the time were susceptible to such siren calls: get rich quick, aspire to great things, break from the restraining tethers of the antiquated past, and anticipate the future.

But in times of economic duress the more specialized occupations were often the most vulnerable and led to quick employment termination. Before government-sponsored unemployment insurance, being fired or laid off was even more devastating than it is now. The effects could be felt the next day. Enlisting in the military for a five-year period was a way of securing a steady (although paltry) income with lodging and board included.

Most enlistees probably took pride in their civilian occupations. At a time of specialization and a cash economy, people took pride in job titles and earnings, representing social position and the satisfaction of making a good product. Workers felt pride in a job well done, playing a part of a larger arena, and doing the best under the constraints of time and funds.

Among recorded occupations for the Seventh Cavalry troopers, the most common previous occupations were laborer (n = 1,413), soldier (n = 983), and farmer (n = 876). Such seasonal and agrarian work may explain the spike in fall enlistments. Next most frequent were clerks (n = 390), teamsters (n = 223), carpenters (n = 203), painters (n = 180), shoemakers (n = 143), blacksmiths (n = 134), and sailors (n = 116).

At the other extreme were the rare civilian occupations. Surprisingly few recruits claimed factory work—or at least called themselves factory workers (n = 2). The most novel civilian occupations included bachelor ([*sic*], n = 1), boot crimper (n = 1), cheese maker (n = 1), dentist (n = 2), glove maker (n = 1), huckster (n = 2), matchmaker (n = 1), Morocco dresser/finisher/tanner (n = 8), photographer (n = 13), physician (n = 3), spring maker (n = 2), submarine diver (n = 2), and veterinary surgeon (n = 4).

Civilian occupations of Seventh Cavalry troopers included a wide spectrum of jobs. These occupations presumably typified those of U.S. male citizens. It is difficult to know how typical these jobs were in the mid-nineteenth century, but the high proportion of civilian laborers has been documented in an 1870s study (Adams 2009:25).

ENLISTMENT AGE

As part of the enlistment process troopers provided their age. And those numbers were written in the Enlistment Records. "No one will ever know how many boys lied about their age in order to enlist, or, consequently, how much effect those discrepancies in official and actual ages had on the army's age statistics" (Coffman 1986:339).

Ordinarily a potential soldier needed to be at least twenty-one to enlist but could not be too old. The acceptable ages in the 1881 regulations were twenty-one to thirty-five years. Enlistees less than twenty-one years old could be accepted, but only with written consent of a parent, guardian, or master [*sic*]. And that person's signature had to be witnessed (Bartholow 1863:158; Coffman 1986:338). These rules seemed to be interpreted loosely to say the least. In a period before birth certificates age was easy to fabricate and distort.

The official exclusion of youngsters less than twenty-one years old was not universal, however. During the 1870s, for instance, the adjunct general and the secretary of war proposed recruiting youths as young as twelve for musicians. Similarly, adolescents had been inducted into the military during the Civil War. This post–Civil War proposal, however, was rejected (Coffman 1986:333).

Several reasons for excluding adolescents existed. Adolescents, it was claimed, were more apt to falter in military life, lining up for sick call and filling hospital beds. Another reason for exclusion was more humanitarian. Youths less than eighteen were thought to have soft cartilaginous bones and soft muscles and still to be full of potential growth. None of these biological systems would mature normally under the rigors of military life—at least so the reasoning went. As such, excluding youths from enlisting was in keeping with the child labor laws that were sweeping western Europe and the United States at that time.

At the other age extreme, men over thirty-five—especially those over forty-five—were also thought to fill hospital bays. Although middle-aged men were officially excluded from first enlistments, troopers of that age could reenlist after a first enlistment—and continue reenlisting.

In the Seventh Cavalry from 1866 to 1884, most soldiers enlisted in their early or mid-twenties (mean 24.52 years) with the most frequent enlistment age being twenty-one (table 5.8, fig. 5.3). It was a young man's army. The age of first enlistment varied between fifteen and fifty years.

The youngest recorded enlistment age was for Winfield Reidfort (or "Piedfort") at the stated age of fifteen. Standing a mere 53 inches tall, he enlisted in 1868 at Fort Leavenworth after being a bugler in civilian life. Serving variously both in Company D and in the band, he fulfilled his enlistment period and exited military

TABLE 5.8. Summary statistics of Post–Civil War Seventh Cavalry ages at enlistment in years

n	Valid	6743
	Missing	1370
	Mean	24.52
	Median	23.00
	Mode	21
	Std. Deviation	4.430
	Skewness	1.371
	Std. Error of Skewness	.030
	Kurtosis	2.140
	Std. Error of Kurtosis	.060
	Range	35
	Minimum	15
	Maximum	50

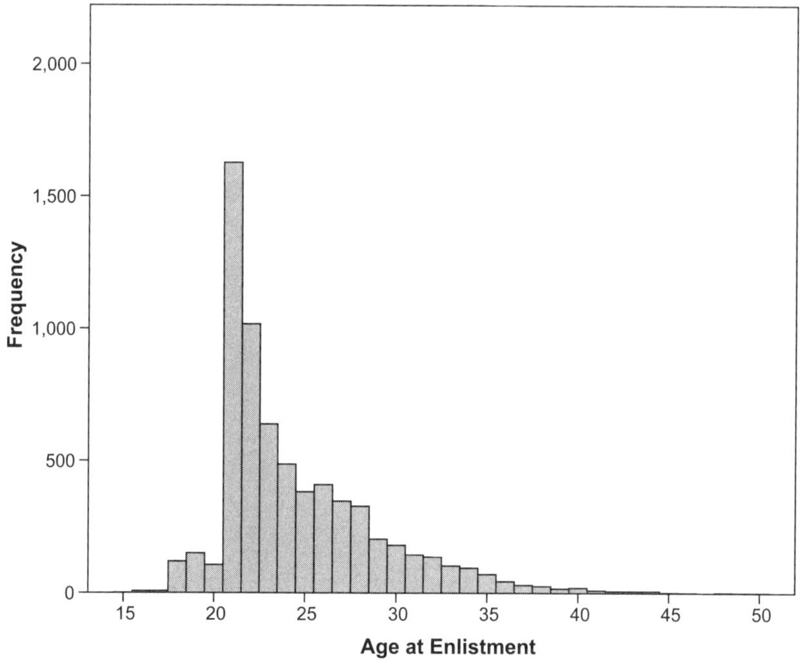

5.3. Age in years of post–Civil War Seventh Cavalry troopers at enlistment.

service as a private five years later, presumably at the ripe old age of twenty. Concerns about youths being unable to withstand the rigors of military duty were unfounded, at least based on Winfield's medical records. He suffered no illnesses.

The oldest enlistee was Irish-born John McGinnis. In 1883, at the near-elderly age of fifty, he enlisted for a fourth time, although for the first time in the Seventh Cavalry. Claiming a previous occupation as tailor, Private McGinnis served his full five-year enlistment period without any medical complaints during his later years.

On the topic of old servicemen, Robert Bartholow (1863:38) claimed: "It is not unusual to find them more than sixty years of age, toothless, almost sightless, rheumatic, and worn out,—suffering, indeed, from the failure of their mental and physical powers, due to the near termination of life." Bartholow's claim is not supported by Private McGinnis's service in the Seventh Cavalry.

STATURE

In addition to age restrictions, being too short or too tall disqualified a potential recruit from enlistment. These stature requirements were largely ignored during the Civil War, as they had been in the French and Indian Wars, War of 1812, and Mexican War. But minimum statures were reestablished after cessation of the hostilities between the states, although they changed from year to year. The minimum height regulation changed nine times from February 1867 through 1874. In December 1874, however, the minimum stature was set at five feet five inches and remained there with relative stability for decades (Ewing 1894:179–80).

Exceptions to the minimum height were permitted. Musicians, who were also exempted from minimum age regulations and might not have completed their growth at the time of recruitment, were exempted.

Exceptions also occurred for teachers and tailors. These desirable trades were apparently needed in the military and did not require full-grown adult size to perform. But in no case were any of these men to be less than a quarter inch below the official minimum (Ewing 1894:180), a scant difference considering measurement errors and an outright violation of the regulations.

Maximum height was of less concern than minimum height. No maximum height rule was established until December 1872 for cavalry enlistments. Then an upper limit of five feet ten inches was imposed (Ewing 1894:180). According to Seventh Cavalry enlistment records (1866 to 1884; n = 6,746), mean height was 67.19 inches (170.7 cm). Mode and median values coincide (67 inches [170.18 cm]; table 5.9).

The stature distribution is slightly asymmetrical (fig. 5.4). The central tendency shifts from shorter heights, toward taller enlistees on the larger end of the distribution. This observation suggests that the minimum stature regulation was enforced more rigorously than the maximum height.

Nonetheless, the distribution shows violation of both minimum and maximum stature regulations. As mentioned, the shortest stature recorded was Winfield Reidfort/Piedfort, who stood a mere 53 inches (134.62 cm) and was only fifteen at the time of

TABLE 5.9. Summary statistics of post–Civil War Seventh Cavalry statures in inches

n	Valid	6746
	Missing	0
	Mean	67.19364
	Median	67.00000
	Mode	67.000
	Std. Deviation	2.018695
	Skewness	.050
	Std. Error of Skewness	.030
	Kurtosis	1.472
	Std. Error of Kurtosis	.060
	Minimum	53.000
	Maximum	77.000

Source: From Enlistment Records.

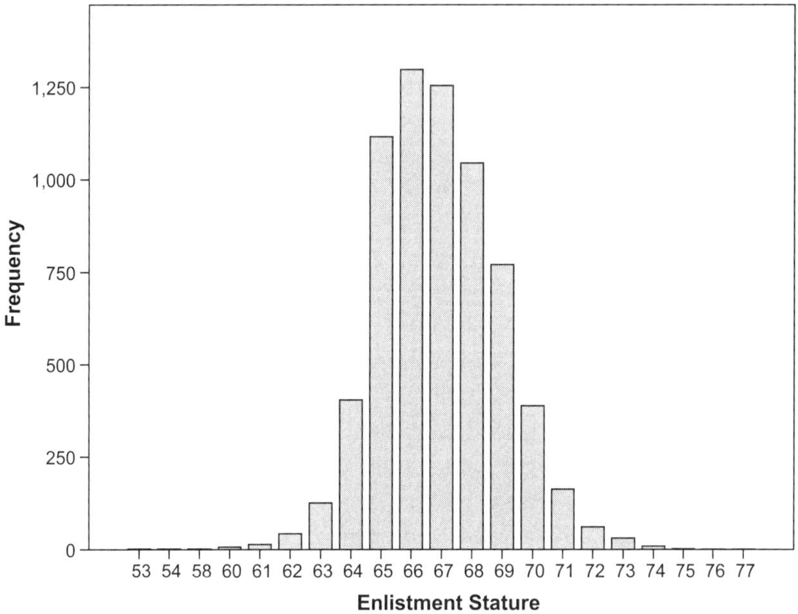

5.4. Statures of post–Civil War Seventh Cavalry troopers from enlistment records rounded to nearest inch.

enlistment. By the time his service period expired in 1873, he may have grown several inches. Exit stature measurements, however, were not recorded.

The tallest enlistee was James Mullins, who stood a whopping 77 inches (195.58 cm) tall. Unlike Reidfort/Piedfort, Mullins lasted only three months in the military and deserted in July 1872. Despite standing out in any nineteenth century crowd—making identification and possible apprehension easy—Mullins disappeared into civilian life without being captured.

The examples of Reidfort/Piedfort and Mullins show that the minimum and maximum stature regulations could be violated. But how frequent were such violations? To examine the stature distribution we employ the minimum standard of 65 inches and maximum standard of 70 inches, ignoring the 0.25-inch waiver. Considering both minimum and maximum violations together, 11.5% of the enlistment records violate height regulations. Most violations occur at the minimum stature (8.9% of all enlistments) and fewer above the maximum (2.6%).

Nearly 9% of the enlistees' statures fall below the 65-inch regulation minimum. Some of these violations may be associated with still-growing recruits. A statistical association occurs between underaged recruits and shorter statures. We examined the ages of 601 recruits with statures less than the regulation minimum of 65 inches (ANOVA F = 10.618, df = 1, 599, $p < 0.001$; Stature = 62.914 + [0.036 × Age]). The younger the recruit, the shorter he was on average. As an additional assessment, the stature difference between recruits aged twenty-one and older versus youthful recruits (under twenty-one) is small—less than an inch (underage $n = 104$, mean 63.21 inches; over 21 $n = 497$, mean 63.89 inches). Nonetheless, the difference is significant ($t = 3.378$, df = 113.945, $p < 0.001$ two-tailed test, equal variances not assumed). These results suggest that an examining surgeon who was likely to disregard one regulation (minimum age, for instance) was also likely to disregard another (such as minimum stature).

Fewer recruits violated the upper stature cap (over 71 inches) than the lower limit. Only 2.6% ($n = 268$) exceeded the maximum. Although some recruits were particularly tall, they were fewer than the shorter regulation violators.

RANK AT DISCHARGE

One measure of a trooper's military success was his rank. Enlisted men normally entered military service as a private or sometimes with a specialized rank (such as trumpeter). From that lowly start the trooper might progress through the ranks. Reenlistees often retained ranks from their previous enlistments.

Ranks included private, corporal, sergeant, first sergeant, commissary sergeant, sergeant major, captain, colonel, major, and veterinarian surgeon. Specialized ranks consisted of blacksmith, wagoner, trumpeter, farrier, bugler, and artificer.

Like most other achieved and acquired statuses, rank was subject to vicissitudes. Soldiers sometimes were busted to a lower rank. But most troopers had attained their highest rank at the time of discharge. And those final ranks were entered on the enlistment records.

Deserters' ranks were not recorded on enlistment records if they successfully escaped service. Ranks of deserters who returned and ultimately exited the service by means other than desertion were usually included in the enlistment records. To examine the association of rank with illnesses and susceptibilities, ranks were combined into categories, presented in table 5.10. Although commissioned officers' health was rarely recorded, they are included here for completeness, not for anticipated analyses.

Although they are excluded from this analysis, medical records exist for some of the future officers of the Seventh Cavalry while they were cadets at the U.S. Military Academy at West Point. Brian Pohanka (1989) analyzed West Point medical records, discovering that cadet George Custer was in the hospital a total of forty times. He was treated for headaches eight times, catarrh seven times, and contusions seven times, as well as for shingles and venereal disease. Marcus Reno was treated for various ailments nineteen times, including catarrh three times, tonsillitis, inflammation of the connective tissues, and a venereal disease. Other future officers with hospital stays or medical treatments included Edward Godfrey, Winfield S. Edgerly, and Benjamin Hodgson, who were all plagued with corns and boils. Henry M. Harrington, John J. Crittenden, and William T. Craycroft were

TABLE 5.10. Military ranks by categories

Rank category	*Ranks*
Commissioned officers	Lieutenants, captains, colonels, majors
Senior noncommissioned officers	Sergeant majors, 1st sergeants, sergeants, chief musicians, chief trumpeters, hospital stewards, commissary sergeants, quartermaster sergeants
Junior noncommissioned officers	Blacksmiths, buglers, corporals, farriers, musicians, saddlers, trumpeters
Rankers	Privates, recruits, wagoners
Others	Civilians, guides, interpreters, packers, teamsters, scouts, surgeons

treated multiple times for sore eyes, headaches, and conjunctivitis. Other future Seventh Cavalry officers treated as cadets were Charles A. Varnum and Luther R. Hare, largely for accidental injuries. The healthier future officers, or at least the ones least treated, included George D. Wallace, James G. Sturgis, Ernest A. Garlington, and James E. Porter. The West Point medical data demonstrate that officers were not immune from medical issues requiring treatment. It is likely that the treatments they received after assignment to the Seventh Cavalry were simply not recorded in the surviving medical records.

NATURE OF DISCHARGE

The nature of the discharge was recorded on the Enlistment Record (table 5.11). They included surgeon's/special orders, general court martial order, government order, act of Congress, expiration of service, and dishonorable discharge. Other discharges indicated a more complex sequence of events: desertions, apprehensions (usually of deserters), and surrenderers. Discharge categories are lumped together for analytical purposes (table 5.12).

TABLE 5.11. Nature of discharges from service for post–Civil War Seventh Cavalry

Nature of discharge	*Overall number (percentage)*	*Number excluding unknowns (percentage)*
Blank, other, or ?	1356 (16.7)	—
Complex (Usually starting with desertion, then apprehended, then whatever follows)	772 (9.5)	772 (11.4)
Unclear (Identified?, AGO, PGO, and dropsy)*	4 (0.0)	4 (0.1)
AOC	3 (0.0)	3 (0.0)
Apprehended, civil authority	2 (0.0)	2 (0.0)
Canceled	28 (0.3)	28 (0.4)
Deserted	2486 (30.6)	2486 (36.8)
Died, died?, drowned, suicide	205 (2.5)	205 (3.0)
Disability	527 (6.5)	527 (7.8)
Discharged, discharged early	11 (0.1)	11 (0.2)
Dishonorable discharge	81 (1.0)	81 (1.4)
Dropped	13 (0.2)	13 (0.2)
Enlistment canceled [see "Canceled" above]	21 (0.3)	21 (0.4)
Expiration of service	1885 (23.2)	1885 (27.9)
General court martial order	22 (0.3)	22 (0.3)
Government order, and government order & surgeon's order [or special order?]	73 (0.9)	73 (1.1)
Insanity	4 (0.0)	4 (0.1)
Killed in action	269 (3.3)	269 (4.0)
Surgeon's orders [or special orders]	338 (4.2)	338 (5.0)
Surrendered	10 (0.1)	10 (0.1)
Transferred	3 (0.0)	3 (0.0)
Writ of habeas corpus	1 (0.0)	1 (0.0)
Total	8114 (99.7)	6758 (100.2)

*Meaning of AGO and PGO unclear.

TABLE 5.12. Nature of discharges by category for post–Civil War Seventh Cavalry

		SEVENTH CAVALRY	
Nature of discharge	*Category discharge types*	*Number*	*Percentage*
Deserted	Deserted	2486	41.6
Died	Died, drowned, suicide	205	3.4
Expiration of service	Expiration of service due to completion of enlistment period	1885	31.5
Killed in action	Killed in action	269	4.5
Left due to Disability	Disability	527	8.8
Others	Act of Congress, apprehended, canceled/enlistment canceled, civil authority, discharged/discharged early, dishonorable discharge, dropped, general court martial order, general order, government order, insanity, surgeon/special order, surrendered, transferred, writ of habeas corpus	610	10.2
Total		5982	100.0

Summary

This chapter reviews two of the three major data sources employed to study the Seventh Cavalry. Regimental Returns and Enlistment Records provide complementary information. The Regimental Returns convey general information about the regiment, including troop strength and number of desertions. Regimental Returns document the number of troops and desertions on a monthly basis. The Enlistment Records give information about specific troopers, including their enlistment dates and biographical information.

The monthly number of Seventh Cavalry enlisted men averaged about 800, with the greatest monthly number in the fall following the Battle of the Little Bighorn and the fewest in late 1881.

Seasonal differences from 1866 to 1884 show a predictable pattern: the greatest trooper numbers in fall and early winter and fewest in summer. Annual numbers fluctuated. The number of soldiers in the regiment by month and year is critical for calculating the overall incidence of disease by month, season, year, and geographic location.

In addition to troop strength, Regimental Returns provide monthly data on the number of desertions. Desertions occurred frequently, at least by modern standards. From 1866 to 1884 the average annual desertion rate was 24%, with much year-to-year variation and a general decline during the period.

Enlistment Records offer a spectrum of information concerning individuals, provided by the enlistee and enlistment examiner and documented by a recorder. For each trooper, the records note where and when enlistment occurred, the trooper's birthplace, occupation, age at enlistment, stature, and complexion. They also deliver information on the trooper's end of enlistment status: specifically, his rank and nature of discharge.

The majority of Seventh Cavalry troopers enlisted in their early and mid-twenties. Most Seventh Cavalry troopers were medium-short in height, averaging 67.19 inches. Altogether 11.5% of enlistees violated enlistment regulations concerning height (8.9% below minimum and 2.6% above maximum). Information on this and the biological as well as occupational backgrounds of the Seventh Cavalry troopers is important for understanding their experience and susceptibility.

We have mentioned some of the problems with the data. Nevertheless, these issues are relatively few and largely surmountable, at least when contrasted with the other records and their interpretations.

The Regimental Returns and Enlistment Records provide the military social and biological backgrounds of the Seventh Cavalry members. They form the foundation for understanding health and life, illness and death, in the post–Civil War mounted corps. The third major source of information is Medical Record, Operation, and Prescription Book forms, which are analyzed and interpreted in subsequent chapters.

CHAPTER 6

Head and Neck Diseases of the Seventh Cavalry

Patrick J. Collison

The battle-related injuries suffered by members of the U.S. Army during the Plains Indian Wars have been the subject of much discussion. This chapter examines much more prosaic afflictions: otolaryngologic (ear, nose, and throat) diseases and related injuries. The data were extracted from the medical records of Seventh Cavalry members who served in the post–Civil War period. An inclusive anatomic approach was taken in selecting the conditions, which were categorized as eye, ear, nose, throat, dental, face and neck, and neurological disorders. Common conditions predominate, such as catarrh (upper respiratory infection), tonsillitis, headache, and traumatic injuries. By correlating the diseases with demographic, seasonal, and geographic information, we can see epidemiological patterns.

Seventh Cavalry Medical Records: The Famous and the Nameless

The material for this chapter was extracted from the medical records of Seventh Cavalry enlisted men, as discussed in chapter 4. Some individuals and events in which they participated are preserved as icons in our national consciousness. Even people from other parts of the world, who know little else of American history, have heard of George Armstrong Custer and the Battle of the Little Bighorn. For the most part this analysis concerns itself with different people and events. These other individuals, with rare exceptions, lived obscure lives. They are long forgotten, except that their names were dutifully recorded by army surgeons and military scribes. The diseases and injuries that affected them are likewise generally not remarkable or spectacular but are the same mundane afflictions that continue to bedevil all of us today.

Although five members of Custer's extended family were killed at Little Bighorn, none of their names appear in the Seventh Cavalry's medical records. But this does not mean that these people were never ill or treated. George Custer, for example, is known to have been treated for illness and injury at West Point during his cadet years, during the Civil War, and during his tenure in Texas before he joined the Seventh Cavalry (Custer 1893:89, 122–23; Welsh 2005). Those events are not recorded in the medical records but appear in other sources, including reminiscences. Perhaps the best-known individual included in the records is Captain Frederick Benteen, who led three companies into battle at the Little Bighorn and survived the hilltop fight along with Marcus Reno. As an officer, his numerous entries in the medical records are an exception, and this listing in itself has significance.

The U.S. Army was (and is) organized as a hierarchical, almost caste-like system (see chapter 1). In the post–Civil War era officers seldom deigned to speak to a private, except in the line of duty. Jenny Barnitz, wife of Captain Albert Barnitz, lamented the vast social gap between officers and men in a letter to her mother from Fort Riley in February 1867: "The officers assume a great deal here. The poor privates are perfect slaves. I do pity them from the bottom of my heart" (in Utley 1977:15). These divisions lessened when the troopers were exposed to extreme weather or the dangers of battle, but they rarely disappeared.

Different treatment by rank extends to the medical records. Demographic information included in the Enlistment Records is generally available only for the privates, noncommissioned officers, and special enlistments, such as farriers, saddlers, and musicians. Results from the Carded Medical Records also indicate that officers are under-represented when compared with enlisted men. This lack of documentation does not necessarily mean that officers were healthier than the enlisted men, although certain perks were available to those of higher rank. Most of the discrepancy in the record is probably explained by differing treatment for sick or injured enlisted men in comparison to officers. Enlisted men reported to "sick call" at seven A.M., and this information was noted by the physician (Utley 1977:158). Officers were able to avail themselves of medical attention in circumstances more of their own choosing Even Joseph Barnes (1870:xxv) noted that "it has been difficult to procure precise narratives of their cases."

This chapter deals with ear, nose, and throat diseases and injuries suffered by members of the Seventh Cavalry between 1866 and 1883 and documented on Medical Record Cards (fig. 6.1). In extracting relevant entries from the database, an anatomically based approach was taken, not only selecting classic ear, nose, and throat (ENT) diagnoses (such as tonsillitis and otorrhea) but expanding the criteria to include all clinical entities from the neck and above. This analysis encompasses dental conditions, eye diseases, headaches, and other anatomically related afflictions. The meaning of some of the diagnoses recorded by late-nineteenth-century physicians is ambiguous or obscure. This ambiguity includes frequently reported conditions, such as catarrh, and rare entities, such as ozena. Current meanings of various nineteenth-century medical terms are provided in the glossary at the end of this volume. SSPS (Green and Salkind 2010) was used for statistical analysis and graphic display of the results.

Diseases and Injuries

In all, 3,272 instances of disease or injury among 2,734 Seventh Cavalry troopers were identified as ENT-related clinical entities, amounting to 1.2 episodes per soldier. For the entire Seventh Cavalry database, 20,511 clinical encounters were recorded among 8,502 soldiers (2.4 episodes per soldier). The difference in the number of medical visits per individual is probably accounted for by the recurrent nature of some of the persistent diseases experienced by the troopers. Malaria, rheumatism, venereal diseases, and alcoholism frequently returned soldiers to the surgeons for the same ailment.

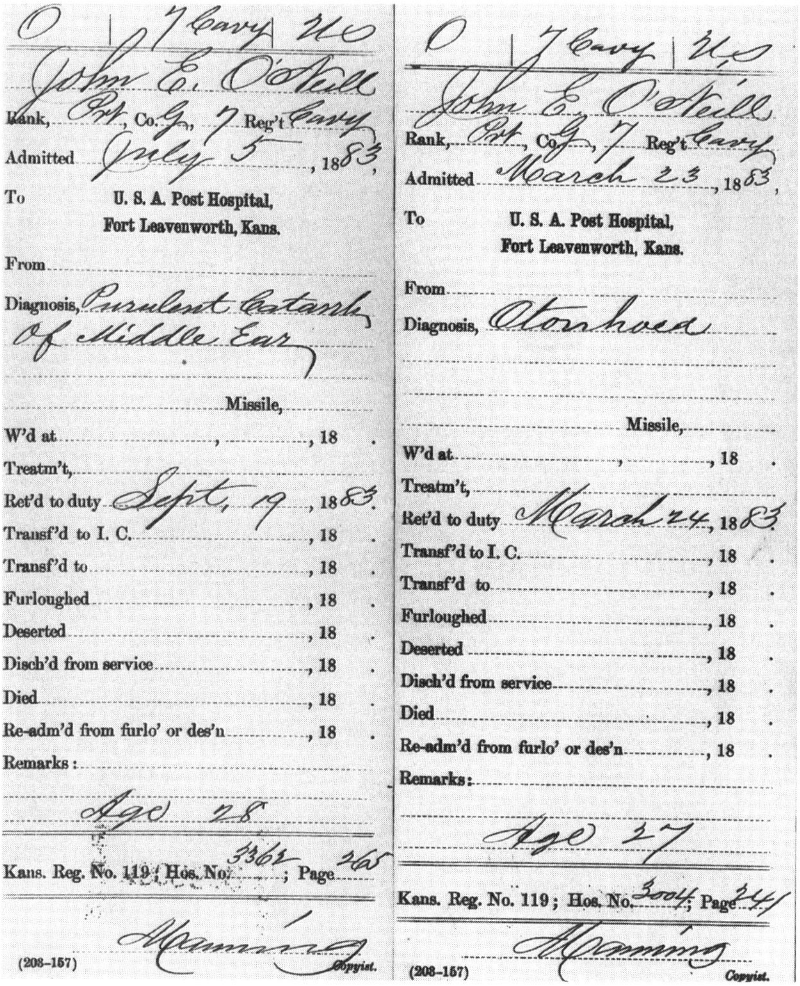

O | 7 Cavy | U.S.
John E. O'Neill
Rank, Pvt., Co. G, 7 Reg't Cavy
Admitted July 5, 1883,
To U. S. A. Post Hospital, Fort Leavenworth, Kans.
From
Diagnosis, Purulent Catarrh Of Middle Ear
Missile,
W'd at , , 18 .
Treatm't,
Ret'd to duty Sept, 19, 1883
Transf'd to I. C. , 18 .
Transf'd to , 18 .
Furloughed , 18 .
Deserted , 18 .
Disch'd from service , 18 .
Died , 18 .
Re-adm'd from furlo' or des'n , 18 .
Remarks:
Age 28
Kans. Reg. No. 119; Hos. No. 3362; Page 265
(208-157) Manning Copyist.

O | 7 Cavy | U.S.
John E. O'Neill
Rank, Pvt., Co. G, 7 Reg't Cavy
Admitted March 23, 1883,
To U. S. A. Post Hospital, Fort Leavenworth, Kans.
From
Diagnosis, Otorrhoea
Missile,
W'd at , , 18 .
Treatm't,
Ret'd to duty March 24, 1883
Transf'd to I. C. , 18 .
Transf'd to , 18 .
Furloughed , 18 .
Deserted , 18 .
Disch'd from service , 18 .
Died , 18 .
Re-adm'd from furlo' or des'n , 18 .
Remarks:
Age 27
Kans. Reg. No. 119; Hos. No. 3004; Page 241
(208-157) Manning Copyist.

6.1. Medical Record Cards showing two instances of ear infection for Private John O'Neill, Company G. Courtesy National Archives and Records Administration, public domain image.

The soldiers' mean age at diagnosis for individual ENT diseases differs little from the mean age for all entries, with a few exceptions. The mean age for tonsillitis was slightly younger (25 years, 1 month) and for carbuncle slightly older (29 years, 4 months) than the average of 26 years, 8 months. The ages of the 103 soldiers involved in "personal affrays" with comrades are also slightly higher than the group mean, at 28 years, 9 months. This observation appears to support the impression that the stresses experienced while serving in the Seventh Cavalry were cumulative with time.

Diseases and injuries suffered by members of the Seventh Cavalry discussed in this chapter are organized anatomically by eye, ear, nose, throat, oral and dental, neck and face, and neurological disorders.

EYE DISEASES AND INJURIES (N = 414)

Ophthalmic conditions suffered by Seventh Cavalry troopers are listed in table 6.1. By far the most common affliction, conjunctivitis, involved inflammation of the mucosal surface of the eyelids and globe. The mean age of soldiers diagnosed with conjunctivitis was 26. Conjunctivitis may be caused by infection, trauma, and allergy as well as by physical, chemical, and thermal irritants.

TABLE 6.1. Eye diseases and injuries of post–Civil War Seventh Cavalry

Disease	*Number of cases*	*Number of soldiers*
Abscess	1	1
Burn	2	2
Cataract	4	4
Conjunctivitis	305	250
Contusion	48	48
Fistula lachrymalis	1	1
Gunshot wound	1	1
Inflammation of eye	25	23
Laceration	9	9
Mydriasis	2	2
Night blindness	8	8
Ophthalmia	6	5
Ptosis	1	1
Presbyopia	1	1
Total		414

Army surgeons may have diagnosed any "red eye" as conjunctivitis, although they appear to have identified specific diseases, such as "iritis" (two cases of which were syphilitic), "ophthalmia" (one case of which was gonorrheal), and "inflammation of the Meibomian glands" (which was probably a stye—an infection of an oil-producing gland at the base of the eyelashes). Conjunctivitis tended to recur, averaging 1.2 episodes per affected soldier. Symptoms lasted 8 days on average (varying from 1 to 152 days). Of these cases, 4 were severe and persistent enough to merit disability discharge. The frequency of conjunctivitis did not vary by season, suggesting multiple etiologies.

Night blindness occurred in 8 cases and if unresolved would have prevented a soldier from serving on nocturnal duty. Classically a symptom of vitamin A deficiency, night blindness may be related to a variety of eye ailments, including myopia, cataracts, and retinitis pigmentosa.

Traumatic eye injuries included 48 contusions, of which 54% were inflicted in fights or brawls, and 9 lacerations, 44% received in a similar manner. Right and left eyes were affected about equally. Some of these injuries must have been severe: the mean duration of disability was 8.1 days, varying from 1 to 97 days for the contusions and as much as 280 days for one laceration. That wound was probably complicated by infection.

EAR DISEASES AND INJURIES ($N = 155$)

As table 6.2 shows, the most common diagnosis of ear disease was otorrhea. Robley Dunglison (1866:596) defines this ailment: "Discharge of purulent or puriform liquid, from the *meatus auditorius externus* . . . It is a symptom of chronic otitis." The data indicate that symptoms were sometimes chronic, lasting as long as 78 days, with a mean duration of 8.7 days. They were often recurrent, as in the case of John O'Neill, who had six episodes of otorrhea, one persisting 47 days. These troopers may have had chronic suppurative otitis media with perforation of their tympanic membrane, or even cholesteatoma, a cyst-like growth that destroys bone in the middle ear and mastoid.

The comment for one case reads "tympanum destroyed." This note probably describes a condition known as "necrotizing otitis

TABLE 6.2. Ear diseases and injuries of post–Civil War Seventh Cavalry

Disease	*Number of cases*	*Number of soldiers*
Abscess of external meatum	1	1
Cerumen impaction	2	2
Deafness	22	22
Dizziness (vertigo)	5	5
Earache	9	9
Frostbite	24	24
Gunshot wound	1	1
Inflammation of ear	4	4
Inflammation of external ear	2	2
Inflammation of middle ear	5	5
Inflammation of internal ear	15	15
Laceration	4	4
Otorrhea	61	51
Total	155	

media," which is now exceedingly rare. It is caused by a virulent form of *Streptococcus* common in the nineteenth and early twentieth centuries. Clinically, the entire eardrum and ossicles dissolve, leaving the patient with severe hearing loss and a chronically draining ear (Ballenger 1977:823).

Deafness was diagnosed in 22 individuals and was always a one-time event. In 7 cases (32%), the condition resulted in disability discharge. Hearing acuity, vision, and speech were screened by medical officers and had to be "perfect" to pass the enlistment physical examination (Rickey 1963:31). Causes of hearing loss are not listed but may have included acoustic trauma from noise exposure, ear infection, and syphilis. One of the dangerous pranks that troopers enjoyed playing on fresh recruits involved substituting 70 grain cartridges for the standard 55 grain gunpowder-charged cartridges fired with their Springfield carbines during target practice. The switch resulted in a startling and sometimes ear-damaging level of noise for the unsuspecting victim (Rickey 1963:211). A significant number of troopers affected by deafness and other forms of sensory deficit were discharged. This disability would have prevented them from performing their duty. Army surgeons probably held a pessimistic view of their prognosis as well as their own ability to treat the conditions.

Cerumen impaction is much less frequent than expected in these records (only 2 cases in 2 soldiers). In contemporary ENT practice, patients with ears occluded by hardened ear wax are seen daily, if not hourly.

NASAL DISEASES AND INJURIES (N = 1366)

The nasal diseases and injuries (table 6.3) include the most common ENT afflictions found in the Seventh Cavalry medical records, catarrh. The term is not currently in general use, but in the 1800s it described conditions characterized by a discharge of fluid from mucous membranes. The term could be applied to almost any organ but generally meant the upper respiratory tract. It was characterized by "cough, thirst, lassitude, fever, watery eyes, with increased secretion of mucous from the upper air passages . . . It is commonly an affection of little consequence, but apt to relapse and become chronic" (Dunglison 1866:186). Variants were recognized by army doctors, who documented "pulmonary catarrh" for

TABLE 6.3. Nasal diseases and injuries of post–Civil War Seventh Cavalry

Diagnosis	*Number of cases*	*Number of soldiers*
Catarrh	1331	1010
Contusion	6	6
Epistaxis	5	5
Fracture	5	5
Frostbite	9	8
Incised wound	2	2
Laceration	4	4
Ozena	3	3
Ulcer of mucous membrane	1	1
Total	1366	

bronchitis and "epidemic catarrh" for influenza. The majority of these cases were viral upper respiratory infections, although nasal allergy could produce a similar clinical picture.

The mean age for contracting catarrh was 27 years 4 months. As expected, duration of symptoms was brief. The mean duration was 4.95 days, but the distribution was skewed to the right (median = 2, mode = 2). The duration distribution (1 to 426 days) shows that some cases persisted (fig. 6.2). The explanation for this temporal pattern is found in the natural history of viral upper respiratory infections. They tend to be self-limited and brief; but bacterial complications, such as sinusitis or bronchitis, may supervene, extending the period of illness. The symptoms (rhinorrhea, nasal congestion, and cough) would have been similar to the inciting viral episode and generally indistinguishable to army doctors lacking radiographic or endoscopic technology.

The seasonal pattern of prevalence for catarrh is striking and indicates that the disease is associated with cold weather (fig. 6.3).

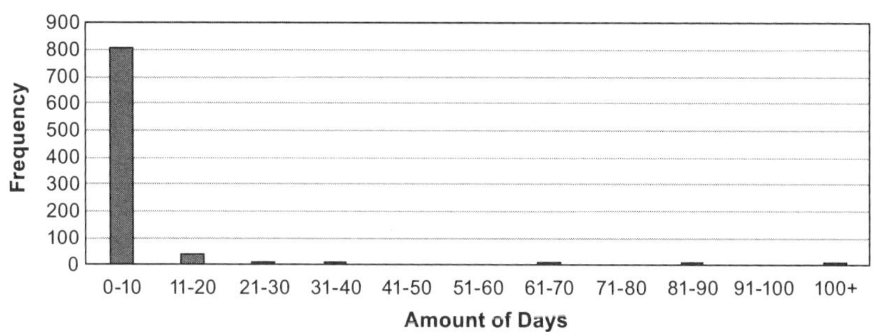

6.2. Duration in days of catarrh in post–Civil War Seventh Cavalry.

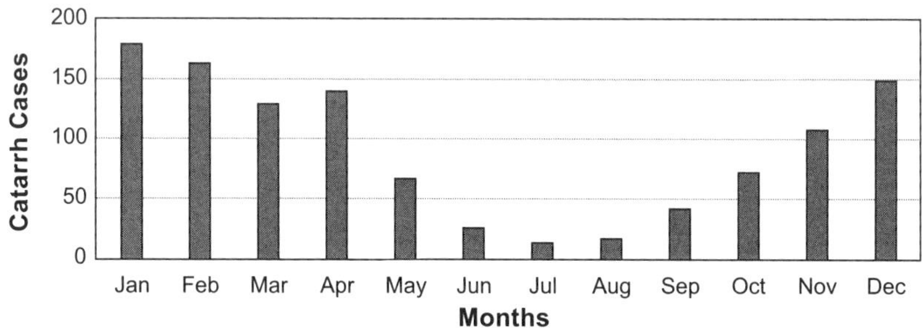

6.3. Monthly distribution of catarrh in the post–Civil War Seventh Cavalry.

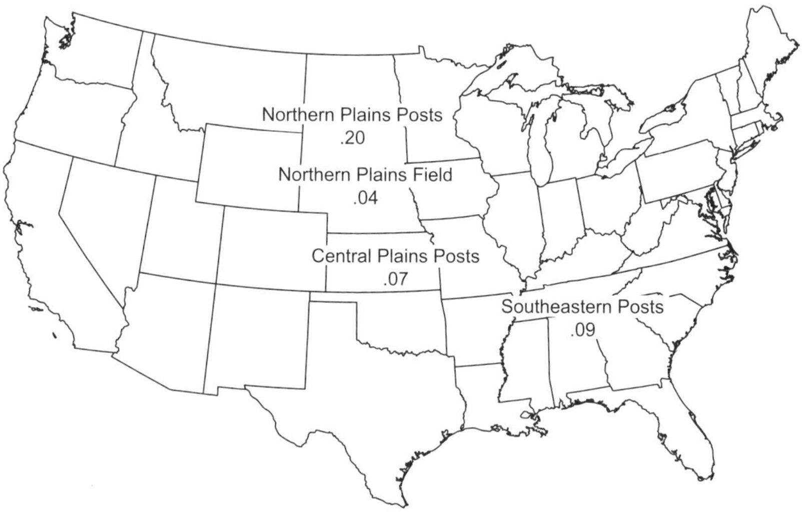

Map 6.1. Catarrh incidence by region and assignment for the post–Civil War Seventh Cavalry. Numbers are cases per soldier. Copyright © 2015, University of Oklahoma Press.

A closer look at the incidence by location (cases/soldier at northern and central plains forts, southeastern locations, and northern plains field expeditions) indicates that crowding associated with winter weather was likely the environmental factor causing seasonal variations in the disease (map 6.1).

Other nasal conditions were much less frequent. Epistaxis (nosebleed) severe enough to require medical attention is recorded five times, and one episode was fatal. Spontaneous bleeding from the larger arteries in the back of the nose (posterior epistaxis) can be profuse enough to cause death from exsanguination or asphyxia. Medical texts from the time indicate that trained physicians understood the anatomy involved and had the tools to deal with such emergencies (Smith 1863).

Ozena is a rare condition involving the mucous membranes lining the nose. The lining may become thin and lose its self-cleansing ciliary function, resulting in the accretion of foul-smelling crusts, bone erosion, and nasal obstruction. Syphilis can cause a similar clinical syndrome, eventually leading to a "saddle-nose" deformity. Dunglison's (1866:700) colorful description notes "a disagreeable odor similar to that of a crushed bed bug."

Nasal trauma (including fractures, contusions, and cuts) was frequently related to interpersonal violence, which was the cause of the injury in 47% of cases. Several nasal fractures were incurred while playing baseball. By the 1860s the sport was already referred to as the "national pastime" and was one of the favorite recreational activities of troopers, along with footraces and boxing (Utley 1977:163, 192).

Frostbite of the nose occurred less often than frostbite of the ear (9 cases versus 24) and was of shorter duration (mean of 4 days versus 15 days). Both organs have a good blood supply, but the nose is warmed by expired air. Frostbite of the extremities, especially the feet, often resulted in gangrene, requiring amputation (see chapter 10).

THROAT DISEASES (*N* = 650)

Pharyngeal and laryngeal conditions are listed in table 6.4. All four entities probably represent viral or bacterial infections. The mean age of the troopers affected by these diseases is slightly below the mean for the entire population at just over 25 years.

Laryngitis was diagnosed 19 times in 18 soldiers, and symptoms lasted for 1 to 29 days (mean duration 6 days). The main symptom was hoarseness, sometimes to the point of aphonia. Likely causes include viral infections and voice overuse.

Pharyngitis, probably characterized by a nonspecific sore throat, occurred 46 times in 45 soldiers. The mean duration of symptoms was 4.73 days, varying from 1 to 24 days. Most of these episodes were probably caused by viruses.

TABLE 6.4. Throat diseases of post–Civil War Seventh Cavalry

Diagnosis	*Number of cases*	*Number of soldiers*
Diphtheria	1	1
Laryngitis	19	18
Pharyngitis (sore throat)	46	45
Tonsillitis	584	483
Total	650	

Tonsillitis was diagnosed 584 times in 483 soldiers, with an average of 1.2 episodes per soldier: 7% of all troopers in the database had tonsillitis. Symptoms lasted 5 days on average, varying from 1 to 78 days. Of these cases, 6 were identified as "quinsy," which is a peritonsillar abscess, resulting from a collection of pus deep to the tonsil that generally requires incision and drainage. One entry reads "[t]onsillitis and tumor left side." The note probably indicates a deep neck abscess, spreading from an infected tonsil and requiring external drainage. One individual died from his acute infection, which began as tonsillitis and progressed to erysipelas, a diffuse soft tissue infection.

Tonsillitis is generally caused by *Streptococcus pyogenes*, although other bacterial and viral agents may produce similar clinical pictures. The signs and symptoms are distinctive enough that nineteenth-century physicians had little difficulty distinguishing tonsillitis from similar disorders and in fact were more precise in their descriptions of diseased tonsils than ENT specialists are now.

Humans are the natural reservoir of *S. pyogenes*, with the nasopharynx and skin being the principal sites of carriage. Transmission is mainly by the respiratory route, facilitated by close personal contact (Hoeprich 1977:240). Like catarrh, the spread of streptococcal infections among members of the Seventh Cavalry was exacerbated by living conditions in posts and in the field. Close physical proximity increased disease transmission, especially for respiratory pathogens. In what was known as the "bunky system," recruits paired in cramped sleeping quarters, where "two men commonly pooled their blankets and slept together for warmth," especially when patrolling the northern plains in winter (Rickey 1963:56). It is important to understand that adequate personal hygiene was often impossible. Soldiers could not even remove their clothing for extended periods in the intense cold. Cavalryman John Larson wrote: "I kept my rubber shoes on my feet for two months and my socks kept my shoes company. If I pulled them off they would have frozen stiff" (in Rickey 1963:255).

The duration and recurrence rates for tonsillitis are worth noting. The mean length of illness is 4.94 days, but the curve is markedly skewed to the right, indicating that a few soldiers were disabled for extended periods. This length of illness conforms closely to historical data. For example, a group of British airmen experienced

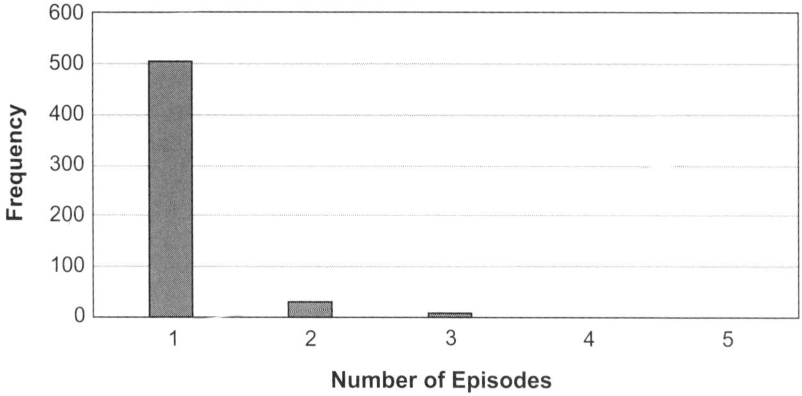

6.4. Number of recurring tonsillitis episodes per year by trooper in the post–Civil War Seventh Cavalry.

epidemic streptococcal pharyngitis at a large Royal Air Force Station in Cyprus in 1957. All were males aged 19 to 30 years and had culture-positive strep infection. They were treated with aspirin (35 cases), sulpha (35 cases), and penicillin (38 cases). The 3 groups experienced no difference in duration of sore throat or fever. Symptoms lasted the same length of time (3 to 6 days) for the soldiers in this study (McDonald 1958:538).

As seen in figure 6.4, the recurrence rate for tonsillitis was low in the Seventh Cavalry. The mean number of episodes per year for those who had tonsillitis was 1.1, and none had more than 4 episodes per year. Thus indications for tonsillectomy for recurrent infection, at least based on today's strict criteria (5 episodes per year), were not met for any soldiers. Complication rates (peritonsillar abscess and deep neck infection) were also low, although one death was recorded, probably from sepsis related to erysipelas. This recurrence rate appears low compared to contemporary populations of young adults undergoing tonsillectomy. Not treating every episode of tonsillitis with antibiotics, contrary to what is done today, may have had the salutary effect of minimizing recurrent episodes by allowing immunity to develop.

Streptococcal tonsillitis did not just give the troopers sore throats, however. Acute and chronic rheumatism was diagnosed 1,056 times in these records. Rheumatic fever, a complication of streptococcal infection, is considered a major cause of severe musculoskeletal pain among Civil War soldiers. The other common cause of rheumatic fever was reactive arthritis following dysentery (Bollet 1991:1197). The Indian Wars and Reconstruction era soldiers of the Seventh Cavalry appear to have suffered the same afflictions. A smaller number of cases of valvular heart disease were also diagnosed by army surgeons in the aftermath of tonsillitis and acute rheumatic complaints. These included 35 cases of "valvular heart disease" and 17 of "hypertrophy." Heart disease was linked to rheumatism as early as 1812, and military surgeons of the mid- to late 1800s were aware of the association, although not the connection to streptococcal tonsillitis (English 1989:34).

Some have argued that rheumatic fever originated in the late 1700s from biological changes in the streptococcal organism and its host, leading to serious cardiac injury and milder musculoskeletal complaints. Thus the catchphrase "strep licks the joints and bites the heart." Clinicians became aware of this association through refinements in observation and technological advances, including the study of large patient cohorts in urban hospitals, frequent use of the autopsy to confirm antemortem physical findings, and general acceptance of the stethoscope. In some nineteenth-century hospitals valvular heart disease ranked second, after tuberculosis, as the leading cause of death (English 1989:43).

ORAL AND DENTAL DISEASES AND INJURIES ($N = 74$)

Table 6.5 lists the conditions that involve the mouth, jaws, and teeth. Soldiers sought care for toothaches 38 times, developed 4 dental abscesses, and underwent 2 tooth extractions. There appears to be a discrepancy between the number of dental problems recorded in the database and the poor oral health evident in the available skeletal material. Scott et al. (1998:297) found evidence of dental disease in the form of numerous caries, abscesses, periodontal disease, antemortem tooth loss, and malocclusion among the casualties at Little Bighorn.

Some of these discrepancies may be explained by the army's lack of a division of dentistry until the 1890s, resulting in an absence of qualified dental care. These duties often fell to the hospital stewards, because physicians were either untrained or uninterested in providing this service (Coffman 1986:383). The United States

TABLE 6.5. Oral and dental diseases and injuries of post–Civil War Seventh Cavalry

Diagnosis	*Number of cases*	*Number of soldiers*
Dental abscess	4	4
Dental caries	1	1
Contusion of jaw, lip, or mouth	8	7
Gunshot wound of maxilla	1	1
Incised wound of lip or mouth	3	3
Jaw fracture	6	5
Lacerated lip	4	4
Parched lips	1	1
Salivary duct fistula	1	1
Sore lips	1	1
Stomatitis	4	4
Toothache (odontalgia)	38	38
Tooth extraction	2	2
Total	74	

Dental Corps was established during the Spanish-American War, too late for these Seventh Cavalry troopers (White 1995:xxxv).

FACE AND NECK DISEASES AND INJURIES (N = 212)

This diverse set of conditions is displayed in table 6.6. They include various forms of trauma, infection, and thermal injury.

A carbuncle is a localized infection characterized by subcutaneous abscess formation and purulent discharge from multiple sinus tracts. It often originates from an infected sebaceous cyst and is included in this review because it is usually located on the back of the neck. The mean age of the soldiers with this diagnosis was 29 years, 4 months, older than most Seventh Cavalry soldiers.

A large number of other localized skin infections (acne, furuncles boils, and carbuncles: 1,174 cases) were also found in these medical records. Most of these conditions are caused by *Streptococcus* or *Staphylococcus* organisms. Poor personal hygiene, often unavoidable

TABLE 6.6. Face and neck diseases and injuries of post–Civil War Seventh Cavalry

Diagnosis	*Number of cases*	*Number of soldiers*
Acne	2	2
Burns and scalds of face or neck	13	13
Carbuncle	13	9
Contusions of face, cheek or neck	68	68
Erysipelas	49	49
Fracture of clavicle	1	1
Gunshot wound to face or neck	8	8
Incised wound of cheek, face or neck	8	8
Laceration of cheek or face	14	14
Mumps	21	21
Neck, stiff, wry or sprain	3	3
Pityriasis	1	1
Rhus poisoning of face, hands or penis	1	1
Roseola	1	1
Scrofula	4	4
Sialoadenitis (parotitis)	2	2
Swollen face	1	1
Thyroid enlargement	1	1
Tumor on forehead	1	1
Total	212	

due to the soldiers' circumstances, contributed to the problem. The recruits' *Customs of Service* contains a section called "Take Care of Your Health," which advises frequent bathing: "Take a plunge in a lake or stream if possible daily and wear clean sox [*sic*] and underwear" (Kautz 2001:253). This ideal was difficult to achieve, as Rickey (1963:43) notes: "Transforming some of the raw recruit material into soldiers necessitated training in personal cleanliness, because many of the new men were not accustomed to weekly bathing."

Erysipelas is a diffuse soft tissue infection of the skin and subcutaneous tissue, generally caused by *Streptococcus*. It is included here because it often arises spontaneously on the face. It can also develop in any area of trauma, however, such as an extremity struck by a projectile. In this setting it can lead to generalized sepsis or gangrene, often with a fatal outcome.

NEUROLOGICAL DISEASES AND INJURIES (N = 401)

The conditions in this last group of ailments involve the central or peripheral nervous system, including injuries to the head and skull (table 6.7). Traumatic injuries to this area were often fatal, particularly penetrating wounds. Of the 11 gunshot wounds to the head, 8 of the patients died. Of the 4 skull fractures, 2 patients died and 1 developed epilepsy.

The records identified 4 cases of peripheral neuropathy involving a single cranial nerve. The first consisted of paralysis of the left side of the face (Bell's Palsy), the second was paralysis and partial aphonia (probably recurrent laryngeal nerve paralysis), and the last 2 involved facial neuralgia (possibly tic doloreaux or trigeminal neuralgia). The first two conditions are thought to be caused

TABLE 6.7. Neurological diseases and injuries of post–Civil War Seventh Cavalry

Diagnosis	*Number of cases*	*Number of soldiers*
Aphonia	4	2
Concussion of brain	6	6
Contusion of head or scalp	27	26
Fracture of skull	4	4
Gunshot wound to head	11	11
Headache	305	270
Incised wound of scalp or forehead	13	13
Lacerated head, forehead, or scalp	26	26
Neuralgia of face	2	2
Paralysis of left face	1	1
Paralysis with partial aphonia	1	1
Total	401	

by viruses, and the third is idiopathic (of uncertain origin). The records showed 4 recurrent cases of aphonia in 2 soldiers. These were likely psychogenic in origin, perhaps a form of conversion disorder.

By far the most common diagnosis in this category was headache, with 305 episodes affecting 270 soldiers. Their mean age is 26 years 6 months, the same as for the entire group. Mean duration of symptoms was 3.8 days, although most cases lasted only 1 or 2 days. For a handful of soldiers headaches were a recurring problem, although the majority suffered only one episode. Today the most common headaches are migraine and tension headaches, with other causes being much less common. The duration and frequency of the disabling headaches suffered by Seventh Cavalry troopers were consistent with migraines in most instances. The men were exposed to two of the most frequently cited risk factors for migraine headache: stress and caffeine. They could hardly have avoided developing an addiction to caffeine, because coffee was often the only form of liquid available: "Strong black coffee was served with every meal" (Rickey 1963:39). Even the *Customs of Service* recommends coffee or tea, rather than water, after strenuous exertion as "an admirable sustainer of strength" (Kautz 2001:250). Given the ubiquity of binge drinking among the troops, many headaches lasting a day or less could have been hangovers.

Discussion

This study has limitations. The information comes from a database derived from various primary sources, generally brief reports handwritten by medical and enlistment personnel over a twenty-year period. Some of the entries are ambiguous, incomplete, or duplicated. Because this chapter focuses on conditions affecting a specific anatomic region (the head and neck) and only includes individuals whose complaints were recorded, it represents a subset of a sample of the entire Seventh Cavalry. Nevertheless, an objective portrayal of the illnesses and injuries suffered by these troopers can be derived from the large number of entries and the concise, uniform style of military record keeping.

It is apparent from examining these medical records that not every episode of illness or injury was documented. For instance, the Seventh Cavalry endured a one-month sojourn in Yankton, Dakota Territory, in the spring of 1873. A severe blizzard ravaged the encampment for forty hours, but there were no reports of frostbite between April 9 and May 12, 1873. Later that month half a dozen troopers were reported to have died and been buried by local townspeople in a Bon Homme County cemetery (Kinsley 2007:40–41), but the medical records remained silent about this incident. No entries are recorded for either event.

Barnes (1870:192) offers an explanation for gaps in post–Civil War medical records: "The regimental officers of the cavalry had particular difficulty in making prompt and accurate returns. When they were . . . dispersed in small detachments, casualties took place of which the regimental surgeon was not cognizant; when they were engaged in expeditions . . . the marches were so rapid that there was little time for clerical work."

Considering how onerous medical documentation can be even under favorable circumstances, this explanation has the ring of truth.

Despite these shortcomings, the data contained in these medical records provide a wealth of information and insight into the diseases affecting the cavalrymen who fought in the Indian Wars and served in the Reconstruction South.

This material is particularly useful for supplementing, confirming, or refuting information obtained from other sources, such as personal accounts, official reports, or skeletal material. For example, John A. Wright is listed as suffering from an accidental gunshot wound to the neck at Fort Hays on July 17, 1869, dying that same day. This documentation in itself is not particularly informative, but an expanded account is available (Otis 1871:21). There the operating surgeon describes Wright's wound in detail. The pistol ball destroyed the upper tracheal rings, thyroid cartilage, and hyoid bone, likely a fatal injury even now. Desperate attempts were made to control bleeding, and Wright's obstructed airway was opened by inserting a "Silver Tube." That device is a metal tracheostomy tube that was available to surgeons during the mid-1800s and nearly identical to the tracheostomy tubes that are currently available.

In another example, on March 16, 1882, four individuals suffered burns to their hands and faces at Fort Leavenworth. Frank Fisher is listed as a blacksmith and Charles Blake as a wagoner. The injuries could not have been severe, because the men all recovered and continued to serve. None received a disability discharge related to this incident. It takes little imagination to reconstruct what took place. The blacksmith and wagoner were probably repairing an iron wagon part at the forge and conscripted the help of two others. All four were injured when they lost control of this heavy piece of equipment.

These examples are particularistic and anecdotal, but the large volume of material in this database can be used to test the validity of individual characterizations of military life and health in the Seventh Cavalry. Elizabeth Custer, for example, gives this rosy assessment of the troopers' well-being at Fort Lincoln in 1875: "I'm sure we could not have been so contented as we were under the circumstances had there not been such perfect health among us all. It was a pleasure to live among so many hundred people and scarcely see anyone who was not perfectly well. Another relief in that life was that we never saw crippled or maimed people, and there were no suffering poor" (Custer 2006:165). The sanguine perspective of this high-ranking officer's wife was contradicted by the medical record. During 1875 there were 434 entries for Fort Lincoln, more than one per Seventh Cavalry soldier stationed there that year. Diagnoses included numerous episodes of upper respiratory infection, dysentery, venereal disease, malaria, alcoholism, and interpersonal violence. They appeared in the same proportions as recorded at other northern plains posts. This is not to say that Elizabeth Custer's memoir, published ten years later, did not reflect the reality that she experienced. As George Armstrong Custer's wife, she presented the perspective of the elite at Fort Lincoln and spent the rest of her life defending and burnishing his reputation.

Several otolaryngologic diseases are noteworthy. Streptococcal infections, such as tonsillitis, erysipelas, and necrotizing otitis media, were common and could have had serious consequences. The infections themselves were sometimes aggressive: rheumatic joint inflammation was disabling and cardiac disease left lasting injury. The antibiotics we have today undoubtedly would have prevented some of these complications, but it appears that they would have had little effect on the duration of infection. In fact they might have increased the recurrence rate.

Several epidemiological features of catarrh or viral upper respiratory infection are evident in these data. Its benign, self-limited nature is apparent, as is a distinct seasonal spike, weaker geographic variation, and increased transmissibility in crowded conditions.

In addition, dental disease was surely more prevalent than these records indicated. The discrepancy between the number of entries and the pathological evidence of tooth decay related to the fact that the Army Dental Corps was not established until after Wounded Knee. Army surgeons lacked training and experience to provide dental care, except perhaps simple extractions. Perceptive troopers would have avoided seeking treatment from incapable or unwilling providers.

One observer described the Seventh Cavalry as "good fighters but mostly heavy drinkers" (Rickey 1963:55). This claim is borne out not only by the frequency of alcohol-related admissions but also by the nature of traumatic injuries. In this sample of head and neck trauma 8.5% of injuries were inflicted in combat and 36.4% in interpersonal violence. In 55% of the cases these injuries were classified as accidental or the cause was not recorded. Because the surgeons seem to have taken note of the circumstances when misbehavior (fighting or drinking) was involved, a canny trooper might report his injury as accidental or simply not volunteer a cause, knowing that such an admission would reflect badly on him and remain in his record. For these reasons the proportion of facial trauma caused by interpersonal violence was probably greater than recorded.

Finally, it is difficult to say anything definitive about the quality of care provided to the Seventh Cavalry soldiers based on these records. Little information is included about treatment or outcomes. Nevertheless, the duration of illness and frequency of complications compare favorably to what would be expected today, with the advantages of modern technology and a systematically reformed medical education system that was unavailable in the late 1800s. At the very least we can say that army surgeons adhered to the Hippocratic principle "Do no harm."

CHAPTER 7

Pulmonary Diseases of the Seventh Cavalry

Patrick J. Collison

This chapter deals with additional diseases affecting a single organ system: the lungs. In the nineteenth century most respiratory diseases were thought to be caused by weather conditions and exposure. In fact our data in part support that contention. They show seasonal incidence of some illnesses (acute bronchitis, influenza, and pneumonia), although others (tuberculosis and asthma) lacked seasonal patterns. We now recognize that these diseases are caused by viral or bacterial infections of various sorts. Although insightful nineteenth-century physicians began to understand that such ailments were related to microscopic organisms that could be passed from person to person, evidence of these entities and proof of their agency came in the 1880s, when the Indian Wars were waning. As an example, the tubercle bacillus was identified by Robert Koch in 1882 and other infectious microorganisms were recognized shortly before and soon after that date. Nonetheless diagnostic practices changed little and treatments hardly at all (Caldwell 1988:159). At the time of its first acceptance, the germ theory advanced neither the hygienic nor the therapeutic controls of infectious diseases (Dubos and Dubos 1996:xxx).

Lacking the advantages of discoveries in microbiology, radiology, and pharmacology, military physicians depended on clinical experience and their powers of observation to diagnose and treat patients. For pulmonary diseases in particular, several important discoveries during the preceding fifty years had advanced their ability to evaluate illness in a cogent, reproducible manner. In nearly all instances progress in the understanding of disease depended on an integration of clinical and autopsy findings. Before these advances in physical examination were promulgated and accepted, physicians depended on a simple assessment of pulse, temperature, and general constitution to determine the underlying causes of their patients' distress.

Two physical examination techniques, percussion and mediate auscultation, were discovered and perfected in the early 1800s, providing a simple yet elegant method of diagnosing chest pathology among living patients. Leopold Arrenbrugger described percussion in *Inventum novum* in 1761. Influenced by his mother's interest in music and observing his father tapping on wine and beer casks to determine the volume of liquid remaining, the Austrian physician learned to interpret tones produced by striking the chest with his fingertips. He described the different sounds heard over the lung cavities in various physiological states: normal, fluid-filled, empty, and so forth. For instance, the shifting fluid levels of a pleural effusion or empyema could be demonstrated by systematically tapping the chest while the patient changed position from recumbent to upright. Arrenbrugger's findings were ignored at the time but revived and finally popularized by the French physician Jean Nicolas Corvisard fifty years later. He was an inveterate researcher who documented the validity of his observations by correlating his clinical notes with findings from over 900 autopsies (Dubos and Dubos 1996:77–78).

The technique of mediate auscultation (listening to breath sounds indirectly) was described by René Laennec in 1818. Direct auscultation, simply placing an ear against the patient's chest, had been employed for millennia. Hippocrates (460–375 BC) described various sounds that signal lung disease: the pleural rub was "a noise like that of rubbing against a leather strap," and the death rattle was "a slight noise like the boiling of vinegar." The method was known but little practiced, because Laennec and others found it impractical in obese individuals. Others objected "for reasons of decorum" to using the technique on large-breasted women. Laennec improvised his first indirect auscultation instrument by rolling up a calling card. He was so pleased with the results that he immediately fashioned the first stethoscope for mediate auscultation of the lungs, a 25 by 2.5 cm tubular wooden device in three detachable parts. The binaural stethoscope, similar to the one used today, was invented in 1851 by Arthur Leared (Dubos and Dubos 1996:80–93).

Armed with his new instrument as well as insatiable curiosity and energy and backing up his findings with clinical and autopsy data, Laennec wrote precise descriptions of the heart and lung sounds produced in various disease states. His systematic observations generated a series of arcane auditory terms that remain indispensable to the clinician's lexicon today.

Some of the "adventitious" breath sounds that may be noted during a physical examination follow. Rales consist of fine high-pitched breath sounds from fluid in small air passages, described as a moist crackling noise like hairs being rubbed together. Ronchi resemble a coarse rattling sound generated by secretions in the bronchi and larger air passages. Wheezes are continuous high-pitched sounds heard during inspiration and/or expiration, depending on the location of airway narrowing. Pectoriloquy, also called whispered pectoriloquy or bronchophony, is an increased loudness of vocalization heard by auscultation over areas of the lung field that display abnormal resonance due to edema or consolidation. Tactile fremitus is a vibration felt on the patient's chest during low-frequency vocalization, perceptible because sound waves are transmitted more efficiently in a fluid or solid medium than in normal, air-containing lung tissue.

As is often the case in the archly conservative world of medicine, Laennec's findings were dismissed and even ridiculed. In time, however, these ideas changed the diagnosis of tuberculosis, pneumonia, emphysema, and other chest diseases to a process based on objective, reproducible physical findings rather than tradition-bound conjecture. Ironically, both Corvisard and Laennec, pioneers of discovery in pulmonary medicine, died of tuberculosis (Duffin 1993:938–42).

By the time the Seventh Cavalry was organized at Fort Riley in 1866, this simple instrumentation and examination technique had become de rigueur for the medical officers and contract physicians who were responsible for providing health care to the troopers. In addition, diagnostic and therapeutic instruments as well as medical and surgical textbooks were available. They were found in the equipment trunks and supply cases that army surgeons carried. Dr. Henry Porter had a supply case with him at the Little Bighorn, which is on display at the State Historical Society of North Dakota in Bismarck (Walker 2008:187). We can be certain that many diagnostic tools and treatment modalities were unavailable to these doctors: for example, X-ray, the tuberculin skin test, and the microscopic and microbiological identification of offending organisms. These advances appeared during the decades at the end of the Indian Wars, and antimicrobial therapy came much later. But some basic surgical procedures, such as tracheostomy and the drainage of pleural fluid, could be performed by surgeons caring for the Seventh Cavalry troopers.

Materials and Methods

The data for this study were obtained from medical and enlistment records of the U.S. Seventh Cavalry from 1866 to 1883. A detailed description of the original databases is included in chapters 4 and 5.

The meanings of the various diagnoses in the context of nineteenth-century medical lexicography are presented in the glossary. In addition, Dunglison's *A Dictionary of Medical Science* (1866) was helpful in understanding the meaning of terms such as pulmonary catarrh, epidemic catarrh, and influenza as well as the difference between terms such as consumption and phthisis. It also is helpful in explaining the difference between nineteenth-century and current medical terminology.

Some of the diagnostic categories are synonymous and are combined for more meaningful analysis. These synonyms include pneumonia and inflammation of the lungs; tuberculosis, consumption, and phthisis; and epidemic catarrh, pulmonary catarrh, and influenza. Based on the duration of illness and outcome, the various conditions can be separated into fairly distinct clinical entities. Acute bronchitis, influenza, and pleuritis were brief illnesses with low morbidity, whereas pneumonia and tuberculosis were more serious and protracted ailments. Asthma and chronic bronchitis were intermediate in severity.

TABLE 7.1. Pulmonary diseases of post–Civil War Seventh Cavalry (by number of cases and duration of illness)

Diagnosis	*Number of cases*	*Number of soldiers*	*Mean duration (days)*
Asthma	13	10	12.5
Bronchitis, acute	714	595	6.5
Bronchitis, chronic	36	32	15
Cough	35	33	6.1
Emphysema	2	2	29
Hemoptysis	8	7	17.4
Hydrothorax	1	1	?
Influenza	68	65	5
Pleuritis	148	147	8.3
Pneumonia	102	100	24
Tuberculosis	63	56	29

Results

Table 7.1 presents the pulmonary diseases found in the Seventh Cavalry records, including number of cases, number of soldiers, and mean duration of illness. Seventh Cavalry lower respiratory diseases totaled nearly 1,200 cases in 1,048 soldiers, about 1.1 episode per individual. Of the 8,500 men listed in these records, 14% experienced pulmonary disease. Although only one organ system was involved, this group of illnesses constituted a diverse assortment in terms of etiology, treatment, and prognosis. They ranged from the benign and self-limited (acute bronchitis and influenza) to life threatening and incurable (consumption). Overall, 22 deaths were attributed to pulmonary diseases (1.8 percent of lower respiratory cases), but many more of the troopers received disability discharges (6%). When upper and lower respiratory diseases were combined, they constituted the third most frequent cause of illness, after diarrheal diseases and intermittent fevers (malaria).

DEMOGRAPHY

The mean age of troopers affected by respiratory ailments was 25 years, similar to the mean age for the ear, nose, and throat diseases (26 years 8 months). Regarding nationality of respiratory patients, 61.1% were born in the United States, and 39% were foreign born. Of these foreign-born troopers, 46% came from the British Isles, mainly Ireland, and 36% from Germany. Most of the native-born soldiers were from the more populous states of the Northeast and Upper Midwest. Only 7% came from states that had joined the Confederacy. This pattern was similar to the pattern of the Seventh Cavalry as a whole (fig. 7.1).

At the time of enlistment, many troopers suffering pulmonary diseases were unemployed, although the majority had been engaged in some form of manual labor. Occupations listed included unskilled laborers (61.2%), skilled manual laborers (18.2%), service workers (8%), craftsmen and artisans (7.4%), artists and performers (3.2%), professionals (1.3%), and businessmen (0.6%). It

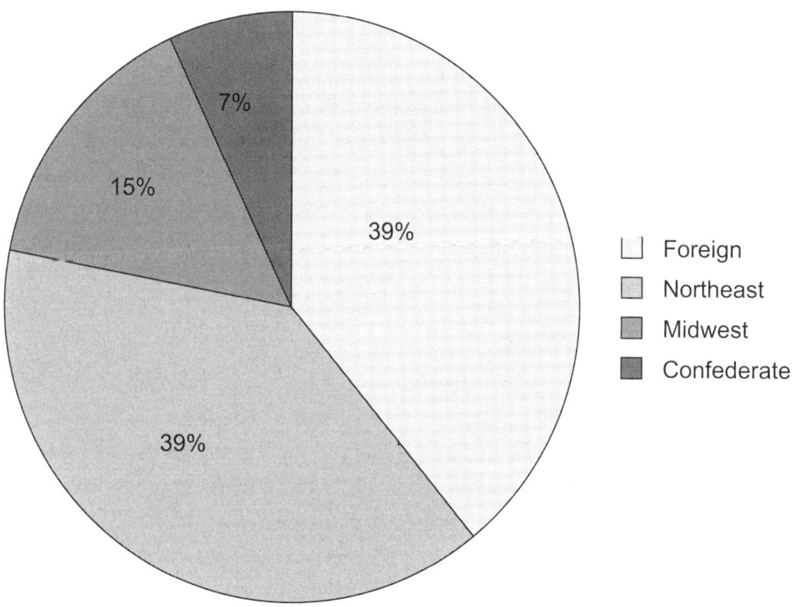

7.1. Nativity of post–Civil War Seventh Cavalry members suffering pulmonary diseases.

is interesting that even musicians and health care professionals enlisted more frequently than businessmen, which was also true of the Seventh Cavalry as a whole.

DISEASES AND TREATMENTS

Asthma

Nineteenth-century physicians were well aware of the signs and symptoms of asthma and attempted to treat it with antispasmodics, such as belladonna (Flannery 2004:119). Anesthetics, narcotics, and counterirritants were also used. If the patient had the means, a "change of air" was recommended. But overall asthma was considered a chronic, probably incurable disease (Dunglison 1866:107).

The records show that 10 soldiers were diagnosed with asthma on thirteen occasions. Their mean age was 29.4 years, significantly older than the average age for all pulmonary diseases. The mean duration of illness was 12.5 days, and one soldier was given a disability discharge based on this diagnosis. The number of cases seems low compared to the 5 to 10% prevalence found today. It is likely that some asthmatics were barred from enlistment and therefore did not appear in military medical records.

Many present-day authorities believe that incidence of asthma has increased since the 1800s, perhaps from higher levels of air pollution. Others speculate that excessive "cleanliness" and reduced exposure to microorganisms from domestic animals related to modernity have caused our immune systems to turn on our own tissues, resulting in an increase in allergies, asthma, and similar conditions.

Bronchitis

Bronchitis is defined as inflammation of the bronchial tubes or large air passages. Nineteenth-century military surgeons recognized cough, mucous production, and dyspnea as the symptoms of bronchitis. They distinguished this relatively mild condition from more serious ones by specific findings on physical examination, including ronchi (large airway sounds) in the absence of rales and other signs found in pneumonia. Chronic bronchitis could be confused with and later identified as tuberculosis but was distinguished by the lack of "hectic" or spiking fever. Treatment of acute bronchitis included antiphlogistics (anti-inflammatory medications), revulsives (counterirritants), and bleeding (Dunglison 1866:150). Specific measures such as cupping, stimulants, expectorants, and potassium iodide were used as well. Chronic bronchitis was treated with syrup of squills, an expectorant obtained from the sea onion (Flannery 2004:123, 132).

Acute bronchitis was diagnosed 714 times in 595 soldiers and described as chronic in 32 troopers. The illness tended to recur, with multiple episodes (2 to 6) in 83 troopers. The duration of confinement averaged 6.5 days (ranging from 1 to 86 days). Although the course was generally benign, significant morbidity and even mortality occurred. Disability discharges were awarded to 17 troopers with bronchitis and 4 others died. In addition, the eventual outcome was recognized as tuberculosis in six cases.

There was a seasonal pattern to the appearance of acute bronchitis among the troops. Nine times as many cases occurred during the winter months as during the summer, regardless of geographic location (fig. 7.2).

The incidence of bronchitis is related to where the troops were deployed. The Seventh Cavalry spent more time on the central and northern plains than in the South during this period (15 years versus 2 years). Taking the duration of deployment into account, bronchitis was diagnosed nearly twice as often on the plains (5.4 cases/100 men/year) as in the more temperate southeastern

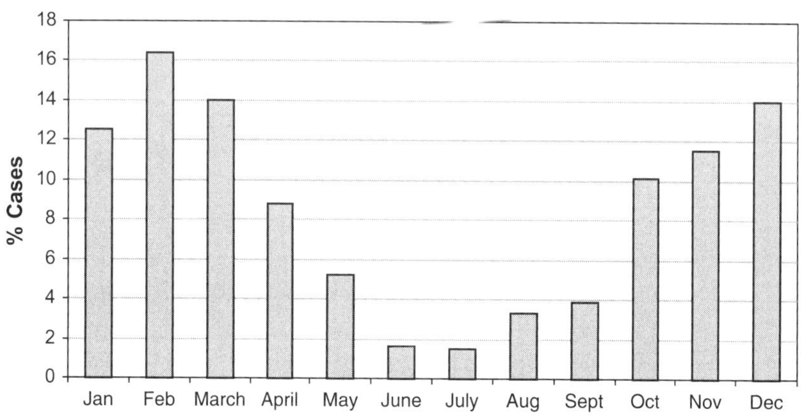

7.2. Monthly distribution of bronchitis in post–Civil War Seventh Cavalry.

area (2.8 cases/100 men/year). The incidence varied from year to year.

The average length of admission for chronic bronchitis was more than twice that for acute bronchitis (15 vs. 6.5 days, respectively). But the designation "chronic" probably applied to patients whose symptoms were never completely resolved. As damage to the bronchial tubes became permanent, pathological changes resulted in bronchiectasis. These hospital admissions would be characterized today as acute exacerbations of chronic bronchitis.

Cough was a separate diagnosis in 35 cases involving 33 soldiers in the medical records. Its mean duration (6.1 days) was nearly the same as for bronchitis. It resulted in no deaths or disability discharges. This entity probably represented a mild form of acute bronchitis.

Pneumonia

Pneumonia is an acute inflammatory condition involving the lung parenchyma (oxygen exchange sacs or alveoli) distal to the terminal bronchioles. Symptoms include fever, cough, chest pain, and dyspnea. Aspiration, inhalation of toxic substances, and bronchial obstruction can cause pneumonia, but most cases result from the inhalation of pathogenic microorganisms, especially *Streptococcus pneumoniae*. Until the 1930s pneumonia was the leading cause of death in the United States (Barry 2004:152–53).

Diagnosis was based on medical history and physical examination. Signs included dullness to percussion over the involved lobes of the lung and auscultatory findings of decreased air entry, rales, whispered pectoriloquy, and altered tactile fremitus (Duffin 1993:938–42). Nineteenth-century clinicians became adept at perceiving and interpreting these subtle physical alterations and used daily changes in their patient to monitor the progression of the disease.

The preferred treatment for pneumonia was tartar emetic (high-dose antimony potassium tartrate) and if it persisted combinations of mercurials, silver nitrate, ipecacuanha, and senegal root (Flannery 2004:317, 119–23).

This category combined inflammation of the lungs (68 cases in 67 soldiers) and pneumonia (34 cases in 33 soldiers), totaling 102 cases. The mean age was 27 and the mean duration of confinement

24 days (ranging from 3 to 96 days). About 20% of the troopers with pneumonia were lost to the service: 11 men received disability discharges, and 8 died. As expected, a seasonal pattern for the disease was apparent, with 65% of cases diagnosed from December through March, similar to the seasonality for acute bronchitis. Most cases of pneumonia probably developed as a complication of viral and bacterial respiratory infections, which also tended to increase in the winter. The yearly distribution appeared to be random.

Pleuritis

Pleuritis symptoms consist of acute, lancinating pain on one side of the chest made worse by inspiration, cough, or pressure and resulting in puerile (short, frequent) respirations. Physical exam reveals a "friction rub" on auscultation or diminished motion and dullness to percussion if fluid is present. Treatment was supportive and symptomatic.

Pleuritis or "pleurisy" was diagnosed frequently in the Seventh Cavalry: 148 cases in 147 soldiers. The mean age was 28, and the illness lasted an average of 8.3 days. It had a relatively high morbidity and even some mortality: 7 soldiers received disability discharges, and 2 died. In these cases the pleuritic involvement was probably an extension of a more serious underlying illness. Surprisingly, contrasted with other acute respiratory disorders, pleuritis exhibited little seasonal difference. The fewest cases appeared in November and December.

Pleurodynia ("false pleurisy") was diagnosed twice in 2 soldiers. This illness was an unrelated condition that involved the intercostal muscles rather than the pleura and is now thought to be caused by a Coxsackie virus.

Influenza

Influenza was defined by Dunglison (1866:516) as a severe form of catarrh occurring epidemically and generally affecting a number of persons in a community. The name comes from the Italian word for "influence," used to describe a phenomenon so vast and overwhelming that it appears to have been generated under the influence of the heavenly bodies. The etiology of the disease is known to be one of three Myxoviruses (A, B, and C), which are RNA viruses. Type A is the one that causes pandemics and exists as subtypes that do not produce cross immunity. The proteins that form the shell of the virus possess a distinctive genetic instability that renders acquired immunity ineffective. This absence of immunity is why vaccination for influenza is necessary every year. Changes take place through mutations and by recombination with other strains as the virus is passed between human groups or between humans and animals, particularly pigs and birds (Barry 2004:98–106).

Influenza has probably existed only since the Middle Ages, making it a relatively new human disease. It has never been absent for more than a few decades since then. During the nineteenth century, three major pandemics have occurred: 1830, 1833, and 1889. Thus the post–Civil War period was a relatively quiescent time for influenza, as our data show.

Typical influenza symptoms include the sudden onset of high fever, sore throat, rhinorrhea, cough, muscle aches, and prostration. Fatalities are usually related to pneumonia, which is the hallmark of the disease. In most outbreaks deaths are restricted to the very young, very old, and infirm. In the majority of these cases pneumonia is caused by a secondary bacterial infection that invades an already compromised patient. Occasionally, as in the worldwide 1918 pandemic, the virus morphed into a more lethal form that targeted healthy young adults (Crosby 1993:807–11).

Nineteenth-century influenza included two other descriptive categories: epidemic catarrh and pulmonary catarrh. Taxonomies from the period presented the three terms as synonyms (Dunglison 1866:516): the symptoms, physical findings, and prognoses were identical.

Combined, influenza was diagnosed 68 times in 65 soldiers. The mean age was 27 years, and the mean duration of illness was 5 days (ranging from 1 to 67 days). For the Seventh Cavalry, as for the rest of the population, influenza was a benign disease. The medical records reported no deaths and no disability discharges. The incidence of influenza by month is striking, with 93% of the cases appearing in January through March (fig. 7.3).

The annual incidence of influenza is interesting. An outbreak with 45 cases took place in the winter of 1867, with minor outbreaks in 1872, 1879, and 1880. Most years were influenza-free. This pattern is consistent with what epidemiologists observe today: the incidence and virulence of the disease varies greatly from year

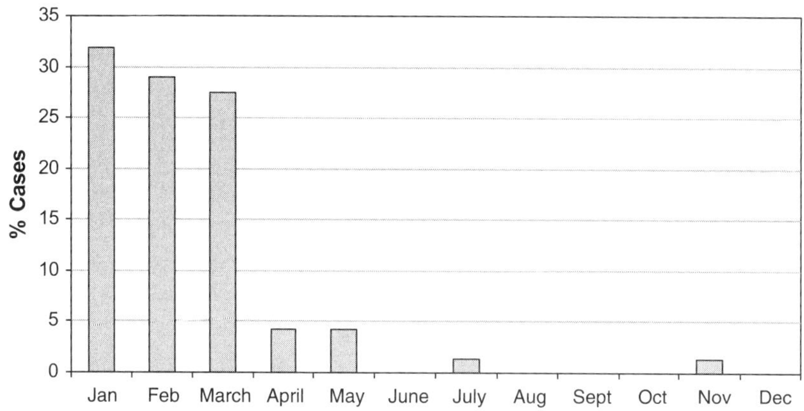

7.3. Monthly distribution of influenza in post–Civil War Seventh Cavalry.

to year, probably due to the ability of the virus to mutate as it passes from one population to the next. Experiments in laboratory animals show that flu is more easily transmitted in cold, dry environments and that certain "epitopes" (essential parts of the virus) subvert human defenses by stimulating an ineffective immune response. This resistance to immunity makes a year-to-year defense difficult to achieve.

During the winter of 1867, only months after enlisting and just before marching with Hancock's expedition on the central plains, 40 soldiers contracted pulmonary catarrh or influenza at Fort Riley. Companies A, D, H, and M were under Custer's command at the fort, and approximately 11% of them suffered the flu. All recovered, but influenza often leaves survivors in a protracted state of fatigue and even depression. In connection with other epidemics, some observers have noted: "The impact on the mental state of the victims would have the most widely noted sequelae" (Barry 2004:238). Perhaps as a result of this condition, a large proportion (63%) of these men deserted in the months that followed the influenza outbreak. Multiple factors have been cited to explain the desertion rate, however, which was particularly high during the years immediately after the Civil War.

Emphysema

Emphysema is characterized by progressive dyspnea, cough, and loss of muscle mass. Physical exam reveals an expanded "barrel chest" with markedly diminished breath sounds. Pathologically, an enlargement in air spaces occurs, caused by destruction of the alveolar walls distal to the terminal bronchioles. Laennec provided precise clinical descriptions of the disease, supported by rigorous autopsy studies, in 1819 (Knudson 1993:708).

This diagnosis was made only twice in 2 soldiers, 1 of whom received a disability discharge. The mean age was 29, above the average age for the whole group. The mean duration was 29 days. The incidence and severity of emphysema increases with age. It is generally associated with smoking, although it has some genetically determined causes, such as alpha-1-antitrypsin deficiency. We know that many of the troopers used tobacco, but probably not long enough for emphysema to become clinically evident.

Tuberculosis

This disease, also called consumption or phthisis during the nineteenth century, was diagnosed 63 times in 56 soldiers. The mean age was 27.5 years, and admissions averaged 29 days (ranging from 1 to 93 days). This infection was the most disabling and life-threatening of the pulmonary diseases, resulting in 7 deaths (12.5% mortality) and 26 disability discharges. It is likely that these young men were considered beyond recovery and sent home to die. In 9 cases the soldiers initially received a more benign diagnosis, usually bronchitis, but were later determined to have tuberculosis. More of the tuberculosis victims were foreign born than U.S. born (48% versus 39%). Also, fewer soldiers who developed tuberculosis had been manual laborers before enlistment than in the rest of the Seventh Cavalry (49% vs. 61%). It is possible that more of these individuals had been city-dwellers. The incidence of tuberculosis was evenly distributed by month (fig. 7.4) and by year.

Pathological, DNA, skeletal, and artifactual evidence indicates that tuberculosis existed in antiquity, but the great epidemics began in the eighteenth century. By the nineteenth century tuberculosis was considered a constitutional disease, meaning that it was related to hereditary and environmental factors that manifested a person's inherent nature. Dunglison (1866:743) expressed the deterministic view of tuberculosis: "This formidable disease occurs accidentally; but, usually, it is caused by a conformation obtained from progenitors." Only after Koch's discovery of the

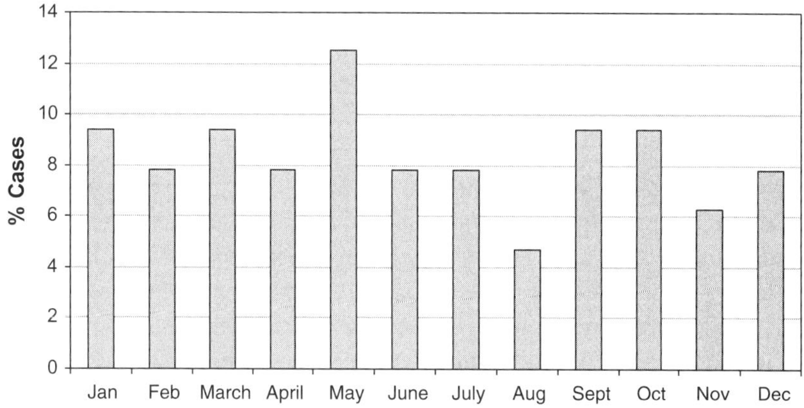

7.4. Monthly distribution of tuberculosis in post–Civil War Seventh Cavalry.

causative organism in 1882 was tuberculosis viewed as something that an individual "had" rather than as the result of an inherent susceptibility or something that an individual "was" (Dubos and Dubos 1996:xxxii).

Phthisis (from the Greek "I waste away, decay") was the most fulminant form of the disease, characterized by a progressive emaciation of the whole body, especially the musculature. Dunglison (1866:744) offers a detailed description of the symptoms and physical findings in three stages:

1. Incipient stage—A sense of unease is accompanied by coughing fits and dyspnea. A lack of free movement of the chest is observed beneath the clavicles and percussive sounds are decreased over the apex of the lungs. At this phase, scattered miliary tubercles are developing throughout the body.
2. Confirmed stage—Purulent expectoration, fever and sweats at night, and a circumscribed redness of the cheeks are noted. A morning cough is troublesome and slight exertion produces dyspnea. Voice and cough become more resonant to auscultation and rales are heard.
3. Last stage—The patient experiences constant spiking fevers, weak pulse, diarrhea, and extreme fatigue. As the tubercles break down and communicate with the

> airways, gurgling is heard, as well as an unusual resonance of cough and voice known as pectoriloquy. Percussion of the chest is tympanitic.

Treatment, at least with the hope for more than palliation, was only possible in the incipient stage. Then the combination of a healthy diet, fresh air, a balance of rest and adequate exercise, and moving to a climate where these benefits could be obtained was considered to offer the best chance for recovery. As the disease progressed, treatment focused on alleviating symptoms: counterirritants for pain, demulcents (sweet or viscous substances) to sooth inflamed mucous membranes, and opiates for cough and diarrhea suppression. Flannery (2004:120) specifically mentions cod liver oil as an alterative thought to be helpful in phthisis. It is interesting that high-fat nutritional supplements (such as Pulmocare) are used today for patients with chronic lung diseases. These formulations are thought to be beneficial to cachectic individuals because fat has a higher caloric content than carbohydrates or proteins and also produces less carbon dioxide, which patients tend to retain. Nineteenth-century physicians seem to have recognized this therapeutic benefit and took advantage of it by administering cod liver oil, olive oil, and other high-fat substances to their patients with chronic lung disease.

Lacking chest X-rays and tuberculin skin tests, military doctors had to rely on medical histories and physical examination, particularly percussion and auscultation of the chest, to diagnose and monitor the progress of tuberculosis.

Hemoptysis and Hydrothorax

These two conditions are listed separately but probably represented manifestations and/or complications of other underlying pulmonary conditions, particularly tuberculosis. Hydrothorax (pleural effusion) is an accumulation of fluid between the visceral (inner) and parietal (outer) layers of the pleura. This illness occurred in 1 soldier, with a fatal outcome. The condition generally develops as a reaction to a serious underlying lung disorder, such as an infection or a tumor. If the fluid buildup becomes large enough, it impairs breathing. Draining the fluid, which these surgeons were capable of doing, provided temporary relief.

The records show 8 admissions for hemoptysis among 7 soldiers. The mean age was 27.6 years, and the duration of hospitalization averaged 17.4 days (ranging from 2 to 71 days). Coughing blood is generally not life-threatening in itself but portends an underlying condition that may be serious. Of the 7 soldiers, 2 received a disability discharge, and 1 died of tuberculosis.

Discussion

On initial inspection the information contained in the medical records of the Seventh Cavalry appears rudimentary and limited, at least compared to the voluminous material found in patients' records today. The data examined here include some basic demographic information, diagnoses, length and date of illness, and brief comments concerning outcome. These simple numerical findings provide objective information that gives us insights into the nature of these ailments, the internal consistency of the diagnostic categories applied by military doctors, and the epidemiology of pulmonary diseases. The severity of these illnesses may be viewed on a continuum from most transient and benign (cough, influenza, and pleuritis); to more severe and uncertain (bronchitis and asthma); to those pulmonary diseases causing the bulk of the morbidity and mortality (pneumonia and tuberculosis). Two conditions are of particular interest, both as historically significant diseases and as current and potentially future public health threats: influenza and tuberculosis.

The influenza epidemics that struck the Seventh Cavalry were typical of outbreaks during the nineteenth century and today. The striking seasonal pattern was concentrated in the winter months, varying in incidence and severity from year to year and causing low mortality among young healthy adults. As noted, a high percentage of the troopers who developed influenza at Fort Riley during the winter of 1867 deserted shortly after recovery. A number of factors were considered as possible causes for desertion.

An unusual syndrome associated with influenza (encephalitis lethargica) was common following the Great Influenza Pandemic of 1918 and was noted during other outbreaks in 1830, 1847, and 1889 (Ravenholt 1993:709). These patients suffered from a localized inflammation at the base of the brain, probably induced by an immune interaction with the influenza virus. Symptoms included somnolence (hence the name "sleepy sickness"), impaired concentration, and impulsiveness that could escalate into violence, especially in young people. Victims may have recovered, but the disease often progressed to a Parkinson-like state, respiratory failure, and death (Vilensky et al. 2007:79–84). The soldiers' medical records showed no neurological disorders following the 1867 epidemic, but depression, lethargy, and behavioral changes after the flu may have played a role. A review of desertion rates for soldiers unaffected by influenza, however, did not support the theory that a form of encephalitis lethargica was responsible. In fact the desertion rate was high for most groups of troopers on the central plains. Rates ranged from 44 percent to 63 percent for soldiers affected by different diseases (diarrhea versus influenza), stationed at different locations (Fort Riley versus Fort Lyon), and under the command of different officers (Custer versus others). In contrast, desertions from Fort Abraham Lincoln (1877–80) were much lower, about 11 percent. The secretary of war, Stephen B. Elkins, reported that one-third of the men recruited between 1867 and 1891 deserted, but the frequency varied, generally declining over time (Rickey 1963:143). A survey of 194 deserters in 1891 revealed that alcohol use and "general dissatisfaction" were the two major causes, tyrannical superiors being the most often reported reason for dissatisfaction. Complaints about poor and insufficient rations, inadequate living conditions, and imperious officers were common during the southern and central plains campaigns. The army did not take "important positive steps" to deal with the desertion problem until the 1880s, but provisions, health care, and wages improved before then (Rickey 1963:144).

The most devastating influenza epidemic of the twentieth century was believed to have started at Fort Riley, Kansas, in the spring of 1918 (Barry 2004:98). U.S. forces massed at the same site where the Seventh Cavalry had formed in 1866 in preparation to engage the Triple Alliance during World War I. Anecdotally, the source of the epidemic was traced to an incident when soldiers burned tons of manure, creating a yellow haze throughout the grounds. The first case appeared on March 11, 1918, and 500 more followed over the next week. After killing about 10 percent of those affected, the sickness seemed to disappear. After 1.5 million Americans crossed the Atlantic, the disease broke out in Europe, where it became more lethal. Then it was transmitted back to the United States, where it traveled from east to west, from one military base to the next. As the draft continued, throngs turned out for parades to support the war effort. The disease spread to the general population. By the time the pandemic had run its course in the fall of that year, 650,000 Americans had died and more than 30 million had succumbed worldwide. Because of its tendency to recombine portions of its RNA with other strains of the virus, this particular version was more deadly, particularly for healthy young adults and children. The cause of this apparent anomaly lies in what has been termed "cytokine storm," an overwhelming inflammatory response generated by youthful and more robust immune systems (Crosby 1993:811).

This devastation is largely forgotten today, and its tenuous connection to the comparatively inconsequential outbreak among Custer's men in 1867 is hard to establish. Yet the Myxovirus responsible for both epidemics, Swine Influenza Type A, is the same organism, probably modified over time by mutations and translocations as it passed back and forth between human and animal populations.

The other condition, consumption, claimed comparatively few Seventh Cavalry victims (0.65 percent) but caused significant morbidity and mortality. Once called the "Captain of the Men of Death," tuberculosis has at times killed more people than any other disease. As late as the 1930s it was the most common cause of death among people aged fifteen to forty-five. Tuberculosis has long been recognized as a "social disease," not because it is spread by sexual activity but in the sense that more than simple exposure was required for transmission. Economic and environmental conditions were also critical. It had profound social effects on the individual and their relatives as well. A tuberculosis diagnosis or death was considered a stigma for the family, associated with hereditary defects or poverty. It also decreased the patients' (most of whom were young adults) prospects for marriage and employment. The great tuberculosis epidemics began in the eighteenth century. During the nineteenth century, it remained a looming presence in the lives of young adults.

A closer look at the data in the medical records provides insight into the effect that tuberculosis had on affected troopers and how the surgeons dealt with it. The incipient stage was often mistaken for chronic bronchitis. In a number of instances this erroneous diagnosis appeared in the records. Nineteenth-century patent medicine promoters took advantage of this phenomenon and the public's fear of tuberculosis by conflating ubiquitous minor symptoms into portents of "galloping consumption" (Young 1961:196). Vast fortunes were made by the purveyors of nostrums, such as Piso's Cure for Consumption, Shiloh's Consumption Cure, and Dr. King's New Discovery for Consumption.

The term "tuberculosis" appeared in print in 1840 and was not in common use until the mid-twentieth century. In only one case was this term applied in the Seventh Cavalry medical records. "Consumption" and "phthisis" were the usual designations, and these terms were used selectively by military doctors. Although both refer to the progressive emaciation that attended pulmonary tuberculosis, phthisis indicated a more advanced or rapid state of wasting and may have signified miliary (from millet seed) or diffuse disease. The duration of confinement before discharge or death reflected this difference, lasting about six weeks for phthisis and three months for consumption. It was clear that medical personnel made an effort to treat their patients who were stricken by tuberculosis with whatever means possible, as some of them remained under care as much as nine months. Treatments became less "heroic" (heavy metals, bleeding, and purgatives) and more supportive and nutrition-based during the later decades of the nineteenth century.

In regard to the other pulmonary diseases listed in the medical records, we are struck by the infrequency of asthma, the seasonality of bronchitis, pneumonia, and influenza, and the lack of seasonal variation of pleuritis and tuberculosis.

Summary

The pulmonary diseases experienced by the Seventh Cavalry consisted primarily of acute and chronic infections that may be divided into three categories in terms of prognosis. The most self-limited and benign category included acute bronchitis, cough, and influenza. Intermediate in severity and of longer duration were conditions such as chronic bronchitis and pleuritis. Pneumonia and tuberculosis caused the most morbidity and mortality. Noninfectious conditions, such as asthma and emphysema, were much less common than today.

Although the medical records say little about treatment, it appears that the military physicians attending the troopers diagnosed and cared for their patients competently under difficult conditions, using the limited resources that they had available to them. Interestingly, the seasonal incidence of influenza corresponded to the incidence today. The tenuous connection to the pandemic of 1918, also originating at Fort Riley, has been noted here.

CHAPTER 8

Malaria Prevalence in the Seventh Cavalry

Colleen Cheverko and Kristina Zarenko

A number of diseases come to mind when we think of illnesses that afflicted soldiers during and after the American Civil War, such as sexually transmitted infections, cholera, and scurvy. Malaria is not often considered, because it is not thought to occur in the United States. Malaria cases today arise in the United States when travelers from Africa, the Pacific, and other regions develop symptoms after their arrival in the country.

Although the *Anopheles* mosquitoes that transmit malaria were present in prehistoric North America, the disease was not. Its appearance in the New World resulted from European settlement and from the African slave trade. Malaria was carried to the United States in the blood of African slaves and then transmitted via the preexisting malaria vectors (Faust 1951; Bretlinger 2006). It soon spread from the Deep South to all regions of the country and remained endemic until the middle of the twentieth century. During the 1950s, malaria was eradicated in the United States through antimalarial drug campaigns and through the reduction of breeding sites for *Anopheles* mosquitoes (Faust 1951).

Despite its eradication in several countries, such as the United States and Canada, malaria remains a global health problem today. Malarial infection can cause loss of hearing, speech, vision, and strength in extreme cases (Bretlinger 2006). In most cases malaria symptoms reduce the health of infected individuals (Bleakley 2010).

Malaria had the potential to disrupt troop strength and performance. This chapter addresses the patterns of malaria in the post–Civil War Seventh Cavalry. Temporal trends in malaria frequency, geographic location where illness occurred, rank, birth location, age at enlistment, and stature are examined.

This chapter continues with a brief discussion of the causes, symptoms, and treatment of malaria from a historic perspective and from a modern perspective. The methods of data collection specific to malaria are presented, along with results.

Historic Perspectives on Malaria

Historic medical discussions of malaria often include "malarial poisoning" listed as part of the miasmic disorders. During and immediately after the Civil War, malaria symptoms accounted for approximately one-quarter of the diseases affecting white troops. During this time, the mortality rate was relatively low, although the morbidity rate was high and likely affected troop performance.

During the Civil War, physicians diagnosed malaria poisoning when a number of symptoms were present: diarrhea, jaundice, dysentery, ulcers, boils, aches and pains, cough, tachycardia, and sweating. Debility, especially due to anemia, was a common symptom. In extreme cases dyspnea, delirium, and coma led to fatalities (Barnes 1888:77–111; Harstad 1960).

Physicians and laypersons made observations about the environmental causes of malaria poisoning, often subscribing to the "theory of organic decomposition" (Barnes 1888:155; Harstad 1960). Similar to what is currently known about the transmission of anthrax, this theory involved the afflicted people being exposed to soils where the malarial spores flourished. The soils thought to transmit malaria were rich in vegetable matter, heat, and moisture, including swamps, marshes, and land near rivers. Water supplies were also associated with malarial poisoning. But the prevailing theories attributed transmission of malaria to water impurity (Barnes 1888:161), similar to present-day understandings of the transmission of cholera.

While water supplies and soil were associated with malarial poisoning, physicians named other predisposing factors that influenced the transmission of malaria. For example, officers during the Civil War thought that land management practices influenced malarial poisoning. They attributed an increase of malaria to clearing brush and disturbing soils, which were necessary steps in establishing a camp or fort. Additionally, enlisted men who were depressed, exhausted, overworked, hungry, and exposed to various weather conditions were more likely to exhibit malaria symptoms.

Because the causes of malaria were not yet identified, treatment and prevention were ineffective in the post–Civil War Seventh Cavalry. Steps to prevent malarial poisoning included access to quality food and water and protection from extreme environmental conditions. Quinine, a prophylactic malaria drug, and willow bark were used as protective agents, although patients taking these substances were often nevertheless stricken with symptoms.

From the late seventeenth century until the early 1940s quinine was used as the primary treatment and prophylactic agent for malaria symptoms. Medical records during the Civil War do not mention the negative side effects of quinine use, although they were certainly present. The only effective treatment during the Civil War was the removal of the affected individual to an environment that did not harbor malaria (Barnes 1888:77–111; Harstad 1960).

Current Perspectives on Malaria

These views of malaria are now outdated. Physicians and laypersons accurately described the transmission environment during the Civil War, but they were unable to identify the causes of malaria. After establishment of the germ theory in the late nineteenth century, *Anopheles* mosquitoes were identified as vectors of malaria transmission. These mosquitoes inhabit the environments described above.

Five types of malaria parasites exist: *Plasmodium falciparum*, *P. vivax*, *P. ovale*, *P. knowlesi*, and *P. malariae*. The United States primarily experienced *P. falciparum* malaria (considered the most serious type) and *P. vivax* malaria. *P. falciparum* was prevalent in the South, while *P. vivax* was more common in northern states (Bretlinger 2006; Autino et al. 2012).

Malaria symptoms include chills, coma, convulsions, fevers, headaches, muscle pain, nausea, sweating, and vomiting. Anemia and an enlargement of the liver or spleen are frequent complications of a malaria infection. The incubation period following initial infection is ten days to four weeks, although symptoms can occur in as little as eight days or as long as one year after infection. Malaria symptoms are cyclical, occurring repetitively every two to three days (Trampuz et al. 2003).

After the recognition of a mosquito transmission vector, a number of therapeutic drugs became available for the treatment and prevention of malaria. The most widespread of these, chloroquine, was one of the most significant public health innovations of its time due to its efficacy against the malaria parasite. However, antibiotic resistance has reduced its effectiveness in the fight against *P. falciparum*. A combination of intravenous and oral antimalarial medications and antibiotics is currently used to treat infections (Trampuz et al. 2003).

Due to the discrepancies between past and contemporary perspectives, a discussion of the methods is necessary. Specifically, the criteria for what is considered "malaria" are described here. Select medical entries that were not included as malaria diagnoses, such as "typho-malarial fever," are also briefly discussed.

Methods

This section presents the methods specific to the examination of malaria prevalence in the Seventh Cavalry. In addition to the more widespread challenges of working with this data set (see chapter 4), malaria investigations present special difficulties. The repetitive, cyclical nature of malaria infections makes the description of the disease challenging. Malaria recurs after the initial infection over a period dictated by the specific strain of the disease, varying from two to three days. The majority of individuals in the military records suffering from what was described as malaria have multiple medical entries, most likely from recurring episodes of the disease.

Multiple episodes for the same individual can occur over time in one location or span several locations. It is difficult—if not impossible—to determine whether multiple records indicate multiple infections or a recurring, ongoing infection. Due to this difficulty, only the earliest reported instance of malaria for each individual is used for the analyses.

For the purposes of this study, malarial cases were organized by individual. The earliest report of malaria for each individual in the records was identified and included in the analyses. Individuals with insufficient information in the medical records or Enlistment Records were excluded from the analyses. Once the individual records were compiled, they were analyzed for the frequency of malaria cases by month and year, state of birth, location of incidence, and age. Chi-square tests examined the relationship between malaria prevalence, rank, and location of birth. Risk ratios were computed to investigate further differences in risk of malaria between officers and rankers and to assess differences between foreign- and native-born individuals. An independent samples *t*-test determined differences in age at enlistment and stature between enlistees with and without malaria.

Due to the uncertain diagnosis of malaria during the period, a variety of terms and classifications were used to describe malaria infection. To identify individuals with suspected cases of malaria, we included complaints of intermittent fever, remittent fever, bilious fever, and malaria. Intermittent fever was sometimes subclassified as quotidian, tertian, or quartan (Barnes 1888). These terms refer to the recurrence cycle of the fevers from the infection. Very few medical records actually listed "malaria" as a diagnosis.

Typhomalarial fever, also called typhoid malarial fever, was excluded from analysis. Despite its name, which refers to a simultaneous infection with both typhoid and malaria, this illness does not exist as a specific disease recognized by modern medicine (Smith 1982:182). Patients diagnosed with typhomalarial fever primarily suffered from typhoid fever, not a combination of the two diseases (Smith 1982:220). The distinction between typhoid and malarial fevers became clear during the late 1800s with an understanding of the diseases' conditions and implementation of diagnostic tests (Smith 1982).

Results

The medical and associated Enlistment Records indicate that 1,331 individuals (about 20% of Seventh Cavalry troopers) were diagnosed with malarial infections. This section presents the results obtained from these records regarding the distribution of malaria by month, season, year, region, rank, location of birth, age at enlistment, and stature.

TEMPORAL DISTRIBUTION OF MALARIA

Malaria was present in the Seventh Cavalry year-round. Despite its constant presence, the rate of primary infection fluctuated by month, season, and year.

Table 8.1 and figure 8.1 show the number of cases of malaria by month. Fewer initial malaria diagnoses occurred from December through July. June presented the lowest instance of malaria in this

TABLE 8.1. Malaria infections by month in post-Civil War Seventh Cavalry

Month	*Number*	*Percentage*
January	83	6.2
February	80	6.1
March	102	7.7
April	81	6.1
May	98	7.4
June	74	5.5
July	90	6.8
August	133	10.0
September	201	15.1
October	196	14.7
November	110	8.3
December	83	6.2
Total	1331	100.0

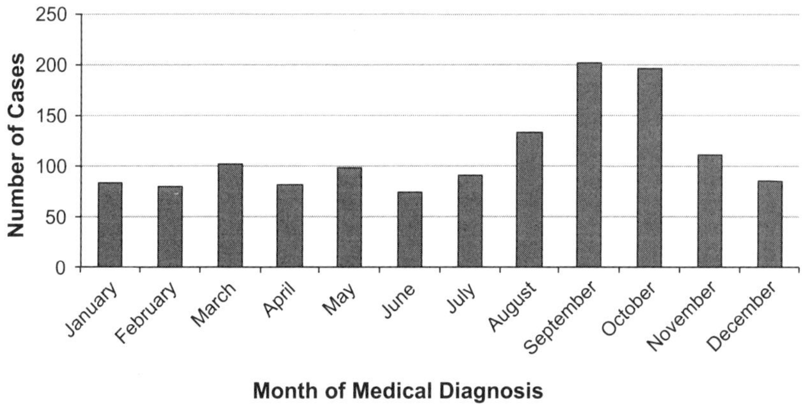

8.1. Malaria cases by month in the post-Civil War Seventh Cavalry.

TABLE 8.2. Malaria infections by season in post-Civil War Seventh Cavalry

Season	*Number*	*Percentage*
Spring	281	21.1
Summer	300	22.5
Fall	504	37.9
Winter	245	18.4
Total	1331	100.0

group and March the highest. A spike in the frequency of malaria occurred in August through October. The highest prevalence was reached in September, followed by October and August.

The distribution of malaria corresponds with seasonal changes. Table 8.2 and figure 8.2 demonstrate that the rates of malaria infections are comparatively stable during spring (March through May) and the beginning of summer (June through August). The frequency of new infections peaks in the fall (September through November) before decreasing during the winter months (December through February).

The greatest differences in the malaria records occur by year (1866 through 1883). Table 8.3 and figure 8.3 show the frequency and percentage of cases by year. The highest incidences of malaria

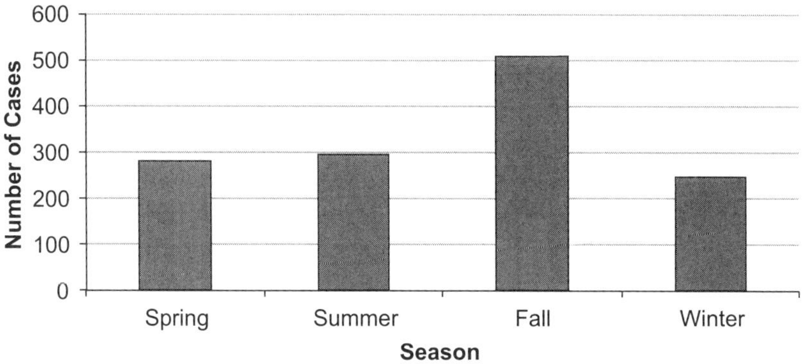

8.2. Malaria cases by season in the post–Civil War Seventh Cavalry.

TABLE 8.3. Malaria infections by year in post-Civil War Seventh Cavalry

Year	*Number*	*Percentage*
1866	100	7.5
1867	140	10.5
1868	94	7.1
1869	40	3.0
1870	88	6.6
1871	135	10.1
1872	129	9.7
1873	66	5.0
1874	22	1.7
1875	111	8.3
1876	69	5.2
1877	36	2.7
1878	61	4.6
1879	55	4.1
1880	40	3.0
1881	22	1.7
1882	65	4.9
1883	58	4.4
Total	1331	100.0

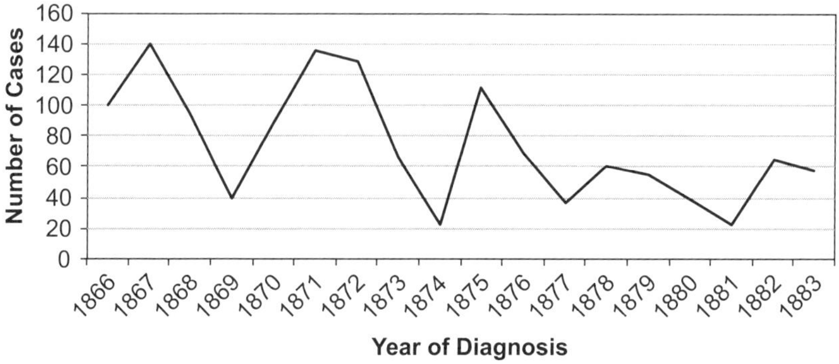

8.3. Malaria cases by year in the post–Civil War Seventh Cavalry.

TABLE 8.4. Malaria infections by geographic region in post-Civil War Seventh Cavalry

Geographic region	*Number*	*Percentage*
Central plains	578	43.4
South	272	20.4
Northern plains	414	31.1
Other and undesignated	67	5.0
Total	1331	100.0

occurred in 1867, when most of the regiment was in Kansas, and 1871 and 1872, when most of the regiment was assigned to the Department of the South. The fewest initial reports of malaria came during 1874, when the regiment was posted to the northern plains, and in 1877 and 1881, when the regiment had been on the northern plains for years.

GEOGRAPHIC DISTRIBUTION OF MALARIA

The data were also examined for trends relating to the geographic location of infection (table 8.4 and fig. 8.4). The location with the highest malaria prevalence was the central plains, with 578 cases (43.4%). The northern plains had 414 cases (31.1%). The region

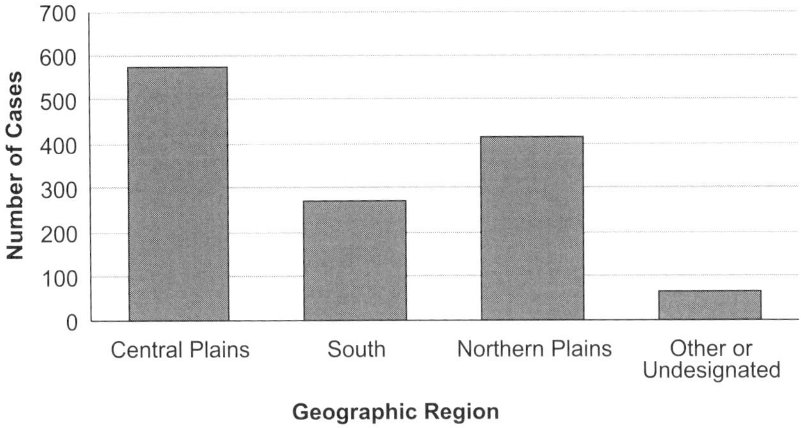

8.4. Malaria cases by region in the post–Civil War Seventh Cavalry.

with the fewest malarial infections was the South, with 272 cases (20.4%).

RANK AND MALARIA

Ranks were assigned to the following groups: commissioned officer ($n = 9$), senior noncommissioned officer ($n = 428$), junior noncommissioned officer ($n = 322$), ranker ($n = 2,233$), and other ($n = 2$). Using these categories, no association between rank and malaria affliction occurred ($\chi^2 = 6.867$, df $= 4$, $p > 0.05$). Further investigation reveals that officers and rankers were equally likely to contract malaria (risk ratio = 1.2).

The results of the examination of rank and malaria affliction were counter to the initial expectation that rankers, due to job assignments, should be affected by malaria more than noncommissioned officers: 25% of rankers developed symptoms of malaria, while 29% of officers developed malaria symptoms.

LOCATION OF BIRTH AND MALARIA

An examination of the relationship between malaria affliction and foreign- and native-born members of the Seventh Cavalry was conducted to determine if a difference in susceptibility to malarial infection existed between the two groups. Approximately 24% of foreign-born enlistees contracted malaria, compared to approximately 21% of native-born enlistees. A significant difference in malaria frequency was found between native-born and foreign-born enlistees in the Seventh Cavalry ($\chi^2 = 7.05$, df = 1, $0.005 < p < 0.05$). Foreign-born enlistees were as likely to contract malaria as native-born enlistees (risk ratio = 1.2), however, indicating that the difference in disease prevalence between the two groups was relatively small.

AGE AT ENLISTMENT AND MALARIA

The age at enlistment for those who were diagnosed with malaria did not differ from the age at enlistment for those who were not ($t = 0.1197$, $p > 0.05$). The age for enlistees with malaria averaged 24.0811 years, while the age for soldiers without malaria averaged 24.0816—a minuscule difference.

STATURE AND MALARIA

The relationship between stature and malaria affliction was also examined. Average stature between the two groups did not differ ($t = -0.176$, $p > 0.05$). The stature for enlistees with malaria was 67.180 inches, while the stature for enlistees without malaria averaged 67.193. As in the case of age at enlistment, the differences in average stature of the two groups were minuscule.

Discussion

These results suggest several generalizations. The personal attributes of the soldiers (birthplace, rank, age at enlistment, and stature) are discussed first. Seasonality and location are then compared with information from other sources from the same period. Finally, the implications of malaria in the Seventh Cavalry are discussed.

The birthplace of the soldiers had little effect on malaria symptoms. Foreign-born enlistees contracted malaria more frequently than native-born enlistees. This difference, however, might be smaller than the statistical test indicated due to the large sample size. The foreign-born enlistees may have had less exposure to the malaria strains present in the United States and therefore might have less acquired immunity to the pathogens. Because *P. vivax* was present in both Europe and the United States, foreign-born soldiers may have been more susceptible to *P. falciparum*. Unfortunately, this hypothesis cannot be tested with the available data.

While the rank of the enlistees was not significantly associated with malaria affliction, noncommissioned officers were more affected by malaria than rankers. This finding did not support the expectation that rankers should have a higher prevalence of malaria because they were likely more often exposed to mosquitoes. The age of enlistment of noncommissioned officers was slightly older than the age at enlistment of rankers, which might account for this result.

Age at enlistment had no effect on whether or not the soldiers contracted malaria. Both soldiers who exhibited symptoms of malaria and those who did not averaged twenty-four years old at enlistment. This finding might be explained by the relatively narrow range of age at enlistment in the Seventh Cavalry.

Stature also did not affect malaria incidence. The stature of soldiers with malaria was similar to the stature of soldiers who did not contract malaria. Both groups of enlistees averaged 67 inches tall.

COMPARISONS WITH OTHER SOURCES

Malaria in the post–Civil War Seventh Cavalry was compared with the incidence of malaria in soldiers during the Civil War. Comparative data came from part 3 of *The Medical and Surgical History of the War of the Rebellion* (Barnes 1888). This volume is the most comprehensive medical source available for the Civil War.

Based on location and stationing, malaria frequency in the Seventh Cavalry should have been highest in the northern plains, then lower in the central plains, and lowest in the South due to the period of their stays in the three regions. But malaria prevalence does not reflect the amount of time spent in each of the regions or the total number of enlistees in the Seventh Cavalry in each of those regions. The Seventh Cavalry was posted in the central plains (43.4 percent of malaria cases) for approximately four and a half years, in the South for only three years (20.4 percent), and in the northern plains for a decade (31.1 percent). These numbers mean that more cases of malaria occurred per year in the South and central plains than in the northern plains. That finding supported data from the Civil War indicating that malaria was more frequent in lower latitudes (Barnes 1888:102).

The seasonality of malaria in the Seventh Cavalry reflected trends observed in Union and Confederate troops as well as civilians during the Civil War (Barnes 1888:102). At that time malaria was most prevalent during August and September and least frequent in February. Similarly, malaria was most prevalent in the Seventh Cavalry during August through October and least frequent in winter months.

IMPLICATIONS OF MALARIA IN THE SEVENTH CAVALRY

Approximately 20 percent of the Seventh Cavalry members exhibited symptoms of at least one bout of malaria during their enlistment. This number excluded the recurring, episodic symptoms of malaria, which could have affected the soldiers for years following their initial exposure to the pathogen. With so many of the troops demonstrating initial malaria symptoms, the overall strength and performance of the troops was affected.

About 10 percent of Seventh Cavalry members who exhibited symptoms of malaria reenlisted in the military at least once following their initial symptoms. The rest of the individuals who exhibited malaria symptoms did not reenlist. Of these, 10 percent were discharged due to disability, and 25 percent deserted or were dishonorably discharged. While a causal relationship cannot be determined between the reasons for discharge and reenlistment, it is possible that "malaria poisoning" affected an individual's decision to stay with the Seventh Cavalry.

Even today malaria is known to decrease productivity in afflicted individuals (Bretlinger 2006; Bleakley 2010). In the American Civil War and other situations of armed conflict malaria could complicate the campaigns of both sides (Bretlinger 2006). Malaria prevalence within the Seventh Cavalry may have impacted the troops' ability to suppress hostilities on the plains and enforce civil rule in the South. Malaria probably afflicted the opposing sides as well.

A slightly higher incidence of malaria may have existed in the Seventh Cavalry than in civilians during the same period. Members of the military are often immunologically, physically, and mentally stressed (Benenson 1984). No comparable civilian medical records during the period are available, however, so contrasts cannot be made. Indians, who may not yet have acquired immunity against malaria, could have been more affected by it, which would have facilitated U.S. military campaigns in the plains regions.

Summary

Historic understanding of malaria differs from what is known about the pathogen today. But the symptoms and some of the treatments of malaria were similar then and now. The environments where malaria was contracted were described in detail in historical reports and accounted for transmission of malaria based on germ theory today because the environments harbored *Anopheles* mosquitoes.

Place of birth affected malaria prevalence, while age at enlistment had no effect on malaria contraction. The seasonal and geographic distribution of malaria in the Seventh Cavalry corresponded to the seasons and locations of malaria diagnoses during the Civil War. Malaria prevalence was highest in the fall and lowest in the winter. The central plains and South had more cases of malaria per year than the northern plains.

CHAPTER 9

Sexually Transmitted Infections in the Seventh Cavalry

P. Willey

Among the many other diseases and injuries that Seventh Cavalry members suffered, including malaria, they were susceptible to sexually transmitted infections (STIs). As today, noteworthy diseases were acquired through sexual acts. At that time none of the STIs were curable. Surgeons merely treated symptoms. We are reminded today of those times not only by HIV/AIDS but by newly emerging infectious adaptations, such as antibiotic-resistant syphilis.

Many different STIs may have afflicted the troopers and their consorts. After providing background on potential sexual contacts and diseases recognized during the nineteenth century, this chapter discusses methods employed with the Seventh Cavalry STIs and the results derived. A discussion and summary follow.

Contrary to what an unfaithful sexual partner might have you believe, STIs do not occur spontaneously, springing forth from filthy toilet seats. They require sexual activity with a partner who is infected. So all of the Seventh Cavalry STIs came from someone.

Consorts of Seventh Cavalry troopers went undocumented, at least in the military medical records. But other historic sources suggested their presence. Some of these relationships involved prostitution and homosexuality.

An implicit institutional relation occurred between the military establishment and prostitution. What appeared to be an overt disavowal by the military often included undercover complicity, including "hog ranches."

Hog ranches, consisting of a saloon and brothel, usually located just outside military reservations, sprouted near posts and camps on the plains. Prostitutes there often included "the vilest and most diseased whores" (Rickey 1963:169). Because enlisted soldiers frequently constituted the lowest grade of customers, the prostitutes they hired similarly occupied the bottom rung of their profession.

In addition, some Indian women on nearby reservations and agencies also played this role. As an example, Indian women were identified as causing STI cases at Fort Buford. That fort's surgeon recommended ending their visits. In fact, from 1870 to 1874, syphilis ranked as the fourth most common infectious disease at Forts Buford, Randall, and Stevenson (Stallard 1978:70, citing Mattison 1954). Association with Indian women apparently contributed to that remarkably high frequency.

Homosexual relations constituted another vector of STIs. Although homosexual acts went largely undocumented in the nineteenth-century military, one example in the Seventh Cavalry stands out. Mrs. Nash, a Seventh Cavalry laundress, married a succession of enlisted men. While married to her third husband, John Noonan, Mrs. Nash died while he was away on campaign in 1878. When preparing her body for burial, Fort Abraham Lincoln's women discovered that Nash was male (Weddon and Huseas 1984; Schneider 1988). Presumably Mrs. Nash had sexual relations with Noonan and her other husbands, and STIs were probably transmitted in that context. We are reminded by this example that even in the nineteenth century the definition of marriage encompassed more than one man and one woman.

One of Noonan's medical records indicated that he reported to sick call with syphilis January 1872 to the post hospital in Yorkville, South Carolina (spelled "Numan"; fig. 9.1). This event happened only weeks after he enlisted in the Seventh Cavalry but well before he married Mrs. Nash. His later (1877) aliments, including orchitis and testicular inflammation, occurred during his married years and may have been related to his 1872 syphilis inoculation.

In addition to such a formal relationship, less formal homosexuality probably occurred among "bunkies." In the immediate

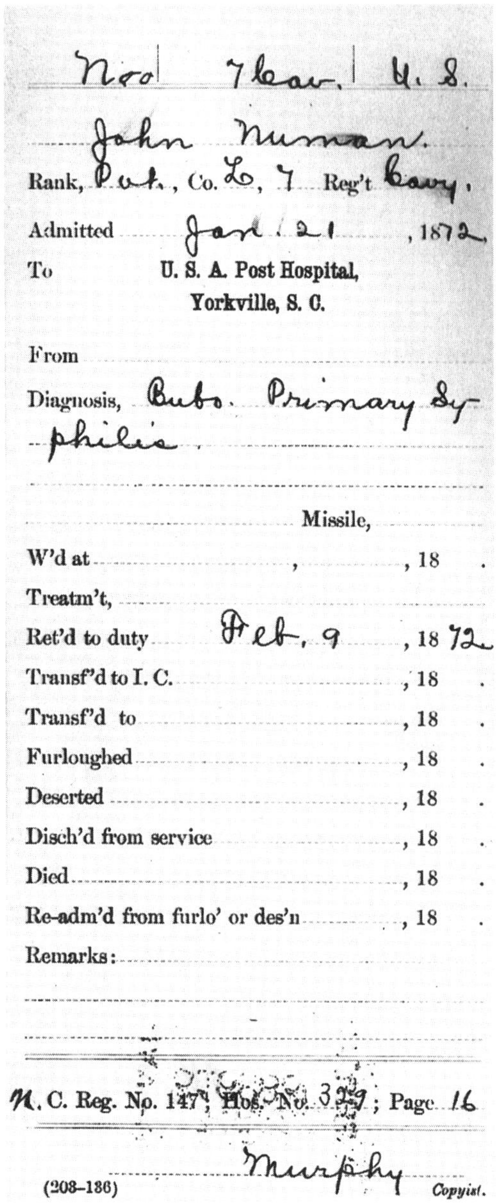

Nco 7 Cav. U. S.

John Numan.

Rank, Pvt., Co. L, 7 Reg't Cavy.

Admitted Jan. 21, 1872,

To U. S. A. Post Hospital,
Yorkville, S. C.

From

Diagnosis, Bubo. Primary Sy-
philis.

Missile,

W'd at , 18 .

Treatm't,

Ret'd to duty Feb. 9, 1872

Transf'd to I. C. , 18 .

Transf'd to , 18 .

Furloughed , 18 .

Deserted , 18 .

Disch'd from service , 18 .

Died , 18 .

Re-adm'd from furlo' or des'n , 18 .

Remarks:

N. C. Reg. No. 147; Hos. No. 329; Page 16

(203-186) Murphy Copyist.

9.1. Medical record of Private John Noonan ("Numan"), Company L, indicating primary infection with syphilis during January 1872 in Yorkville, South Carolina. The Seventh Cavalry displayed increased STIs while stationed in the South. Noonan later married Mrs. Nash, who, on her death in 1878, was discovered to be male. Courtesy National Archives and Records Administration, public domain image.

post–Civil War period bunkies experienced close sleeping arrangements: two men to a bed. Sexual conduct may have occurred. Single bunks became standard issue, replacing the double bunks starting about 1872 (Greene 1981). That transition, like most military changes, required several years to implement.

These more unusual relationships belie the more traditional routes of acquiring STIs, including married couples, love affairs, and rapes. In more conventional relationships laundresses constituted the only females with standing in the nineteenth-century U.S. Army. Although their social status was low, their attentions were often sought by enlisted men. Marriage sometimes ensued.

The medical records regarding STIs focused on the enlisted men who sought treatment, like most of the other medical conditions analyzed in this volume. However, officers were not exempt from STIs. For example, Lieutenant James Sturgis was treated for gonorrhoeal orchitis on November 5, 1875.

Two other Seventh Cavalry officers were treated for venereal diseases while they were cadets at the U.S. Military Academy at West Point. George Custer was treated for gonorrhea from August 29 to September 3, 1859, in the West Point hospital. A few years earlier Marcus Reno had been treated for syphilis twice, once on July 5, 1856, and again on October 28 (Pohanka 1989:5).

Infections passed from outside sources into the Seventh Cavalry, within the Seventh Cavalry, and from the Seventh into surrounding communities. But what STIs did the surgeons recognize that originated from these contacts?

Diseases

The STIs that the Seventh Cavalry suffered from may have included, among others, chancroid, chlamydia, genital lice, gonorrhea, herpes simplex, human papillomavirus, scabies, syphilis, and viral hepatitis (Hepatitis B). Today such infectious diseases are identified based on germ theory principles and laboratory assessments. That theory asserts that distinct microorganisms cause infections and produce symptoms, even if the symptoms caused by different microorganisms are similar. Before adoption of the germ theory and its requisite diagnostic laboratory tests, however, symptoms constituted the diagnosing hallmarks of diseases. So symptoms separated one STI from another. Using symptoms as the diagnostic parameter, nineteenth-century military surgeons identified two STIs: syphilis and gonorrhea. Those diseases combined for approximately 5 percent of the diagnoses in the Seventh Cavalry medical records.

Syphilis and gonorrhea had been recognized and diagnostically separated by symptoms starting in the late eighteenth century. They had been considered different manifestations of same disease until the distinctions were established in the late 1700s. The causative venereal agents were identified only later. Bacterium *Neisseria gonorrhoeae* was recognized as causing gonorrhea in 1879. The identification of the causative agent of syphilis (the bacterium *Treponema pallidum*) did not occur until 1905. Concurrently with that discovery, salvarsan was developed as a relatively effective arsenic-based treatment. At about the same time the definitive Wasserman blood test made it possible to identify the bacterium. Only in the 1940s did penicillin appear as a truly effective means of combating both syphilis and gonorrhea (Aufderheide and Rodríguez-Martín 1998:157–64; Ortner 2003:278–97; Powell and Cook 2005:20–24). Until then a gonorrhea or syphilis diagnosis constituted a lifetime sentence. Treatment of those diseases in the nineteenth century involved managing symptoms rather than curing the ailment. This strategy compares to treating incurable HIV/AIDS today. Before presenting the impact of STIs on the Seventh Cavalry, the two STIs diseases are described.

SYPHILIS

Venereal syphilis is the first of the two STIs recognized in the nineteenth century. It appears in two forms: acquired venereal syphilis and congenital syphilis. Only the first form is relevant here.

Acquired venereal syphilis spreads by sexual interaction. Following contact with syphilis, a three-week incubation period occurs. Then the first symptoms of syphilis appear, usually consisting of painless lesions (chancres). Once chancres emerge—most commonly on the genitals—they persist for three to six weeks. Then they disappear. For the next six to eight weeks a period of quiescence occurs as the bacteria disseminate to other anatomical locations and provide a foundation for the next symptoms. At that point a skin rash and/or mucus membrane inflammation may happen. These symptoms continue for two to four weeks, followed by a second, longer and more variable period of dormancy.

About one to ten years after initial infection the tertiary phase of venereal syphilis may commence. This stage is eclectic in its expression and anatomical distribution. Many different anatomical systems may be affected. Organs of the skeletal, cardiovascular, and nervous systems constitute the most vulnerable ones, but there are many other targets. Until diagnostic laboratory tests developed, diagnosis of syphilis in this third phase remained fickle. Hence earlier physicians dubbed syphilis the "great imitator." It mimicked the symptoms of many other diseases, proving difficult to diagnose. As if that chameleon characteristic of the disease were not bad enough, some infected people showed no symptoms and unknowingly spread the disease to their partners.

In the nosology of the day nineteenth-century military surgeons identified syphilis in Class Zymotic and Order Enthetic, noting whether it was primary or constitutional syphilis. In their usage, both secondary and tertiary phases seem to be included in their constitutional category.

Nineteenth-century treatment of venereal syphilis included administration of a variety of herbal remedies and small doses of mercury. Mercurial treatment often involved oral administration as well as employing salves placed directly on the chancres. Such management continued until the patient's gums became painful and tender. At that point mercury administration ceased until the detrimental conditions moderated. When symptoms did ameliorate, treatment began again and continued until the associated complaints reappeared (Chuinard 1979:134). Mercury was an ineffective treatment for most syphilis victims. Its uselessness gave rise to the saying "A night with Venus, a lifetime with mercury." It was an important adage but often ignored by young men.

The distribution of the disease in a population (epidemiology) is an important consideration. Syphilis infection peaks in early adulthood (twenty to twenty-five years), when people tend to be most sexually active. The rate of venereal syphilis infection in pre-antibiotic days was estimated to be between 5 to 10 percent in urban areas (Aufderheide and Rodríguez-Martín 1998:157–64; Ortner

2003:278–97; Powell and Cook 2005:20–24). And the infection frequency of some groups was much greater. For instance, some California Civil War troops had syphilis rates as high as 50 percent (Murphy 1985).

GONORRHEA

Gonorrhea was the other STI recognized in the nineteenth century. Here the modal course of the disease is provided first, followed by nineteenth-century treatment of its symptoms and nineteenth-century military nosology and epidemiology.

The earliest symptoms of gonorrhea appear two to five days after contact. Primary complaints usually involve inflammation of the urethra. Females often experience a burning sensation while urinating or an abnormal vaginal discharge. Males may complain of a urethral discharge of fluids or a burning sensation while urinating. But many infected people show no symptoms. After this initial stage gonorrhea may spread to the cervix or prostate or follow the reproductive structures upstream, affecting other associated organs. Gonorrhea may also cause inflammation in systems other than reproductive structures, such as synovitis.

To treat the symptoms of gonorrhea during the nineteenth century the urethra was irrigated with solutions. In the early nineteenth century such concoctions included saccharum saturni (sugar of lead, lead acetate) and balsam of copaiba (Chuinard 1979:159) as well as saltpeter (Chuinard 1979:156). Later in the nineteenth century treatments incorporated mercury and silver nitrate. They continued to be used until effective antibiotics developed in the 1940s.

Gonorrhea shows similar age-related epidemiological incidences as syphilis. In the United States it is most frequent among sexually active young adults, usually fifteen to twenty-nine (Communicable Disease Center 2012). So by age, occupation, and period the post–Civil War Seventh Cavalry young adult males represented a group especially vulnerable to STIs.

Seventh Cavalry surgeons documented the presence of gonorrhea in medical records. In their nosology they identified it in Class Zymotic and in Order Enthetic. They noted whether it was "plain" gonorrhea or more exactly identified the symptoms, such as inflamed testes (gonorrheal orchitis), a severe, pus-producing inflammation of the eye (gonorrheal ophthalmia), or narrowed urethra (gonorrheal stricture).

Methods

Using those nineteenth-century military categories as well as other diagnoses attributed to these diseases, the Seventh Cavalry data base was searched for diagnoses indicating STIs. Listings included bladder infections (when attributed to gonorrhea), buboes (when secondarily identified as syphilic, gonorrheal, or venereal), chancres, chancroids, enlarged inguinal glands (when attributed to gonorrhea), gleet, gonorrhea, iritis (when attributed to syphilis), ophthalmia (when attributed to gonorrhea), orchitis (when attributed to gonorrhea or syphilis), urethra stricture (when associated with gonorrhea), syphilis, ulcers (when attributed to syphilis of mouth), locomotor ataxia (thought to be associated with tertiary syphilis), and rheumatism (when associated with syphilis). Other illnesses that could be less certainly attributed to STIs were excluded from this analysis.

Results

Seventh Cavalry medical records were analyzed for evidence of the manifestation and distribution of syphilis and gonorrhea. This section also considers distributions of STIs by time, space, nativity, age, height, and rank.

SYPHILIS

Among the nearly 1,000 STI complaints in the Seventh Cavalry medical records, almost 60% documented syphilis (n = 585; some discussed below have multiple specifications and identifications). More than 40% of the syphilis diagnoses indicated the primary stage (n = 256). In addition, some records showed chancres or chancroids (n = 13), often the first symptom of syphilis. About a third of the syphilis complaints identified ongoing progress of the disease. Some syphilis records documented secondary syphilis

(n = 21), and more indicated constitutional or tertiary syphilis (n = 169). A scattering of the other marginal comments mentioned syphilitic buboes (n = 8), rheumatism (n = 4), ulcer (n = 3), iritis (n = 3), and periostitis and orchitis (n = 1 each). The other nearly 20% of the syphilis diagnoses lacked qualifying details, remaining unstated and unspecified.

GONORRHEA

Gonorrhea constituted nearly of all of the other 40% of STI records (n = 392). The vast majority of the gonorrhea records lacked additional details, remaining unstated, unqualified, and unspecific. Among the minority gonorrheal records that included marginal notes, the greatest number indicated orchitis (n = 68), stricture of the urethra (n = 14), buboes (n = 5), gleet (n = 2), and ophthalmia (n = 1).

OTHER

In addition to the syphilis and gonorrhea accounts, a solitary record noted a "venereal bubo" without further elaboration.

All STIs (syphilis, gonorrhea, and venereal bubo) are combined in the following sections, which examine STIs by time, geographical location, nativity, enlistment age, height, and rank.

TEMPORAL DISTRIBUTIONS

The STI complaints remained fairly constant during the shorter time intervals (months and seasons) but not the longer one (annual). On a monthly basis (table 9.1), STIs fell evenly, averaging 81.2 each month. The greatest number occurred in February (n = 100) and fewest in May (n = 63). On a seasonal basis (table 9.2) temporal uniformity continued. The seasons averaged 243.5 STIs, with the greater incidences in fall (n = 265) and winter (n = 250) and lower numbers in spring (n = 229) and summer (n = 230).

Despite the poet's claim: "In the Spring a young man's fancy lightly turns to thoughts of love" (Alfred, Lord Tennyson's "Locksley Hall"), spring did not have such an effect in the

TABLE 9.1. Monthly STIs in post–Civil War Seventh Cavalry

Month	*Number*	*Percentage*
January	73	7.5
February	100	10.3
March	89	9.1
April	77	7.9
May	63	6.5
June	80	8.2
July	83	8.5
August	67	6.9
September	82	8.4
October	96	9.9
November	87	8.9
December	77	7.9
Total	974	100.0

Note: Three medical records lack admission dates and are omitted from this summary.

TABLE 9.2. Seasonal STIs in post–Civil War Seventh Cavalry

Season	*Number*	*Percentage*
Spring	229	23.5
Summer	230	23.6
Fall	265	27.2
Winter	250	25.7
Total	974	100.0

Note: Three medical records lack admission dates and are omitted from this summary.

nineteenth-century Seventh Cavalry, at least as indicated by STI frequencies. Spring had the fewest STIs of any season.

Unlike monthly and seasonal STI occurrences, annual incidences of STIs displayed marked differences (table 9.3, fig. 9.2). They averaged about 55.7 cases/year (excluding the partial year 1866). The fewest instances of STIs happened in 1874 (n = 19), followed closely by 1869 (n = 21). The greatest number of STI complaints were sandwiched in 1871 (n = 140) and 1872 (n = 112).

TABLE 9.3. Annual STIs in post-Civil War Seventh Cavalry

Year	*Frequency*	*Percent*
1866	26	2.7
1867	58	5.9
1868	77	7.9
1869	21	2.2
1870	37	3.8
1871	140	14.3
1872	112	11.5
1873	93	9.5
1874	19	1.9
1875	61	6.3
1876	55	5.6
1877	27	2.8
1878	53	5.4
1879	47	4.8
1880	26	2.7
1881	48	4.9
1882	34	3.5
1883	39	4.0
Total	973	99.7
Missing System	3	.3
Total	976	100.0

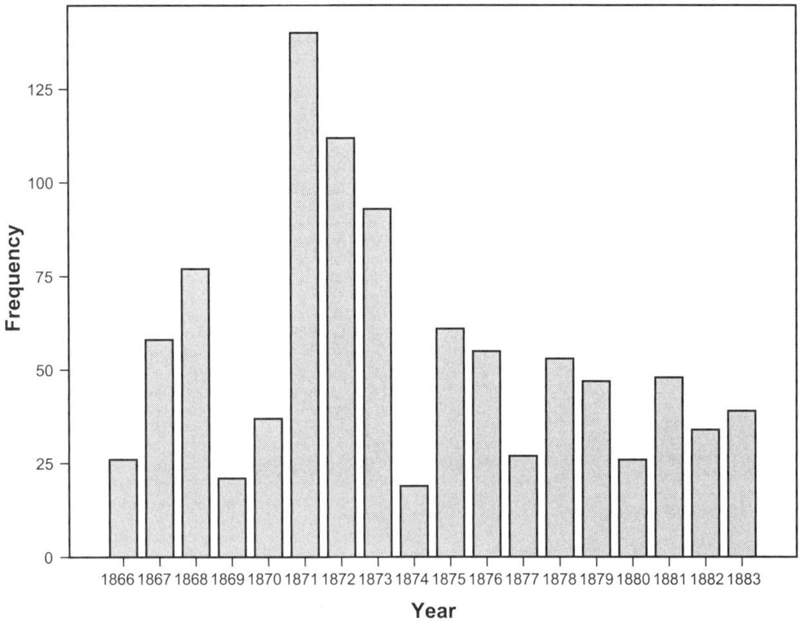

9.2. Annual frequency of sexually transmitted infections (STIs) in post–Civil War Seventh Cavalry. Note lows in 1869 and 1874 and highs in 1871 and 1872.

That greatest frequency amounted to more than seven times the lowest count. What was special about 1871 and 1872?

POSTING REGION

Posting locations hold the explanation to the temporal spike. In the post–Civil War period the Seventh Cavalry was first stationed in the central plains (part of 1866 to 1870), followed by assignment in the South (1871 to 1873), and finally transferred to the northern plains (1873 to the end of the study period).

Taking those locations in chronological order (table 9.4, fig. 9.3), the central plains had a relatively infrequent STI annual average (approximately 55 records per year). STI complaints in the south spiked (averaging approximately 125 per year). And in the northern plains STI diagnoses dropped even below those of the central plains (averaging approximately 32 per year). The annual STI rate in the

TABLE 9.4. Geographic location of STIs in post–Civil War Seventh Cavalry

Geographic locations	*Frequency*	*Percent*
Central plains	246	25.2
South	348	35.6
Northern plains	351	35.9
Other and undesignated	32	3.3
Total	977	100.0

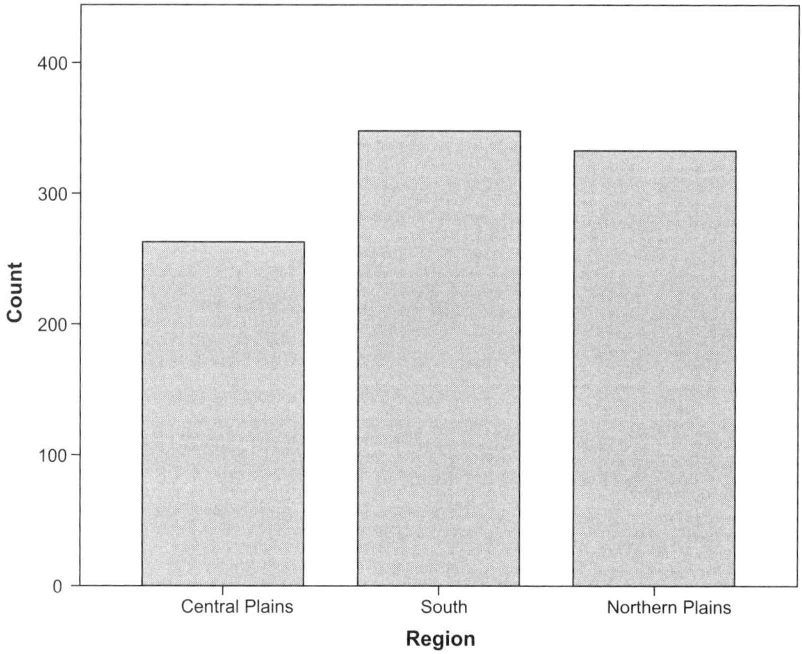

9.3. Distribution of STIs in the post–Civil War Seventh Cavalry by geographic location. Note that this chart distorts annual average STI records because the Seventh Cavalry was posted in the central plains for about four and a half years, in the South for less than three years, and in the northern plains for a decade. So the average annual STI rate was greatest in the South and less in the central and northern plains.

South amounted to more than double that in either of the other two posting regions. This irregular distribution begs for an explanation.

While stationed in the south troopers probably had greater access to sexual contacts than when posted in the plains. The South was a more developed region with a denser population during the Reconstruction period than the plains. In contrast, both the central and northern plains retained frontier-like characteristics, including less settled, smaller populations and probably fewer potential sexual partners. Plains postings were described as a "chain of bachelor communities strung out across the West" (Butler 1985:126), thus minimizing heterosexual opportunities.

BIRTHPLACE

Among the STI sufferers, 573 included enlistment information concerning nativity. Comparing foreign-born and native-born soldiers with and without STI records, the distribution displays statistical significance ($\chi^2 = 5.59$, df = 1, $0.025 > p > 0.01$). Foreign-born soldiers reported STIs more frequently than native-born soldiers. Perhaps foreign-born soldiers took greater risks than U.S.-born soldiers. The native-born vs. foreign-born STI rates differed, but what about troopers within those groups?

Within the list of U.S.-born enlistees, the three states with the most enlistees and most STI cases (New York, Ohio, and Pennsylvania) were examined. No differences in proportions of STIs occurred among troopers from those three states. For the three foreign countries with the greatest number of enlistees and STIs (England, Germany, and Ireland), the distribution approaches—but does not achieve—statistical significance ($\chi^2 = 5.16$, df = 2, $0.10 > p > 0.05$). Germans reported proportionally fewer STI cases and Irish more. So the only nativity difference in STI frequencies indicated that foreign-born troopers were more likely to report STIs than U.S.-born troopers.

AGE AT ENLISTMENT

Were young soldiers more likely to show STI symptoms than older men? Did youth and its associated increased testosterone produce reckless moments?

To see if those stereotypes hold for the post–Civil War Seventh Cavalry we examined the age at enlistment for troopers reporting STIs and those not reporting them. There was a difference ($t = -5.514$, df = 752.688, $p < 0.000$, two-tailed test, equal variances not assumed). Younger men tended to have a higher STI rate than older men, although the difference between means was only about one year (STI mean age = 23.6884 years, without STI mean age = 24.5952 years).

HEIGHT AND RANK

Using the enlistment records we also examined the relationship of STIs, height measured at enlistment, and rank at completion of service period. Stature differences between troopers with and without STIs was not statistically significant ($t = -0.745$, df =705.093, $p = 0.457$, two-tailed, equal variances not assumed). Size apparently did not matter, at least in terms of contracting STIs.

Rank recorded at the conclusion of the trooper's enlistment period provided a means of assessing whether enlisted men's military status affected STI frequencies. All three ranks (senior noncommissioned officers, junior noncommissioned officers, and rankers) had the same STI frequencies ($\chi^2 = 3.84$, df=2, $0.25 > p > 0.10$). Rank apparently did not have its privileges among the post–Civil War Seventh Cavalry enlistees, at least in terms of STIs.

Discussion

Like other ailments, STIs showed patterns by time, place, and trooper characteristics among the post–Civil War Seventh Cavalry enlisted men. These results, however, were based on some assumptions that may have caused distortions. We consider first those assumptions then STI severity.

ASSUMPTIONS

It is tempting to believe the numbers presented in the results section under-represented the actual incidence of STIs among the post–Civil War Seventh Cavalry. Several lines of reasoning support this, including (1) STIs masked by symptoms and not identified by surgeons as STI-caused, (2) STIs recognized but deemphasized in diagnoses, (3) STIs not reported to the surgeon because sufferers ignored or self-medicated, and (4) STIs present but lacking symptoms.

First, STI symptoms might not have been associated with venereal diseases by surgeons. But they were venereal nonetheless. Recall that adoption of the germ theory and definitive tests for gonorrhea remained embryonic until late in the study period. In these medical records diagnosis was based on symptoms.

Examples of additional symptoms that may have indicated STIs but were not noted as such in medical records include abscesses of the scrotum, inflammation of testicles, debility, heart disease, herpes and other skin diseases, synovitis, ecthyma, dysuria, prostatitis, and retention of urine. And these symptoms were not the only ones. Some urethral strictures and buboes were identified as gonorrheal or syphilitic, and others as nongonorrheal or nonsyphilitic. But some urethral strictures and buboes went unqualified. Thus they may have represented STIs but necessarily were excluded here based on lack of further documentation.

Second (and related to the first possibility), the surgeon may have recognized STI symptoms but excluded them from the diagnosis, considering them of lesser or secondary importance. As an example, in July 1881, Private Henry Haack was diagnosed with melancholia and transferred to the Government Asylum for the Insane. Buried in the secondary notes is surgeon R. J. Hill's comment: "There is also a history of Syphilis of many years duration." Possibly Haack suffered from tertiary neurosphyilis, causing his mental derangement. But none of Haack's other three medical records mention syphilis. So using medical records that emphasized a primary diagnosis may have masked the causative STI in Haack's case as well as in others.

Third, some troopers probably ignored symptoms or self-medicated for STIs. As a consequence the symptoms did not come to the surgeon's attention and of course went undocumented in the medical records.

Finally, some STI-infected victims may have lacked symptoms—the STI "Typhoid Marys" of the Seventh Cavalry. Take gonorrhea as an example. Asymptomatic gonorrheal rates vary tremendously, depending on the group being tested. Asymptomatic gonorrhea victims ranged from as low as 0.2% in a twentieth-century male military sample, through 14% in a small sample of males visiting a venereal disease clinic, to a high of 26% in males with recent contact with infected partners (summarized in Thatcher et al. 1969). Without STI symptoms nineteenth-century physicians would not have diagnosed STIs.

Based on these four lines of evidence, the Seventh Cavalry STI rates presented here appear to be a minimum figure. The actual frequencies of STIs may have been much greater than represented.

But the Seventh Cavalry medical records may have over-represented the number of infected soldiers. Many of the STIs recorded appeared to be ongoing cases and development of a single infection, not new infections. Of the total number of STI cases (n = 976), the majority of instances (n = 504, 51.6%) involved recidivists. Of the 201 individuals with multiple entries (table 9.5), most repeaters had 2 cases (n = 130, 64.7%); the greatest number for a single person consisted of 6 cases (n = 1, 0.50%).

For those histories with enough information and detail, three possibilities existed (note, however, that more than half of the histories lack such details).

First, serial STIs may have resulted from the same infective event, representing development of an infection during a few days or weeks ($n \sim 30$). These records showed no apparent major

TABLE 9.5. Post–Civil War Seventh Cavalry members with two or more records of STIs

Number of repeat STIs by individual	*Frequency*	*Percent*
2	130	64.7
3	47	23.4
4	20	10.0
5	3	1.5
6	1	.5
Total	201	100.0

development of the disease course. Some serial primary syphilis records probably demonstrated ongoing symptoms of a single infection, documented in multiple medical records within a few days or weeks of one another.

Second, in other instances the same recidivist suffered different infections ($n \sim 80$), clearly indicating different infectious events. As an example, a gonorrheal infection in one record might be followed by primary syphilis in a later record, demonstrating that the trooper suffered two separate infections. These infections clearly were different diseases caused by different inoculations.

Third, some serial STI records may have represented continuing, developing symptoms from a single infection over longer periods ($n \sim 110$). As an example, primary syphilis could have developed over weeks or months into secondary and then tertiary syphilis. Many records of constitutional syphilis probably documented the ongoing progress of the disease without reinfection.

So, according to this contrary line of evidence, STI recidivists suggest inflation in STI counts, not under-representation as claimed earlier. Based on these two conflicting perspectives it is unclear whether the medical records demonstrated over-representation or under-representation of Seventh Cavalry STI rates. Probably both. But how these conflicting processes impacted the records and our understanding of STIs is unclear due to lack of requisite diagnostic details.

Could the last explanation for STI inflated rates (continuing syphilitic infections) explain the spike in STIs in the South contrasted with STI frequencies found in the central and northern plains? Should the region be renamed the "Syphilitic South"?

To test that suggestion proportions of the two diseases (gonorrhea and syphilis) were compared by posting regions (central plains, South, and northern plains). That distribution was statistically significant ($\chi^2 = 13.13$, df = 2, $0.005 > p > 0.001$), but not in the predicted direction. The gonorrhea-syphilis ratio in the South was about what would be expected by the overall frequencies. The central plains, in contrast, showed high rates of syphilis, while the northern plains had high incidences of gonorrhea. So ongoing, developing syphilis symptoms do not explain the high rates of STIs in the South.

SEVERITY

How severe were the STI diseases? Some were severe enough to terminate enlistment periods before normal expiration of service dates. At least eleven services ended due to STI disability. But considering all terminations of service due to disabilities, few identified STI as the reason (2.1 percent). As ubiquitous and problematic as STIs were among the post–Civil War Seventh Cavalry troops, few such diseases terminated service early.

Of course other reasons for disability dismissal may have involved venereal disease. These may have included urethra stricture, testicle inflammation, and bladder inflammation, but they lacked STI details in the enlistment termination information. So as it stands STIs apparently caused a small loss of men and potential service.

One particularly severe STI case and its treatment is noteworthy. Private Henry Lehman of Company I was diagnosed with a venereal disease by acting assistant surgeon James B. Ferguson at Fort Totten. Lehman first underwent treatment for venereal disease on March 12, 1874. The doctor noted that the disease had originated years earlier, before Lehman emigrated from Germany. Suffering with pain through his chest and shoulders, Lehman was admitted to the hospital with a large node on the front of the sternum. He was placed on a mercurial course of treatment alternating with large doses of potassium iodide and tonics. The node was opened and contained purulent matter. An attempt was made to heal it from inside-out with the potassium iodide and tonics. Apparently the treatment was successful, because Lehman returned to duty on April 13.

Lehman later accompanied the Northern Boundary Expedition and was readmitted to the hospital in September when he returned to his post with the old symptoms in an aggravated form. Ferguson diagnosed a tumor of the sternum as large as a closed fist that fluctuated to the touch. An incision was made with a sharp-pointed bistoury through the tumor down to the bone. In some places the bone was found to be soft and carious, and a raspatory was used to remove the superficial softened layer. The inside of the tumor was painted with a strong solution of carbolic acid and packed with lint saturated in a weaker solution of the same. The chest was painted with tincture of iodine. Lehman was placed on a treatment course of corrosive chloride of mercury in combination with potassium chloride and extract of Geuhaud. Ferguson noted that he believed the mercury treatment to be the best in such cases and that it was well proven (NARA, Medical History of Fort Totten, RG 94, vol. 48). Today such a treatment is known to cause heavy metal toxicity in patients. In any case Lehman's disease terminated with his death on June 25, 1876, at the Battle of the Little Bighorn, not from the infection.

In conclusion, we should be mindful that during the nineteenth-century STI diagnoses constituted lifetime sentences. Some men carried STIs into service when they enlisted. Other troopers acquired them during service. But whether they were infected before enlistment or during service, all STIs persisted into their postmilitary lives.

Summary

This chapter presents sources of STIs, kinds of STIs recognized in the nineteenth century, their temporal and regional variation in the Seventh Cavalry, and differences in trooper rates by nativity, age, height, and rank.

Various sources for sex (and STIs) were available. They included laundresses, prostitutes, and Indian women. Of course the transmissions of STIs were not unidirectional. Troopers were vectors as well as recipients of infections.

Some sexual contacts resulted in STIs, two of which were recognized in the nineteenth century: syphilis and gonorrhea. Syphilis constituted approximately 60 percent of the Seventh Cavalry's STI diagnoses and gonorrhea the other 40 percent.

The number of STI diagnoses varied depending on time and place. Monthly and seasonal STI rates fell flat, showing no temporal differences. But annual STI rates fluctuated wildly. The lowest annual counts occurred in 1869 and 1874, the highest in 1871 and 1872. Those years with the greatest STI frequencies corresponded with the shorter time that the Seventh Cavalry spent in the South.

The lower counts came while the Seventh Cavalry occupied the central and northern plains.

Differences in STIs by nativity and age were found. Foreign-born troopers suffered more frequent STIs than U.S.-born Seventh Cavalry members. And younger troopers displayed more frequent STIs than older ones. No height or rank differences in STI proportions were evident.

CHAPTER 10

Cold Injuries in the Seventh Cavalry

Katie Cohan

As the American Civil War came to an end, the hardships of serving in the nineteenth century United States military continued. When the war ended in 1865, the public wearied of conflict. This sentiment had an effect on military funding. Congress appropriated funds for a reduced military, and army provisions issued by the Quartermaster Department were tolerable and meager at best. Thus the men of the post–Civil War army, including the newly formed Seventh Cavalry, often faced extreme weather conditions with inadequate equipment. Cold injuries (or frostbite injuries) were common afflictions. "Cold injury" refers to bodily damage from exposure to cold temperatures, primarily affecting the extremities and parts of the face. Frostbite only occurs at temperatures below freezing, although exposure time and temperature vary from person to person and from one circumstance to the next (Giesbrecht and Wilkerson 2006:74).

Methods and Materials

A cold injury data set was established for the Seventh Cavalry and analyzed to determine intrinsic and extrinsic factors associated with frostbite injuries. To establish a cold injury list, the post–Civil

War Seventh Cavalry health records (see chapters 4 and 5) were transferred into Excel 2007 and the cold injury cases listed in the Carded Medical Records were extracted. Trooper identification numbers were matched with Enlistment Register data: complexion, stature, nativity, rank, and other biographical information. Among the thousands of medical complaint records, 227 individuals experienced cold injuries. Many troopers experienced multiple instances of cold injury, and some had multiple enlistment periods. To approximate the individuals' status at the time, the Enlistment Register information used for these troopers came from the enlistment period when the individual experienced the cold injury. The data were further assessed using PASW Statistics 18 (SPSS 2009). Only the cold injuries recorded in the health records were employed in this study. Some minor frostbite cases undoubtedly were self-treated and were never reported to the surgeon. These other cases can only be learned from anecdotal sources. Such sources were excluded from the cold injury statistical analysis but were considered to amplify the narrative discussion.

Additional explanations are needed concerning complexions and their analysis. Enlistment Records note the complexion (color and appearance of skin) of each trooper. Table 10.1 presents terms used to describe the Seventh Cavalry troopers' complexions. The definitions of those terms are assessments, compiled after reviewing definitions in Webster's *Third New International Dictionary* (Gove 2002).

Table 10.2 shows that some complexions were more frequent among the troopers than others. Nearly half of the men had fair complexions (43.9%), while 23.5 percent had dark complexions. The majority of enlisted men had one or the other of these two complexions (67.4%).

For analytical purposes complexions were combined into a few categories. Most individuals were lightly pigmented (56.9%), while 23.6% were darkly pigmented (table 10.3). A small percentage (1.1%) had medium pigmentation, and 18.4% had complexions for which pigmentation levels could not be categorized. Individuals with undetermined pigmentation levels were excluded from consideration in the complexion analysis.

TABLE 10.1. Complexion terms and descriptions

Complexion term	*Definition*
Black	Very dark in color
Brown	Not excessively dark or light in color, dusky or intermediate in hue
Dark	Brown or close to black in color
Fair	Light in color
Florid	Reddish or rosy in color
Freckled	Having a noticeable amount of freckles on the skin
Fresh	Appearing healthy or youthful in complexion
Fush	Possibly a misspelling of fuchsia, meaning purplish-red in color Also possibly a misspelling of fresh (Seventh Cavalry Codebook)
Light	Of a light hue in color
Medium	Not excessively dark or light in color, intermediate in hue
Olive	Dull greenish-yellow
Pale	Light in color, lacking color
Pockmarked	Having small scars or pits on the skin
Red	Reddish in color
Robust	Appearing healthy or strong
Ruddy	Healthy or reddish in color, possibly feverish
Sallow	Sickly yellowish in color
Sandy	Light yellow to brown in color
Sulley	Possibly a misspelling of sully, meaning soiled or dirty Also possibly a misspelling of sallow (Seventh Cavalry Codebook)
White	Very light in color, lacking color

Source: After Cohan 2011:44, table 6.

TABLE 10.2. Frequencies of complexions in post–Civil War Seventh Cavalry troopers

Complexion	*Frequency*	*Percent*	*Percent present*
White	5	0.1	0.1
Pale	1	0.0	0.0
Fair	2960	36.5	43.9
Light	874	10.8	13.0
Sandy	45	0.6	0.7
Medium	22	0.3	0.3
Brown	9	0.1	0.1
Dark	1588	19.6	23.5
Black	4	0.0	0.1
Olive	2	0.0	0.0
Ruddy	901	11.1	13.4
Red	1	0.0	0.0
Florid	189	2.3	2.8
Fuchsia	12	0.1	0.2
Sallow	111	1.4	1.6
Robust	2	0.0	0.0
Fresh	13	0.2	0.2
Sulley	5	0.1	0.1
Freckled	1	0.0	0.0
Pockmarked	1	0.0	0.0
Total	6746	83.1	100.0
Missing	1373	16.9	
Total	8119	100.0	

Source: After Cohan 2011:64, table 23.
Notes: Percent: The percentage of total entries in this category, including individuals lacking information ("Missing" row).
Percent present: The percentage of total entries in this category, not including missing data. This percentage best represents the information because it only accounts for entries with available data.

TABLE 10.3. Categories of complexions in post–Civil War Seventh Cavalry employed in cold injury analysis

Complexion category	*Frequency*	*Percent*	*Percent present*
Lightly pigmented	3840	47.3	56.9
Medium pigmented	76	0.9	1.1
Darkly pigmented	1592	19.6	23.6
Pigmentation level unclear	1238	15.2	18.4
Total	6746	83.1	100.0
Data N/A	1373	16.9	
Total	8119	100.0	

Source: After Cohan 2011:64, table 24.
Notes: Percent: The percentage of total entries in this category.
Percent present: The percentage of total entries in this category, not including missing data. This percentage best represents the information because it only accounts for entries with available data.

Background

Before discussing the factors related to cold injuries, this section reviews the geographical location of the Seventh Cavalrymen. During the study period, the regiment occupied three regions. From 1866 through 1873 the Seventh Cavalry was stationed on the central plains and in the South. Even in late spring troopers were exposed to freezing temperatures and harsh weather conditions on the plains. In the spring of 1873 the regiment moved to the northern plains, where winters were long and brutal. From 1873 through the early 1880s cavalrymen dealt with these conditions, resulting in many cold injuries. Table 10.4 shows posting locations where cold injuries occurred among Seventh Cavalry troopers.

At these locations troopers were exposed to the elements when on guard duty, march, and campaign. Figure 10.1 depicts cattle in a blizzard on the Colorado Plains in the late 1800s. Many cavalrymen endured similar unforgiving conditions while on campaign, often lacking adequate gear and shelter.

TABLE 10.4. Regions and posts of post–Civil War Seventh Cavalry cold injuries

Region	*State/territory (post)*
Central plains	Colorado (Fort Lyon)
	Kansas (Fort Dodge, Fort Harker, Fort Hays, Fort Leavenworth, Fort Riley, Fort Wallace)
	Nebraska (Camp Sheridan, Fort Kearney)
	Indian Territory (Camp Supply)
Northern plains	Dakota Territory (Field, Fort Abercrombie, Fort Abraham Lincoln, Fort Buford, Fort Meade, Fort Rice, Fort Seward, Fort Totten, Fort Yates, Standing Rock–Sioux Reservation)
	Montana (Camp Poplar River)
South	Kentucky (Taylor Barracks)
Other	"Field"

Source: After Cohan 2011:11, table 2.

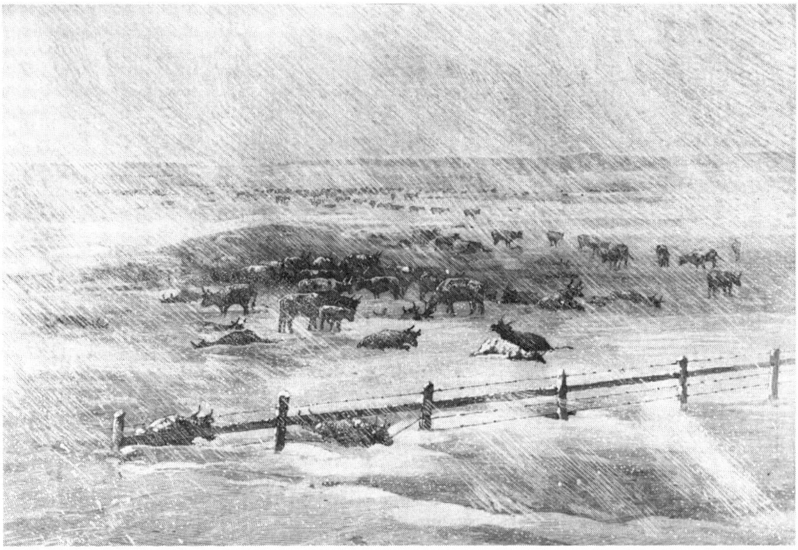

10.1. *Cattle in a Blizzard on the Plains* shows cattle enduring a severe storm. Source: Drawing by Charles Graham from a sketch by H. Worrall in 1886. Courtesy Department of the Denver Public Library Western History and Genealogy Department, Call no. Z-156.

The Post–Civil War Army Uniform

The first line of defense against cold is clothing. The military uniform exemplifies a cultural adaptation to changing environments. From the 1860s through the 1870s, however, the gear issued to soldiers failed to provide adequate protection from cold injuries, especially for men stationed in Dakota Territory (McChristian 1995:23). To understand the effects of cold exposure, it is necessary to recognize how these uniforms made soldiers vulnerable to the cold.

By the 1870s military opinion was divided regarding what uniforms and equipment the army needed. Surplus uniforms from the Civil War were issued to postwar troopers. Knee-length sky-blue kersey coats were also issued to help protect the body from cold. Officers wore long overcoats called cloak coats. Cavalrymen were also issued capes that ended at the wrist with body linings of various materials, such as burlap or flannel. For extra protection the body lining and overcoats included cuffs that could be extended over the hands as mittens. For additional protection members of the Seventh Cavalry started to line their overcoats with wool blankets. In 1871 blanket-lined overcoats began to be issued to posts above 42° latitude (McChristian 1995:21–23).

Flaws in many of these materials, overlooked during wartime, were noted in the peacetime military. In 1867 Corporal Cyrus Reed highlighted the difficulties of marching in Wyoming: "The ice across the Platte was not strong enough to hold us, so we broke the ice with the butts of our muskets and forded the river up to our arm pits in the icy water. A few days later, we staggered into Fort Laramie, that is what was left of us, our feet wrapped in our torn blankets, as our shoes were gone" (Rickey 1963:256).

Based on these inadequacies, troopers often modified army gear to mitigate extreme temperatures on the plains (McChristian 1995). Soldiers working in temperatures below zero often donned as much clothing as possible while attempting to maintain mobility. Captain Simon Snyder documented the difficulties of staying warm in November 1876:

> I am now wearing two flannel and a buckskin shirt, one pair of drawers, trousers of buckskin and a pair of army

> trousers, two pairs woolen socks, a pair of buffalo overshoes and big boots, a heavy pair of blanket leggings, a thick blouse and heavy overcoat, a heavy woolen cap that completely covers my head, face and neck except nose and eyes and still I am not happy . . . when I am all fixed out I am a sight to behold and have all I can do to mount my horse. (Rickey 1963:256–57)

Some soldiers added their own alterations, while others found or purchased extra gear, such as buffalo or bear fur coats. In 1876 Second Lieutenant Henry H. Bellas, near Fort Reno, Wyoming, described extra gear and modifications made: "Frozen noses, fingers and feet were general. The old buffalo robes which we had taken from the Cheyenne village, were cut up and made into shoes, leggings and caps, to afford protection from this truly Arctic weather" (Greene 1993:184).

In the early 1870s buffalo hide overshoes began to be issued at posts in the north, but they did not always keep the feet dry. These overshoes kept the soldiers' feet warm in dry conditions, but in wet conditions they made things worse. When wet, or even damp, the overshoes could cause the feet to freeze (McChristian 1995:77). Many troopers bought additional shoes or improvised gear by covering their feet with materials such as burlap. In the 1860s inadequate winter headgear was provided, so some soldiers purchased their own heavy caps. Others added earflaps to their forage caps.

In the late 1870s official uniforms began to be altered to minimize cold exposure. In 1876 a sturdier kersey overcoat was issued. This same year new arctic overshoes were distributed. Made of vulcanized rubber, these overshoes were waterproof and much easier to dry than buffalo overshoes. Woolen mittens were also issued. In 1877 buffalo overcoats were sent to northern posts. In 1878 muskrat caps and gauntlet gloves began to be used. Some men started to use felt boots, although this footgear was short-lived because the boots had limitations similar to those of the buffalo overshoes (McChristian 1995:174–77, 2007:170–77). Figure 10.2 shows band members (not Seventh Cavalrymen) at Fort Keogh donning the aforementioned buffalo overcoats, muskrat caps, and arctic overshoes.

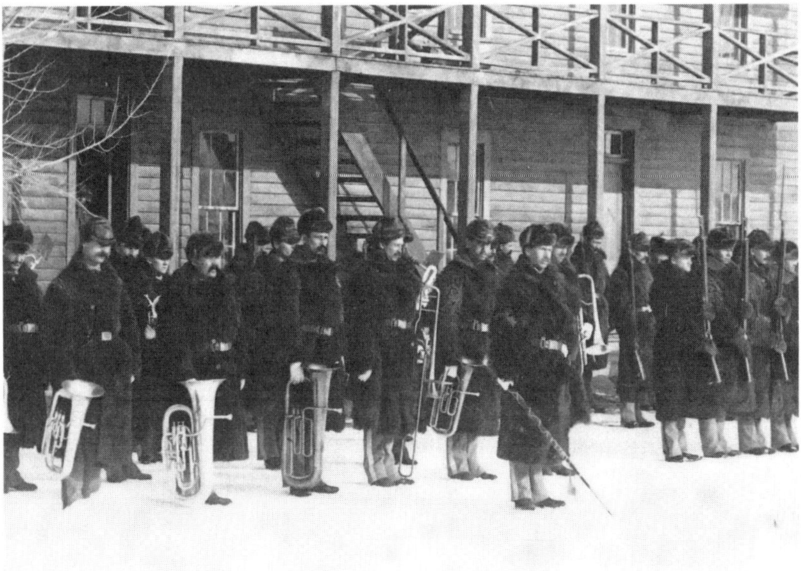

10.2. Band members at Fort Keogh, Montana Territory, wearing buffalo overcoats, muskrat caps, and arctic overshoes. Courtesy of Little Bighorn Battlefield National Monument, National Park Service, Bowen_749A, public domain image.

Following the sharp decline in buffalo herds by the early 1880s, other materials had to be used for winter uniforms. The Miles Overcoat, named for General Nelson A. Miles, consisted of blue canvas with a flannel lining. Cords drew the cape tight around the head and neck. A canvas belt around the waist maintained warmth. The 1883 Miles Overcoat was made of brown duck with a canvas belt (McChristian 2007:170–77), the last major innovation during our study period.

After the Civil War many uniform changes were available in limited quantities, so not all members of the Seventh Cavalry may have been issued the same protective clothing. Because gear and equipment were gradually altered for better cold protection during this period, however, it was hypothesized that cold injury levels decreased over time from improvements in material efficacy and greater attention to clothing quality. This hypothesis is discussed further below.

Harsh Weather and Inadequate Gear

During the period of study, many campaigns were conducted in the winter months to catch immobilized tribes by surprise. For instance, the Seventh Cavalry fought the Battle of the Washita, in present-day Oklahoma, during November 1868 (Hoig 1979). Even in times of relative calm the weather on the plains required caution. Elizabeth B. Custer (1885:104), wife of Lieutenant Colonel Custer, described the daily life of the Seventh Cavalry on the northern plains in the 1870s in her journal:

> The weather seemed to grow colder and colder as the winter advanced—from 20° to 30° below zero was ordinary weather. . . . When the thermometer went down to 45° below zero, the utmost vigilance was exercised to prevent the men from being frozen. The general took off all the sentinels but two, and those were encased in buffalo overcoats and shoes, and required to walk their beat but fifteen minutes at a time.

The temperature could reach such extreme lows that available technology ceased to function. General Miles included descriptions of the weather and thermometer readings in his notes:

> During the winter campaigns of 1876 and '77 all the mercurial thermometers we had with us were frozen solid. The following winter a spirit thermometer registered between 55 and 60° below. . . . Even when the air was perfectly still and all the moisture of the atmosphere was frozen, the air was filled with little frozen jets, or shining crystals. . . . The [men] made woolen masks that covered the entire head . . . and nearly all had buffalo overcoats. This command of more than four hundred men looked more like a large body of Esquimaux than like . . . United States soldiers. (Miles 1969:218–19)

Because of these conditions cold injuries were frequent in the post–Civil War army on the plains. Besides normal cold exposure, sudden changes in weather and especially the severe conditions in the northern plains affected the health, energy levels, and morale of troopers. Higher-ranking service members often had previous experience operating in harsh military environments. Therefore many officers and experienced enlisted personnel knew how to cope with these conditions better than new recruits.

Nineteenth-Century Treatment of Cold Injuries

Cold injuries in the military occurred frequently while troopers were on march and sometimes simply resulted from brief exposure to the elements. Treatment of those injuries often had to wait until troopers reached a post, and remedies were not always effective. Some men had body parts amputated. Others died from their injuries.

In 1812 Baron Dominique Larrey, Napoleon Bonaparte's military surgeon, recorded the treatment of frostbite on those wounded during the retreat from Moscow. The wounds were massaged with snow to warm the area (Larrey 1814). This method was used throughout the nineteenth century, continuing until 1956. Then it was discovered that rapid rewarming followed by treatment with aloe vera and painkillers was more effective (Murphy et al. 2000).

Post–Civil War treatment, however, followed this earlier technique. Affected areas were often treated with various solutions for days before amputation was deemed a last step. For instance, in Wyoming in December 1870, Private Richard Bowen, Thirteenth Infantry, came to the post hospital with frozen feet. Nurses rubbed his feet and ankles with snow and attempted to restore circulation. His feet were subsequently wrapped in cloth doused in whiskey, and he was given morphine. Whiskey and a mixture of quinine and iron chloride were applied to the feet in the days after the injury. Because some of the skin was missing from Bowen's feet, lime water and olive oil liniment were applied. He was ordered to drink milk punch and beef tea. Nonetheless, Bowen died after a few days (Otis 1871:167).

As another example, Sergeant William Earl of the Seventh Cavalry was admitted to the hospital in December 1870 after being discovered outside following a night of heavy drinking. His feet and left hand were severely affected. These areas were rubbed with snow and soaked in ice water. Olive oil and lime water were later applied to the wounds. Carbolic acid was also applied. He was ordered to drink milk punch and beef tea. He was given opiates so that he could sleep. Earl's legs began swelling, and he became increasingly melancholic and delirious as the days passed. Surgeons decided that an amputation was necessary. Nonetheless, Earl died on December 31, 1870 (Otis 1871:168).

Factors Associated with Cold Injury Vulnerability

Previous anthropological and military studies suggest that intrinsic and extrinsic factors contribute to cold injuries (Blair et al. 1957; Candler and Ivey 1997; Burgess and Macfarlane 2009). As mentioned earlier, an analysis of the relationship between cold injury frequencies and many of these variables was possible using the information available in the Seventh Cavalry enlistment and medical records (table 10.5).

It should be noted that the severity and anatomical location of troopers' cold injuries were listed in the extrinsic category because these variables were not inherent to each individual. A discussion of the variables that were related to cold injuries is presented below.

TABLE 10.5. Extrinsic and intrinsic variables and cold injury frequencies

Variable type	*Variables associated with cold injuries*	*Variables not related to cold injuries*
Extrinsic	Geographical location of injury	Rank at the time of discharge*
	Time of year and climatic events	Nature of discharge
	Activity during the time of injury	Change over time (uniform improvements)
	Rank at the time of discharge*	
	Severity of cold injury	
	Anatomical location of injury	
Intrinsic	Stature	Nativity
		Age at the time of enlistment
		Complexion

*Although rank at the time of injury was not significant, it approaches significance.

GEOGRAPHICAL LOCATION AT THE TIME OF COLD INJURY

It was hypothesized that geographical location affected cold injury frequencies in the Seventh Cavalry. Of the variables examined here, the relationship between geographical location and cold injury frequencies was the most unmistakable. Three of the four forts with the highest percentages of cold injuries (Forts Abraham Lincoln, Totten, and Yates) were located in areas where the low temperature in January averaged 9.9° Fahrenheit or less. The exception was Fort Lyon, Colorado, where the low averaged 10 to 19.9° Fahrenheit. Only one man was admitted for frostbite in the South (Taylor Barracks, Kentucky). Maps 10.1, 10.2, and 10.3 show the geographical distributions of cold injuries.

There was a relationship between fort locations with the lowest temperatures in January and increased levels of frostbite, resulting from severe temperatures and weather patterns in these regions.

But why were so many cases of frostbite recorded at Fort Abraham Lincoln? Perhaps the most obvious answer is time. According to Scott Larkin, interpretive director of the Fort Abraham Lincoln

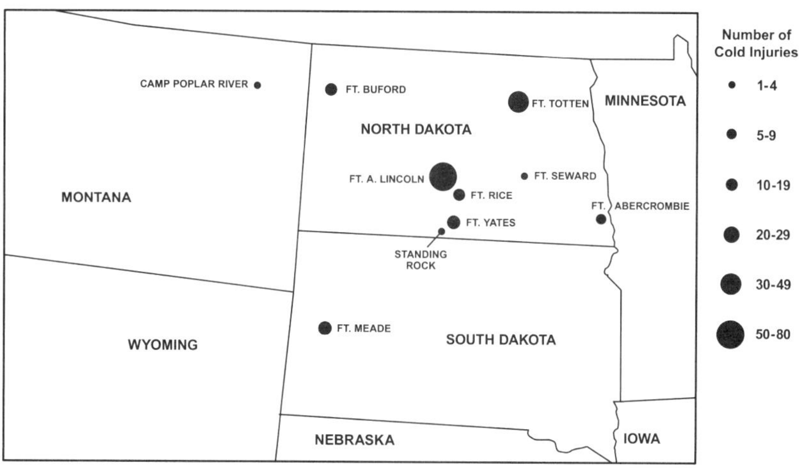

Map 10.1. Postings where cold injuries occurred in the post–Civil War Seventh Cavalry on the northern plains. The greatest frequency of cold injuries occurred at Fort Abraham Lincoln and Fort Totten. Copyright © 2015, University of Oklahoma Press.

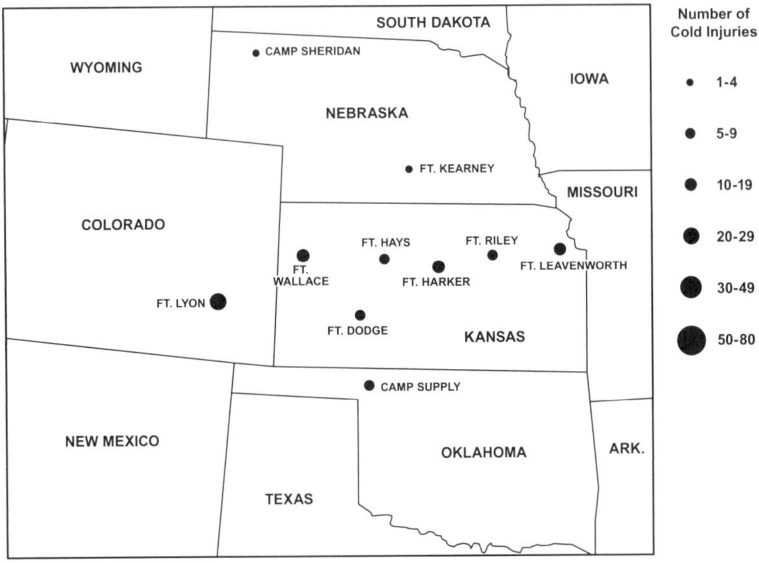

Map 10.2. Postings where cold injuries occurred in the post–Civil War Seventh Cavalry on the central plains. The greatest frequency of cold injuries occurred at Fort Lyon and Fort Leavenworth. Copyright © 2015, University of Oklahoma Press.

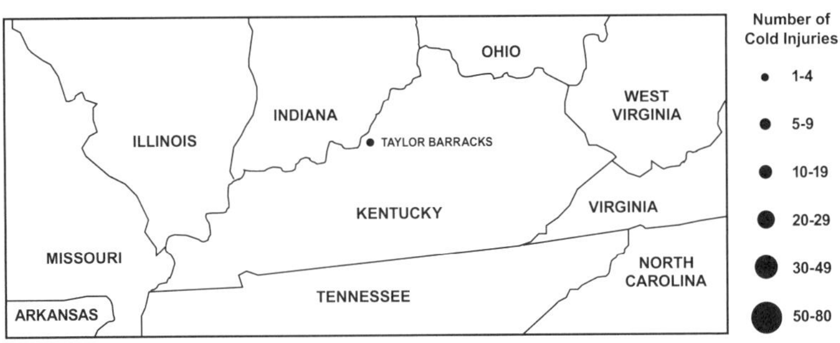

Map 10.3. Posting where cold injury occurred in the post–Civil War Seventh Cavalry in the South. Only one injury happened in this region, at Taylor Barracks. Copyright © 2015, University of Oklahoma Press.

Foundation (personal communication, February 24, 2011), the Seventh Cavalry spent approximately nine years (from 1873 to 1882) stationed primarily at Fort Abraham Lincoln. Thus the Seventh Cavalry spent half of the seventeen years in the study period headquartered at Fort Abraham Lincoln. This could account for

TABLE 10.6. Seventh Cavalry cold injuries at Fort Abraham Lincoln by year and troop strength

Year	*Frequency*	*Troop strength*	*Percentage of troopers affected*
1873	2	10462	0.0
1874	11	10218	0.1
1875	8	8842	0.1
1876	22	10628	0.2
1877	10	11707	0.1
1878	1	8675	0.0
1879	16	8902	0.2
1880	2	8950	0.0
1881	4	7900	0.1
Total	76	86284	0.1

Source: After Cohan 2011:108, table 57.

the high frequency of injuries recorded there. Troopers also arrived at Fort Lincoln after serving in southern locations, so the men may have been unprepared for the harsh Dakota winters and suffered increased injuries as a result. To clarify this issue table 10.6 shows the distribution of cold injuries at Fort Abraham Lincoln by year.

Contrary to this explanation, rather than most cold injury cases occurring at the beginning of the Seventh Cavalry's stay at Fort Abraham Lincoln, the peak number of injuries occurred later in 1876 and 1879. The greatest number of injuries recorded at Fort Abraham Lincoln during the course of a single month was eight, reported in December 1876. One explanation for the increase in cold injuries is that many new recruits joined the regiment after the Battle of the Little Bighorn the previous summer. As mentioned previously, it was hypothesized that some of these new troopers were unaccustomed to operating in the extreme cold of the northern plains or lacked suitable uniforms. Interestingly, three of the injuries in December 1876 affected recruits who had enlisted earlier that year, so it is possible that these men had not adjusted to the lifestyle or the climate at the time of their injuries. To clarify

TABLE 10.7. Bismarck, Dakota Territory, mean temperatures, fall 1876 and winter 1877

Year	*Month*	*Mean temperature*	*Highest temperature*	*Lowest temperature*
1876	October	40.75°	74°	14°
1876	November	18.30°	67°	−15°
1876	December	6.84°	62°	−23°
1877	January	6.32°	44°	−30°
1877	February	26.40°	60°	−5°

Note: Temperatures in Fahrenheit.

why there was such a high frequency of injuries in December 1876, microfilm copies of the *Bismarck Weekly Tribune* (1876–77) were consulted to determine mean temperatures before and after this month (table 10.7).

The high frequency of cold injuries in December 1876 might be due to the very low mean temperature (6.84° F) in the area that month. But the mean temperature in January 1877 was even lower (6.32° F), so low temperatures alone cannot account for the increase in cold injuries during December.

The absence of vegetation to serve as a windbreak exacerbated the conditions. On arriving in Yankton in present-day South Dakota, Elizabeth Custer (1885:8) recalled that the ground was "perfectly bare of every earthly comfort." She soon learned why many people said the region had eight months of winter each year. Figures 10.3 and 10.4 illustrate the desolate environment troopers experienced at Fort Abraham Lincoln.

The only cold injury in a summer month occurred at Fort Abraham Lincoln in June 1877, when Conrad Bombach suffered frostbite to both of his feet. Blizzards, wind, and cold weather were common in this region, exposing troopers to cold injuries even in spring and summer. In fact, during the spring when the Seventh Cavalry was moving toward the Little Bighorn in 1876, troopers experienced cold winds and heavy snowfall from May 31 through June 2, 1876 (Wiche 2006).

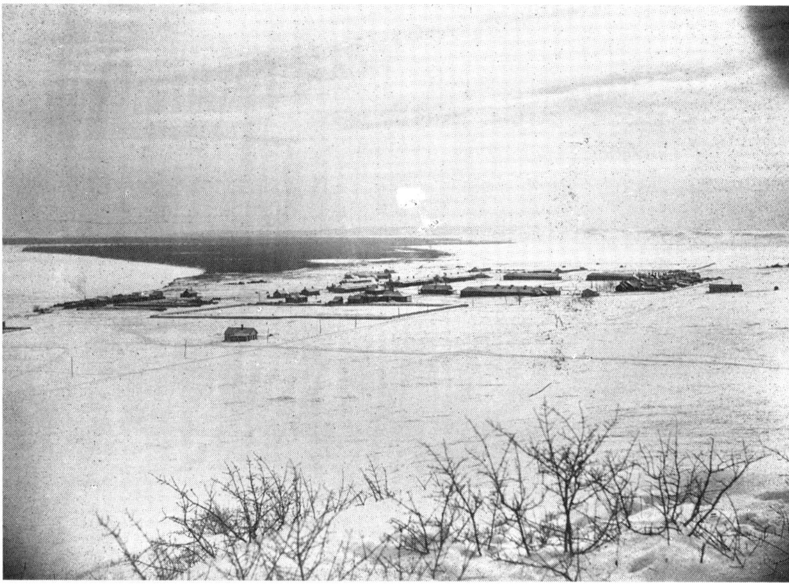

10.3. *Fort Abraham Lincoln, General View, Winter* shows the Missouri River and buildings (stables, barracks, officers' houses, and so forth) and was noted in the records as an image of a "barren landscape." Source: David Frances Barry, taken between 1874 and 1879. Courtesy Department of the Denver Public Library Western History and Genealogy Department, Call no. B-838.

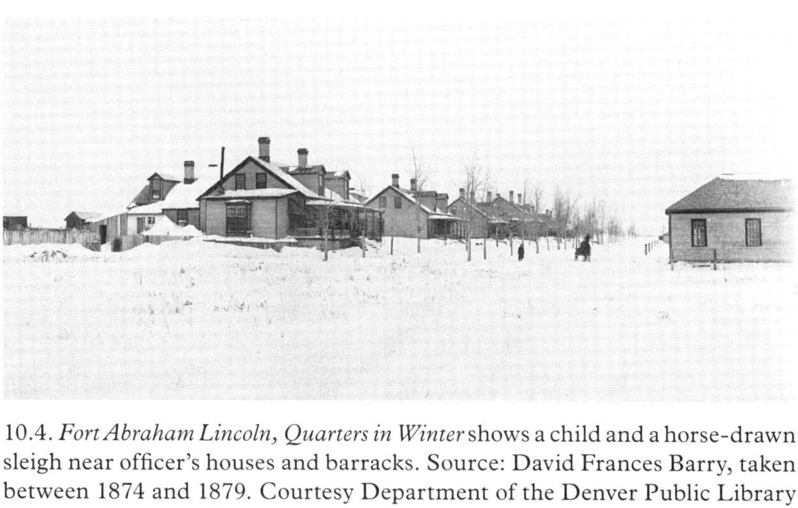

10.4. *Fort Abraham Lincoln, Quarters in Winter* shows a child and a horse-drawn sleigh near officer's houses and barracks. Source: David Frances Barry, taken between 1874 and 1879. Courtesy Department of the Denver Public Library Western History and Genealogy Department, Call no. B-251.

TIME OF YEAR AND CLIMATIC EVENTS

Not surprisingly, the majority of cold injuries (75.1 percent) occurred during the winter months (December through February), and 86.2 percent of all cold injuries happened between December and March. These data correspond with the observations of David DeGroot et al. (2003), who found that 86 percent of all cold weather injury cases happened from December through March in a late-twentieth-century sample. This distribution of injuries was expected in the Seventh Cavalry sample because temperatures were lowest during these months.

The two months when the most cold injury cases occurred were January 1881 (fifteen recorded cases) and December 1868 (fourteen recorded cases). In January 1881 six injuries were recorded at Fort Buford, four at Fort Yates, three at Fort Abraham Lincoln, and two at Fort Meade. All three forts were located in Dakota Territory, areas still known for their harsh winters. In December 1868 seven injuries were recorded in Indian Territory and seven at Fort Lyon. Interestingly, four of these seven cold injuries recorded in Indian Territory were dated between December 1 and 9. Not only did these injuries occur in a winter month in present-day Oklahoma, but they probably corresponded with the Seventh Cavalry's involvement in the Battle of the Washita (discussed further below).

ACTIVITIES AT THE TIME OF COLD INJURY

Auxiliary medical record annotations show that troopers participated in a variety of activities when their cold injuries occurred. For instance, some men were in the field or on duty, while others were hunting, chopping wood, or working with a chisel or axe. Direct contact with metal objects caused severe cold injuries because metal conducts heat quickly and freezes skin at a rapid rate (Giesbrecht and Wilkerson 2006:74). William Candler and Hazel Ivey (1997) noted that touching metal led to cold injuries in their Alaskan sample.

As further documented in the medical records, some men were prisoners when they sustained cold injuries, and another individual was scouting. Both of these situations left troopers exposed to the elements. One man received frostbite on his right middle finger after "imprudent exposure of his hand," and yet another was intoxicated at the time of his injury.

It has been observed that being in the field or in battle increased cold injury vulnerability because soldiers were exposed and were often required to stay in one position for long periods (for example, DeGroot et al. 2003). Lieutenant Colonel Custer (1874:153) described men donning additional clothing when they realized that they were heading into the field during the 1868 winter campaign without appropriate shelter or fire during the "bitter, freezing hours of night." This troop action took place just before the Battle of the Washita at the end of November. Men frequently left for the field hastily or in undesirable conditions to overtake Indian groups. Troopers were often exposed to extreme cold and wind during these times. Seventh Cavalry cold injuries indicate this vulnerability; eleven men in the sample suffered cold injuries while in the field.

During the study period, one of the Seventh Cavalry's major engagements happened in cold weather. As mentioned earlier, four cases of frostbite occurred in Indian Territory from December 1 through 9, 1868, after the Battle of the Washita on November 28, 1868. The frozen landscape was snowy, and temperatures fell below zero (Custer 1874; Hoig 1979). Interestingly, Custer (1874:184, 189) reported that the cavalry returned to Camp Supply in Indian Territory by November 30 and was on campaign again by December 7, 1868. Therefore it is likely that the injuries recorded from December 1 through December 9 were associated either with the Battle of the Washita or with the subsequent return to the field in Indian Territory.

STATURE

A relationship between cold injuries and trooper stature was found ($t = -2.667$, df $= 6730$, $p = .008$), with cold injury patients being 0.37 inches taller than non–cold injured men. Although this relationship is interesting, a more effective way of determining the influence of human size on cold injury susceptibility would have been possible only if the weights of the troopers had been recorded. Unfortunately, weights were not available for the Seventh

Cavalrymen. It can only be stated that the cold injury patients were slightly taller than the non–cold injured patients, possibly because increased height was associated with increased energy loss. Mean differences in heights between the non–cold injured patients and the cold-injured patients were small, so this difference may have resulted from the large sample size (over 8,000 men).

RANK AT THE TIME OF DISCHARGE

Rank at the time of discharge is marked with an asterisk in table 10.5: although the relationship between rank and cold injuries was not significant, it approached significance ($\chi^2 = 5.390$, df = 2, $p = .068$) and warrants discussion. Comparable to other observations (for example, DeGroot et al. 2003), most men in the Seventh Cavalry who experienced cold injuries were rankers (all privates and one wagoner). More rankers experienced cold injuries than expected. Thus it is possible that these lower-ranking men were injured more frequently because they had less experience operating in the cold and were less prepared for military activity than the higher-ranking officers. Furthermore, fewer junior noncommissioned officers had cold injuries than expected.

SEVERITY

The average length of hospital stays for a cold injury was 16.69 days, with a median of 6.5 days. According to DeGroot et al. (2003), the average time for an individual to be hospitalized in their sample of late-twentieth-century U. S. soldiers was 6 days, the median being about 3 days. Because their sample was from 1980 through 1999, it is likely that this decrease in hospitalization time from the 1800s to the 1980s demonstrates improvements in treatment or less severe cold injuries. Both sets of results appear to be skewed positively, however, probably reflecting outliers (the most severe cases in each sample).

ANATOMICAL LOCATION OF INJURY

As noted by Gordon Giesbrecht and James Wilkerson (2006:74) and in historical accounts, frostbite most often affected the extremities and parts of the face. The distribution of cold injuries in Seventh Cavalry patients reflected this pattern. Over 99 percent of cold injuries in the sample affected the feet, toes, hands, fingers, ears, nose, or face of the patient. This result corresponded with Candler and Ivey's (1997) study, where the majority of injuries affected the service members' hands, feet, ears and noses. One trooper suffered from frostbite to his genitals. Six men in the Seventh Cavalry sample were affected in more than one anatomical location (for example, fingers and toes, hands and feet, or face and hands). Although the results showed an expected distribution of cold injuries, these injuries also reflected the inadequacies in the clothing issued, as discussed earlier.

Discussion of Additional Variables

UNIFORMS AND EQUIPMENT

Although each of the variables in table 10.5 was investigated, not all of them related to cold injury vulnerability. Recall earlier accounts of soldiers who wore layer upon layer of clothing and had difficulty performing the simplest tasks. Because uniforms and equipment were modified to improve cold protection, it was hypothesized that cold injury levels would decrease from 1866 to 1883. Surprisingly, rather than finding a decrease in cold injuries, injuries increased and decreased irregularly from 1866 through 1883. Uniform and equipment improvements (such as rubber overshoes or gloves) did not diminish overall cold injury frequencies.

CHANGE THROUGH TIME

As noted, although the number of cold injuries varied from 1866 through 1883, no decrease in cold injuries occurred during the period. This finding differs from what would be expected with improved equipment. As an example, during the first year (1866), 0.1 percent of all enlisted troopers experienced a cold injury, while the final year (1883) showed that 0.2 percent of all enlisted men were affected. Improvements in equipment, gear, and military methods did not have a significant mitigating effect on cold injury frequencies, although the Seventh Cavalry's access to the new cold weather clothing and footwear is not clearly documented in the historic record.

NATURE OF DISCHARGE AND TERMINATION FROM SERVICE

More men who experienced cold injuries left service due to disabilities than would be expected ($\chi^2 = 11.295$, df = 2, $p = .004$). It is clear that some cases of frostbite were severe enough to merit disability discharge. However, less than half of the disability discharges received by cold-injured soldiers (9 of 22) resulted from cold injuries.

Some men deserted the army following cold injury. As an example, Albert Baker experienced frostbite on January 19, 1883, and returned to service from hospitalization on February 5, 1883. Baker deserted that same day. Similar cases appeared in the record. It is possible that some men who suffered from frostbite were either exhausted or traumatized by the experience and chose to desert rather than stay and risk frostbite again.

NATIVITY

Other researchers (for example, DeGroot et al. 2003) have investigated the relationship between nativity and cold injuries. It was hypothesized that individuals born in the coldest climates were better adjusted to low temperatures and thus suffered fewer cold injuries than men who were born in warmer climates. The results were not significant ($\chi^2 = 5.300$, df = 3, $p = .151$), however. Therefore this hypothesis was not supported.

AGE AT ENLISTMENT

Previous authors (such as DeGroot et al. 2003) have studied the relationship between service members' age and degree of cold injury. DeGroot et al. (2003) discovered that soldiers from seventeen to twenty-one years old suffered cold injuries more frequently than older soldiers. The majority of injured troopers served in the military for less than five years. Thus it was hypothesized that the younger Seventh Cavalrymen would sustain more cold injuries because they had less military and field experience. It was also believed that older individuals could instead be more vulnerable due to overall weakening of their bodies. However, no relationship between cold injury and age was found (t = .029, df = 6732, p = .977). The results of this test suggested that trooper age did not influence cold injury susceptibility.

COMPLEXION

In addition, this study tested the relationship between cold injury and skin pigmentation to determine whether or not post–Civil War Seventh Cavalry data supported or rejected the cold injury hypothesis. Previous researchers (for example, Daanen 2003) suggested that African Americans showed more debilitating biological responses to cold than other service members. Based on this research, skin pigmentation levels might influence cold injury vulnerability. It was hypothesized that Seventh Cavalrymen with the darkest complexions in the sample would experience more cold injuries and more severe cold injuries.

There was no relationship between complexion category and cold injury frequency (χ^2 = 1.194, df = 2, p = .550). Despite Hein Daanen's (2003) research and the suggestion by Peter Post et al. (1975) that variation in skin pigmentation levels was related to cold injury susceptibility, the Seventh Cavalry data did not support this finding. Men with medium and darkly pigmented skin were as vulnerable to cold injury as men with light skin. After analyzing the data in several ways, the cold injury complexion hypothesis was rejected.

Additional Effects of Cold

Frostbite was not the only affliction caused by exposure to cold temperatures in the Seventh Cavalry. Medical records showed that lacerations occurred from slipping on or being cut by ice. For instance, in December 1878, Joseph Halpin experienced a chest contusion after falling on the ice. Also documented in the Seventh Cavalry medical records are ice-related sprains and fractures.

Exposure to extreme cold and blizzard conditions could cause men to become disoriented and sometimes lose their way while on march. The cold could be so bitter that men did not even want to continue to safety. Furthermore, residual pathologies can occur after frostbite injuries, resulting in pain long after the initial cold injury (Blair et al. 1957). When considering the Seventh Cavalry troopers' experiences, it is important to remember that many likely suffered such symptoms and probably felt the effects of their injuries years later.

Dietary information was not analyzed here, but the cold certainly took a toll on trooper diet. During the Indian Wars, troopers were issued field rations consisting of bacon, hardtack, and coffee (Fisher and Fisher 2011:91). These rations were supplemented by locally available fish and game or pemmican. This diet provided soldiers with inadequate nutrition and thus affected their susceptibility to illness and disease. Men exposed to extreme cold had a harder time eating and drinking because their provisions could freeze, as exemplified by Indian Wars correspondent Robert Strahorn's account of bacon and bread that were "frozen solid" (Cozzens 2004:214).

Challenges Illustrated by This Study: Under-Representation of Medical Problems and Missing Data

While conducting this study, it became apparent that cold injuries were under-represented in the Seventh Cavalry records. Brief descriptions of medical problems were sometimes recorded by physicians in prescription books while on march or in the field. It was likely that these books were used when it was convenient, but not all medical problems in the field were recorded when they occurred. And if a medical issue was recorded in the prescription book, it was often an incomplete entry.

An example of this possible under-representation was found in accounts of the Yankton blizzard, from April 13 through 18, 1873. Elizabeth Custer (1885:13) remembered this storm and the effects of the blizzard on troopers. After taking in six men who had been caught in the blizzard on the evening of April 14, she recalled: "The frozen men were in so exhausted a condition that they required immediate attention. . . . I saw symptoms of that deadly stupor which is the sure precursor of freezing. . . . Poor fellows! They afterwards lost their feet, and some of their fingers also had to be amputated."

Despite this account describing frostbite, no corresponding cold injuries were found in the medical records during the spring of 1873 that could be associated with this blizzard. If Custer remembered correctly, then this lack of documentation indicates an under-reported number of cold injuries. In contrast, some historical accounts may have been exaggerations, so that the absences of such cold injuries in the medical records were correct.

Also contributing to the low frequency of recorded cold injuries in this instance is the fact that many cavalrymen found shelter in Yankton during this blizzard. Some troopers found refuge with the Custers and in Yankton hotels. Yankton townspeople also opened their homes to stranded soldiers (Custer 1885).

If cold injuries were under-reported in the medical records, then some of the relationships between different variables and cold injuries or changes in cold injury frequencies might be reflected poorly in the statistical analyses in this study. This problem is a limitation of historical records that cannot be resolved. When combining statistical analyses with background research and the study of personal accounts, experiences of these individuals may be documented with greater accuracy. Personal accounts must be considered cautiously, however, because many individuals recorded their experiences long after the events occurred.

Summary

Post–Civil War Seventh Cavalrymen faced many challenges during their time in the military. Being stationed in frigid climates on the central and northern plains, especially at Fort Abraham Lincoln, exposed troopers to the elements and made them vulnerable to cold injuries. Serving in colder months and performing outdoor activities often increased troopers' chances of suffering from frostbite. Although improved cold-weather gear was issued, these uniform changes failed to decrease frostbite incidences. Often troopers adjusted to the cold by modifying their uniforms, attempting to eat frozen food, and doing whatever they could to keep warm and stay alive.

CHAPTER 11

Other Injuries in the Seventh Cavalry

P. Willey

The Seventh Cavalry is known for its epic battles with Indians, most notably at the Battle of the Little Bighorn. Such encounters caused injuries and traumatic deaths. But there were many other sources of Seventh Cavalry injuries. They involved more mundane, day-to-day vulnerabilities and traumatic occurrences, as chapter 10 on cold injuries reveals.

Whether from accidental events, errors, or intentional interpersonal violence, injuries constituted a substantial portion of the Seventh Cavalry's recorded ailments. Almost 20 percent of the Seventh Cavalry medical records noted trauma as the cause of visits to the surgeons. That proportion should not be surprising. Consider, if you will, the youthful, male, risk-taking group involved. In addition, regions where the Seventh was posted during the post–Civil War period (the West and South) had violent reputations.

Chapter 10 focuses on one such issue—cold injuries. This chapter investigates the Seventh Cavalry's other injuries. The first part shows how the Seventh Cavalry medical ailments fit the nineteenth-century injury categories introduced in chapter 3 and describes extrinsic and intrinsic associations with those injuries. Employing the medical records' marginal notes for additional insights, three major causes of injuries are then explored. These involve injuries associated with transportation-related events, from interpersonal violence, and from battle encounters.

Basic Materials

Based on Seventh Cavalry medical records, injuries are separated from other illness categories. Identification of injuries is fairly simple, consisting of readily identifiable categories.

Recorded injuries total 3,974 instances. The more frequent injury categories include (in alphabetical order) abrasions, arrow wounds, bites, burns and scalds, concussions, contusions, dislocations, fractures, gunshot wounds, incised wounds, lacerations, poisonings, punctures, sprains, and sunstroke (table 11.1).

More durable materials rubbing, skittering, or scraping across soft tissues caused abrasions. They were usually superficial. The Seventh Cavalry's medical records included 6 abrasions. Many more were likely self-treated.

Arrow wounds happened when propelled projectiles pierced tissues. The Seventh Cavalry medical records included 11 instances of arrow wounds. All happened on the central plains in 1867 and 1868, none later or elsewhere. Perhaps the most graphic example was Sergeant Frederick Wyllyams of Company G, who was killed near Fort Wallace, Kansas, in 1867 (fig. 1.1). This temporal and geographic distribution likely indicated a shift from Indians employing traditional bows and arrows to their use of firearms introduced by Euro-Americans. Treatment of embedded arrows involved identifying anatomical structures and extraction of arrows with forceps, followed by draining and bandaging the wound (Mays et al. 1994)

Bites resulted from teeth causing damage to tissues. Various animals produced 9 bites in the Seventh Cavalry's medical records, including 3 bites of "serpents," presumably rattlesnakes, copperheads, or cottonmouths. Horses and dogs delivered several bites, 2 had unidentified origins, and others were received in fights. (For more about human-bites-human, see the last section of this chapter.) Bites were probably under-represented in the medical records. Many bites, such as those by horses, may have resulted in a primary diagnosis of laceration or contusion, not listed as the causative "bite."

Tissues exposed to excessive heat resulted in burns and scalds. The Seventh Cavalry's medical records documented 95 burns. As one example, Charles A. Warner was burned on January 20, 1878,

TABLE 11.1. Post–Civil War Seventh Cavalry injuries for entire sample (all injuries and subsets)

	ALL INJURIES		TRANSPORTATION-RELATED INJURIES		INTERNECINE VIOLENCE-RELATED INJURIES		BATTLE-RELATED INJURIES	
Kind of Injury	*Frequency*	*Percent*	*Frequency*	*Percent*	*Frequency*	*Percent*	*Frequency*	*Percent*
Abrasions	6	0.2						
Arrow wounds	11	0.3			7	3.8	4	3.3
Bites	9	0.2	1	0.2	4	2.2		
Burns and scalds	95	2.4			3	1.6		
Concussions	10	0.3	2	0.4	1	0.5		
Contusions	1855	46.7	357	67.5	64	34.6		
Dislocations	45	1.1	6	1.1	2	1.1		
Fractures	130	3.3	29	5.5	11	5.9		
Gunshot wounds	246	6.2			37	20.0	99	80.5
Incised wounds	318	8.0	4	0.8	11	5.9		
Lacerations	269	6.8	44	8.3	33	17.8		
Poisonings	57	1.4						
Puncture wounds	62	1.6			1	0.5		
Sprains	775	19.5	78	14.7	9	4.9	1	0.8
Sunstrokes and insolations	15	0.4						
Others*	71	1.8	8	1.5	2	1.1	19	15.4
Total	3974	100.2	529	100.0	185	99.9	123	100.0

*The category "others" consists of unusual or eclectic diagnoses, including foot injury, horse/mule kicks, chafes, amputations, blisters, dizziness ("in the head"), drowned, traumatic erysipelas, fall, injury, KIAs, neuralgia, strains, struck in side, sunburn, ulcer, and wound.

at Standing Rock, Dakota Territory, falling on a stove while fighting. He returned to service the next month.

Concussions resulted from sudden impact of the head and/or spine, which caused damage to tissues surrounding the brain and often involved loss of consciousness. The Seventh Cavalry's medical records included 10 concussions from various causes. If the concussion was severe, the patient was wrapped in hot blankets with hot water bottles, administered purgatives, and given bed rest (Barnes 1870:65).

Crushing of soft tissues led to contusions (bruises), most frequently from blunt force. The Seventh Cavalry's medical records documented 1,855 contusions. Most of these records lacked additional comments. Among the cases with ancillary notes, however, accidents were frequently mentioned. They often involved being kicked by, stepped on, thrown from, falling from, or wrenched by horses. Other means of conveyance caused contusions too, including wagons, sleighs, carts, saddle pommels, and even "car seat while en route," likely referring to a rail car seat. (For more about those transportation-associated injuries, see below.)

In one particularly elaborate blunt force incident, Private Joseph Harwood received a fractured skull in August 1871 in Elizabethtown, Kentucky. He was described as being "[o]n a drunken spree. Caused by a stone thrown by a negro." Surgical intervention was required. "About one inch square of the parietal bone was removed and the depressed portion of the occipital bone was replaced in its normal condition." Harwood survived the injury and surgery but subsequently suffered problems with epilepsy.

Severe displacement of a joint resulted in a dislocation (luxation), usually involving torn tendons, ligaments, and/or disruption of joint capsules. The Seventh Cavalry's medical records reported 45 dislocations. Most records indicated the dislocated joint (such as shoulder or ankle), and a few noted the cause of the dislocation. As an example, Private John Brown dislocated his arm into his armpit during a fall in July 1872 at Elizabethtown, Kentucky. The joint was reset "by gentle traction on the hand and arm." No sequelae were recorded.

Breaks, splits, or separations of a bone from the bone's adjacent portions constituted fractures. The Seventh Cavalry's medical records documented 130 fractures. Nearly all fracture records indicated the bone broken (for example, right humerus), and many mentioned the fracture's complexity (simple, comminuted, or compound). Approximately one-third of the fracture records noted the cause of the fractures. Like contusions, many fractures were associated with unfortunate encounters with horses and wagons. For example, Farrier John Rivers fractured his right acromial process (of the scapula) when he fell from a wagon on May 10, 1880, while stationed at Fort Abraham Lincoln. Although no procedures were documented in his case, the normal treatment would be to set the body part, stabilize it, and provide time for healing. Rivers returned to service the healing-appropriate six weeks later.

Propelled bullets, pellets, and other firearm-related discharges resulted in gunshot wounds. The Seventh Cavalry's medical records documented 246 gunshot wounds. Almost all of these included the location of the wound (for example, both thighs), and many documented treatment of wounds. A few mentioned the nature of the injury (such as whether it was accidental or received in action against hostiles). For example, Private Engelbirt (elsewhere Englebert) Saylor on August 11, 1873, while in action on the Yellowstone River Expedition, received a gunshot wound from a Henry rifle to the upper third of his right radius. He transferred from the field, returning to home forts on the Missouri River for recovery. Although it was not recorded in Saylor's records, treatment generally involved probing to identify the location of missile, extracting it, bandaging the wound, and permitting it time to heal.

Gunshot and other combat-related wounds were under-reported because soldiers killed in action or dying of wounds but not receiving medical treatment were not documented in the medical records. For instance, the 268 combat-related deaths sustained at the Battle of the Little Bighorn on June 25 and 26, 1876, mostly resulted from gunshot wounds. But only the 3 men who died of gunshot wounds under a physician's care had such documentation (Scott et al. 1998:287).

Blades produced incised wounds, resulting in cut, chopped, or sliced flesh. The Seventh Cavalry's medical records documented 318 incised wounds. Supplementary notes often indicated the location of the wound (for example, left foot), and few offered additional details. As an example of a particularly detailed account on

October 7, 1879, while at Fort Meade, John Bergman received an incised wound from a saber during a brawl. He returned to service several days later.

Lacerations resulted from tearing, mangling, or ripping soft tissues. The Seventh Cavalry's medical records documented 269 lacerations. Many records noted the injury location (for example, right hand), some mentioned the instrument involved (such as a sharp stick, wood saw, or horse kick), and a few identified what action caused the wound (for example, an accident).

Poisonings occurred when toxic substances contacted skin or were ingested. The Seventh Cavalry's medical records documented 57 cases of poisoning. Most involved contact with plants of the genus *Rhus*, the genus that then encompassed poison ivy, poison oak, and poison sumac. But a few cases of poisoning resulted from ingesting opium, contacting cactus spines, and being stung by insects.

Piercing and penetrating instruments produced puncture wounds. The Seventh Cavalry's medical records included 62 puncture wounds. Most such records noted the injured part (for example, left foot), fewer indicated what object or action caused the wound (such as stepped on nail), and even fewer included the cause of the wound.

Sprains (subluxations) resulted from joints being wrenched, pulled, or twisted with partial breaking or ripping of ligaments or other joint attachments. The Seventh Cavalry's medical records listed 775 sprains. The records occasionally mentioned the sprain's location (for example, wrist) and less frequently how the injury occurred (such as a fall from a wagon). As an example, Sergeant W. H. Clark sprained his left ankle when he was thrown from a horse in July 1883 at Fort Meade. He returned to service five days later.

Sunstroke resulted from excessive exposure to heat. Symptoms included elevated body temperature and convulsions. In addition to its modern meaning, during the nineteenth century sunstroke sometimes was associated with mental derangement. The Seventh Cavalry medical records documented 15 instances of sunstroke and insolation.

To review these physical insults, the greatest frequency of injuries consisted of contusions (46.7% of all injuries), although others were common, including sprains (19.5%), incised wounds (8%), lacerations (6.8%), and gunshot wounds (6.2%). The other kinds of injuries constituted the remaining small proportion (about 12%).

General Injuries

This section examines the Seventh Cavalry's medical records for a broad perspective on all injuries. Topics include general considerations (temporal trends and geographic regions) and intrinsic variables (birthplaces, ages, and heights). The next three sections discuss injuries associated with transportation and interpersonal violence.

TEMPORAL DISTRIBUTION OF INJURIES

The analysis of temporal patterns of general injuries starts with the monthly distribution then proceeds to seasonal and annual frequencies. To test for differences in monthly distribution, injuries are analyzed using admittance months. Fewest injuries occurred in August, and most in January (table 11.2 and fig. 11.1). This monthly distribution achieves statistical significance ($p < 0.000$).

To test the possibility that more injuries occurred in some seasons than in others, the months were combined into the four seasons. Using the seasons of all years in our study period, a mean of 992.25 cases of injury-related events occurred in each of the four seasons (table 11.3 and fig. 11.2). The minimum number happened in summer (n = 808) and maximum in winter (n = 1,176). Assuming injuries should have been randomly distributed by season, a significant divergence of injuries by season existed ($\chi^2 = 34.82$, df=3, $p < 0.001$). Under-representation of summer injuries and over-representation of winter injuries contributed most to this.

This spike in winter injuries may reflect being cooped up during cold months, with resultant "cabin fever" and increased antagonisms. In addition, winter presented challenges beyond those associated with milder seasons, including cold and ice (see chapter 10).

As an alternate explanation, perhaps injuries were equally distributed by month and season but documented differently. In winter, according to this explanation, troops were under the watchful

TABLE 11.2. Admittance month of injuries in the post–Civil War Seventh Cavalry for entire sample (all injuries and subsets)

	ALL INJURIES		TRANSPORTATION-RELATED VIOLENCE-RELATED		INTERNECINE INJURIES	
Month	*Frequency*	*Percentage*	*Frequency*	*Percentage*	*Frequency*	*Percentage*
January	441	11.1	49	9.3	13	7.0
February	357	9.0	31	5.9	16	8.6
March	379	9.5	32	6.0	9	4.9
April	328	8.3	44	8.3	10	5.4
May	305	7.7	56	10.6	8	4.3
June	280	7.0	47	8.9	21	11.4
July	299	7.5	39	7.4	18	9.7
August	229	5.8	35	6.6	19	10.3
September	289	7.3	38	7.2	16	8.6
October	300	7.6	61	11.5	17	9.2
November	384	9.7	49	9.3	17	9.2
December	378	9.5	48	9.1	21	11.4
Total	3969	99.9	529	100.0	185	100.0

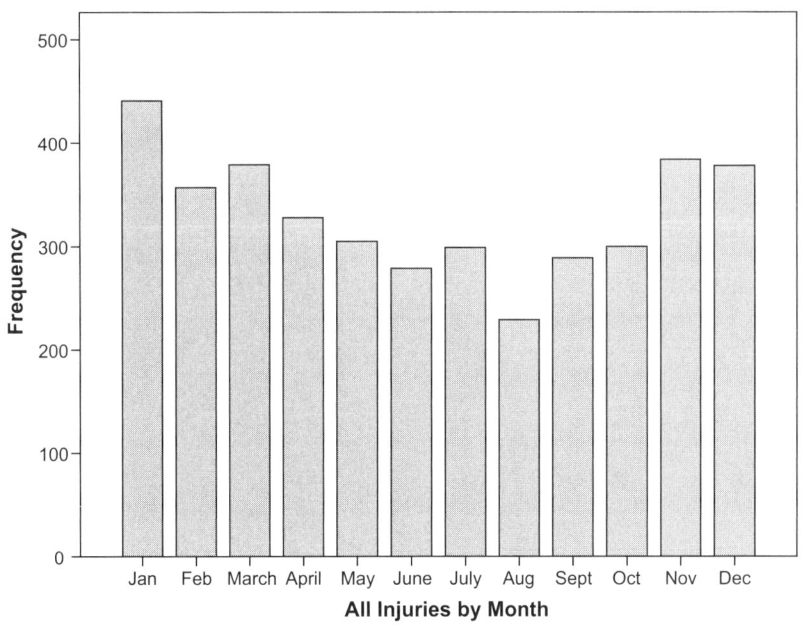

11.1. Admittance month of all injuries in the post–Civil War Seventh Cavalry. Note greatest frequency in January and least in August.

TABLE 11.3. Admittance season of injuries in the post–Civil War Seventh Cavalry for entire sample (all injuries and subsets)

	ALL INJURIES		TRANSPORTATION-RELATED INJURIES		INTERNECINE VIOLENCE-RELATED INJURIES	
Season	*Frequency*	*Percentage*	*Frequency*	*Percentage*	*Frequency*	*Percentage*
Spring (March–May)	1012	25.5	132	24.9	27	14.6
Summer (June–August)	808	20.4	121	22.9	58	31.4
Fall (September–November)	973	24.5	148	28.0	50	27.0
Winter (December–February)	1176	29.6	128	24.3	50	27.0
Total	3969	100.0	529	100.1	185	100.0

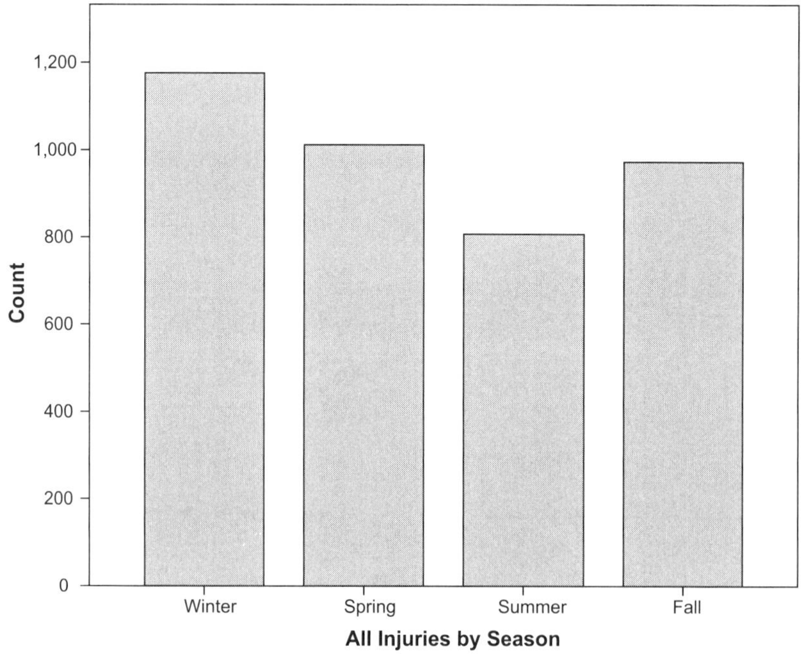

11.2. Admittance season of all injuries in the post–Civil War Seventh Cavalry. Note greatest frequency in winter and least in summer.

eye of medical professionals. Thus complaints then were more likely to be documented in the medical records than during warmer months and seasons, when companies tended to be deployed in the field and on marches, away from the post hospital.

Years of injury among the Seventh Cavalry's medical records were examined to determine whether there was a temporal trend from 1867 through 1883 (table 11.4, fig. 11.3). A methodological note is in order: the partial years 1866 and 1884 are omitted from these statistical analyses (although shown in the tables).

The annual injury totals showed spikes (1868 and 1878) and troughs (1869, 1873, and 1874). The fewest injuries (n = 132) occurred in 1873, midway in our study period. The maximum number of instances (n = 365, averaging about one injury each day of the year) happened five years earlier, in the leap year 1868. On average 233.4 injuries occurred each year. And the overall annual distribution deviated from a random pattern (1867 to 1883, χ^2 = 251.88, df = 16, $p < 0.000$).

When the total number of enlisted men and number of injuries were compared by year, the results remained significant (χ^2 = 247.20, df = 17, $p < 0.001$). Injuries increased most in 1868, probably related to more patrolling and the Battle of the Washita. And injuries remained high in 1877, when the Seventh Cavalry chased hostiles and fought engagements at Canyon and Snake Creeks. Injuries decreased in 1869, however, probably due to comparatively light duty escorting and mopping up after the Battle of the Washita. Injuries were also infrequent in 1873, when the Seventh Cavalry moved from the South to the northern plains and provided railroad escort along Yellowstone River. In addition, injuries were low in 1874, when the Black Hills Expedition took place.

POSTING REGIONS: CENTRAL PLAINS, SOUTH, AND NORTHERN PLAINS

This section turns to the distribution of injuries by geographic regions to determine whether the frequency of injuries was distributed evenly across the Seventh Cavalry's posting locations or whether some geographic regions were more injury-prone than others. The Seventh Cavalry was deployed first on the central plains (1866 to 1870), then transferred to the South (1871 to 1872),

TABLE 11.4. Admittance year of injuries among post–Civil War Seventh Cavalry members for entire sample (all injuries and subsets)

	ALL INJURIES		INTERNECINE TRANSPORTATION-RELATED INJURIES		VIOLENCE-RELATED INJURIES	
Year	*Frequency*	*Percentage*	*Frequency*	*Percentage*	*Frequency*	*Percentage*
1866	73	1.8	5	.9	0	
1867	235	5.9	2	.4	14	7.6
1868	365	9.2	1	.2	8	4.3
1869	141	3.5	0		2	1.1
1870	265	6.7	1	.2	1	.5
1871	213	5.4	8	1.5	9	4.9
1872	247	6.2	23	4.3	7	3.8
1873	132	3.3	14	2.6	8	4.3
1874	144	3.6	24	4.5	7	3.8
1875	247	6.2	46	8.7	3	1.6
1876	237	6.0	28	5.3	14	7.6
1877	285	7.2	56	10.6	11	5.9
1878	301	7.6	74	14.0	14	7.6
1879	252	6.3	53	10.0	24	13.0
1880	215	5.4	45	8.5	21	11.4
1881	222	5.6	46	8.7	18	9.7
1882	219	5.5	62	11.7	10	5.4
1883	172	4.3	41	7.8	13	7.0
1884	2	.1	0		1	.5
Total	3968	99.9	529	100.0	185	100.0

Note: The earliest year in the study (1866) was partial and has been omitted from statistical assessments; only whole years are tabulated. The year of one apparent typo (1886) also has been omitted.

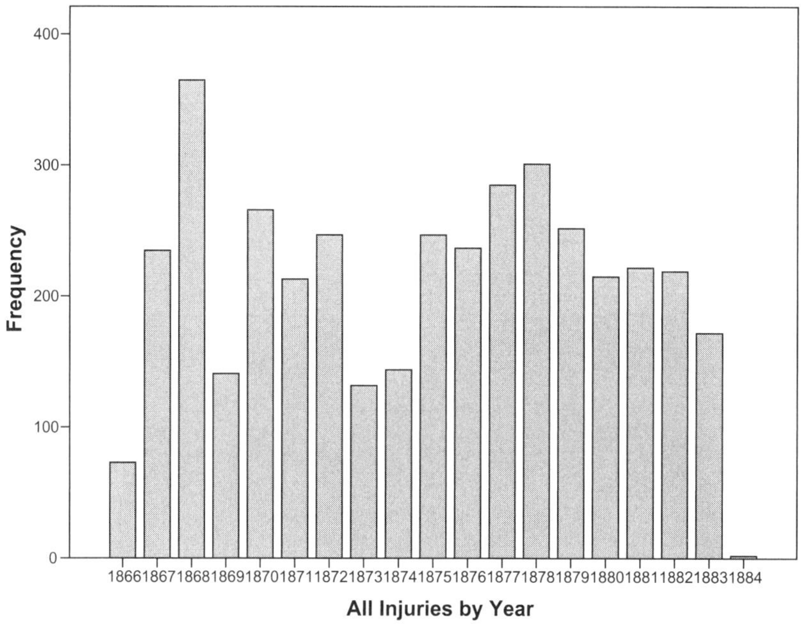

11.3. Admittance year of all injuries in the post–Civil War Seventh Cavalry.

and finally stationed in the northern plains (1873 to the end of the study period).

The raw count of injuries by geographic region is examined first and then compared to proportions of injuries and number of soldiers in those locations. Excluded from this tally are cases outside the three principal regions (for example, Fort Columbus, New York, and Washington, D.C.) as well as unstated or unclear locations. Taken together, the omitted injury records are a small proportion (1.8%) of geographic-specific injuries and should have little effect on geographic patterns of the remaining records.

Overall (table 11.5), the Seventh Cavalry sustained fewer injuries while stationed in the South (14.1% of injury total) than when posted in the central plains (30%). Outnumbering both of these regions combined, the majority of injuries occurred while the Seventh Cavalry was deployed in the northern plains (55.9%). The raw frequencies tell only part of the story, however.

What about the proportions of violent episodes per year in those regions? The Seventh Cavalry, after all, was stationed in the

TABLE 11.5. Geographic region where post–Civil War Seventh Cavalry injuries occurred for entire sample (all injuries and subsets)

	ALL INJURIES		TRANSPORTATION-RELATED INJURIES		INTERNECINE VIOLENCE-RELATED INJURIES	
Region	*Frequency*	*Percentage*	*Frequency*	*Percentage*	*Frequency*	*Percentage*
Central plains	1191	30.0	11	2.1	20	11.5
South	560	14.1	42	7.9	17	9.8
Northern plains	2221	55.9	465	89.9	137	78.7
Total	3972	100.0	518	100.0	174	100.0

northern plains longer than in the central plains and South combined. As it turns out, Seventh Cavalry annual injuries averaged less in the northern plains than in the central plains and South combined.

BIRTHPLACES

We now turn to intrinsic influences on injuries, including nativity, age, and stature. Were soldiers of some nationalities or from some states more likely to be injured than others?

Overall, the birthplaces of the sufferers of 2,208 instances of injuries were documented (table 11.6). U.S.-born troopers reported more injuries (n = 1,225, 55.5%) than foreign-born ones (n = 983, 44.5%). When the nationality (foreign-born vs. native-born) of those who suffered injuries was compared with the nationality of those who did not suffer injuries, a proportional difference emerges ($\chi^2 = 24.57$, df = 1, $p < 0.001$). Native-born troopers displayed proportionally fewer injuries, while foreign-born troopers reported proportionally more injuries.

Did variation within these two broad birth locations explain the difference between them?

Foreign-born trooper nationalities with the greatest number of injuries were Irish (n = 357 injuries), German (n = 323), English (n = 106), and Canadian (n = 60). Comparing these nationalities

TABLE 11.6. Birthplaces of post–Civil War Seventh Cavalry members suffering injuries for entire sample (all injuries)

Birth location	*Selected nativities (number)*	*Number*	*Percentage*
Foreign-born		983	44.5
	Ireland (357)		
	Germany (323)		
	England (106)		
	Canada (60)		
U.S.-born		1225	55.5
	New York (247)		
	Pennsylvania (220)		
	Ohio (157)		
	Massachusetts (102)		
Total		2208	100.0

of soldiers with injuries to those from the same countries without injuries, no difference in the distributions occurred ($\chi^2 = 0.64$, df $= 3$, $0.80 > p > 0.90$). So these foreign nationalities all reported similar proportions of injuries.

Among native U.S.-born troopers, the four birth states with troopers reporting the greatest number of injuries were New York ($n = 247$ injuries), Pennsylvania ($n = 220$), Ohio ($n = 157$), and Massachusetts ($n = 102$). All four states were eastern or Great Lakes states with large populations and constituted large proportions of Seventh Cavalry troopers. Comparing overall number of troopers from those four states who suffered and did not suffer injuries, no relationship was found ($\chi^2=2.50$, df $= 3$, $0.50 > p > 0.30$). Injuries among native-born troopers by birth state appear equally distributed.

So the difference between troopers sustaining injuries and number of enlisted men by birthplace occurred between foreign- and native-born solders, not among foreign nationalities or among U.S. home states. Foreign-born soldiers were simply more likely to be injured than U.S.-born soldiers.

AGE

Were soldiers of all ages likely to suffer injuries? Authorities have claimed that young adult males (risk-taking individuals in the throes of hormonal surges, lacking adequate interpersonal skills, and quick to anger) were more likely to engage in risky acts and to be involved in fights and accidents (Courtwright 1996a, 1996b). If those claims are true, then younger Seventh Cavalry members should show more injuries than older troopers.

The enlistment age of injured Seventh Cavalry soldiers contrasted with the age of uninjured troopers hits significance (t = 3.300, df = 6740, $p < 0.001$, two-tailed, equal variances assumed). The difference, however, is not what we expected. The average age of injured troopers (24.77 years) is slightly older than the average age of uninjured troopers (24.39 years), not younger.

Two possible explanations and an observation are in order. The first possibility is that older soldiers may have been more antisocial and remained in the military in part because they fit civil society poorly. These ornery older soldiers may have been quicker to anger and more prone to violence and accidents, resulting in injuries.

The second possibility is that older soldiers were similarly injury-prone as their younger counterparts but slower, weaker, and less well coordinated. Older soldiers lost fights and lost balance and thus were more likely to suffer injuries. If this explanation is correct, youth did have its advantages.

Finally, as a general comment, although injured troopers average older than uninjured troopers, that difference is minuscule. Less than half of a year separates the means of the two groups, a difference whose significance is questionable.

HEIGHT

The last intrinsic variable is stature. Although the injured soldiers' mean stature (67.16 inches) is slightly taller than the uninjured mean (67.21 inches), heights of troopers with and without injuries show no statistically significant differences ($t = -0.891$, df = 6740, $p = 0.373$).

Transportation-Related Injuries: Ungulates, Wagons, and Trains

This section and the following ones deal with subsets of the Seventh Cavalry injuries: conveyance-related injuries and two kinds of violence-related injuries. These discussions rely on marginal notes written on Seventh Cavalry medical records to identify the cause of injuries, not essential scripted information documented on all records. This reliance on notes may inject methodological limitations.

About one-third of the injury medical records have marginal notes concerning circumstances or causes of injuries, while the other two-thirds lack such documentation. So the majority of records are incomplete in this respect. For example, it is likely that some injuries noted as resulting from falls may have been falls from horses. But with no marginal notes specifying the tumble's circumstances, such cases were omitted from this consideration of conveyance-related injuries. Similarly, some kicked chins may have resulted from antagonistic actions by other persons. But lacking specific details related to cause, we omitted them from that specialized discussion.

First, we consider transportation and its dangers. Horses, wagons, and other means of transport formed the lifeblood of the cavalry, the military, and civilian society in general. Mobility was essential to the cavalry's function as well as the military's movements and supportive functions.

Mobility, however, came with baggage. Such dependence meant close association with potentially damaging vehicles and animals. Transportation technology caught the post–Civil War Seventh Cavalry near the apex of horse and mule use, at a time of continuing ship operation and the ascendancy of railroads (Wilson and Chen 2008). Additional changes have occurred since then. Similar vulnerabilities continue today, most often as vehicular accidents. They have a tremendous impact on the U.S. population.

During the most recent two decades (1990–2009), more than 10 million Americans were involved in motor vehicle accidents annually, resulting in 36,000 to 47,000 deaths each year (U.S. Census Bureau 2012:693, table 1103). If other transportation-related deaths were included in this count (for example, those involving bicycles, skateboards, and horses), fatalities would have been even greater.

Influences increasing the likelihood of accidents today include distracted and intoxicated drivers and excessive speed. Demographic variables also affect the probability of accidents. If you have any doubts about this assertion, add a teenaged driver to your automobile insurance policy. Drivers less than twenty-five years old are twice as likely to be involved in accidents as the population as a whole. And males have greater fatalities at all ages than females (Chang 2008; U.S. Census Bureau 2012:698, table 1114). Risk-taking, intoxicated young adult males are particularly vulnerable to bravado and vehicular accidents.

In the nineteenth century, before the self-serve internal-combustion engine ascended to supremacy, reliance on horse power and steam power constituted major risks. Such was the case in the post–Civil War Seventh Cavalry. Its medical records included 529 injuries related to transportation, nearly 13.3% of all injuries. This section summarizes those injuries by kinds, causes, actions, anatomical locations, year, geographic regions, and trooper ages and other intrinsic variables.

KINDS OF INJURIES

Table 11.1 shows the kinds of transportation-related injuries. Contusions constitute the majority of the conveyance-associated injuries (more than two-thirds). Sprains trail contusions, at approximately 15%. And lacerations follow with about 8%. Less frequent transportation-related injuries include fractures (n = 29), dislocations (n = 6), incised wounds (n = 4), concussions (n = 2), and a bite (n = 1). Other documents identify the culprit or wound (for example, "horse kick," amputation, and fall) but fail to indicate the kind of injury in the normal nineteenth-century nosology categories.

CAUSES

Ungulates and wagons caused most of the conveyance-related injuries. Among all causes in this category, horses were responsible for the majority (more than 80%), although mules (n = 22) and even a cow emerged as perpetrators. The vehicles that produced injuries (about 10%) consisted mostly of wagons, carts, carriages, ambulances, and an omnibus. Other moving objects that caused injuries included wheels ($n = 5$), railway cars (possibly $n = 4$), and sleighs ($n = 3$).

ACTIONS

The most frequent action that caused transportation-related injuries was being kicked by an animal (approximately 43% of recorded causes). As an example, Terrence Cavenaugh got a contused left leg, "occasioned by kick of horse," while at Yorkville, South Carolina, in January 1872. Next most frequently, falls from ungulates and vehicles constituted more than one-third of the injuries in this category. As an example, Gustave Koehler received a lacerated lip when he was "thrown by a fractious horse" at Fort Yates in October 1882.

Less frequent causes of conveyance-related injuries involved ungulates, including being stepped on ($n = 21$), being fallen on or falling with ($n = 16$), and being bitten ($n = 11$). The last cause includes James Sayers, who received a lacerated hand from the "bite of an officer [*sic*] horse" at Fort Meade in 1883. Sayers served as farrier at that time, so the steed was likely biting the hand that shoed it.

Even less frequently, a few conveyance-related injuries resulted from being run over ($n = 8$); pulled, wrenched, or jerked ($n = 4$); and hurt while catching a horse ($n = 2$). Hitting also caused a few injuries ($n = 2$). As an example, Frederick Tobey fractured his right little finger while "striking his horse with his fist" at Fort Lincoln in December 1878. We wonder what injury (if any) his horse sustained.

ANATOMICAL LOCATIONS

Anatomical locations of transportation-related injuries show a pattern. The majority of them affected the lower appendages (thigh, knee, lower leg, ankle, foot, and toe; approximately 55%). Next most frequently, injuries occurred to the upper appendages (arm, forearm, wrist, hand, fingers; about 15%), followed by the torso (back, side, breast, chest, and epigastric region; approximately 12%). The head (scalp, brain, face and lip; $n = 36$); shoulder ($n = 24$); genitals, groin, and testicles ($n = 14$); and hip ($n = 11$) showed fewer injuries.

Those are the descriptive parameters. Now we compare and contrast transportation-related injuries with variables that are extrinsic and intrinsic to the individual soldier.

TEMPORAL FREQUENCIES

Transportation-related injuries are considered in a temporal context, organized by month, season, and year. Injuries were greatest in October and May, fewest in February and March, averaging 44.08 injuries per month (table 11.2 and fig. 11.4). The monthly differences were significant ($\chi^2 = 21.74$, df = 11, $0.05 > p > 0.02$).

Although transportation-related injuries generally peaked in fall and fell in spring, that distribution failed to achieve statistical significance ($\chi^2 = 3.48$, df = 3, $0.50 > p > 0.30$).

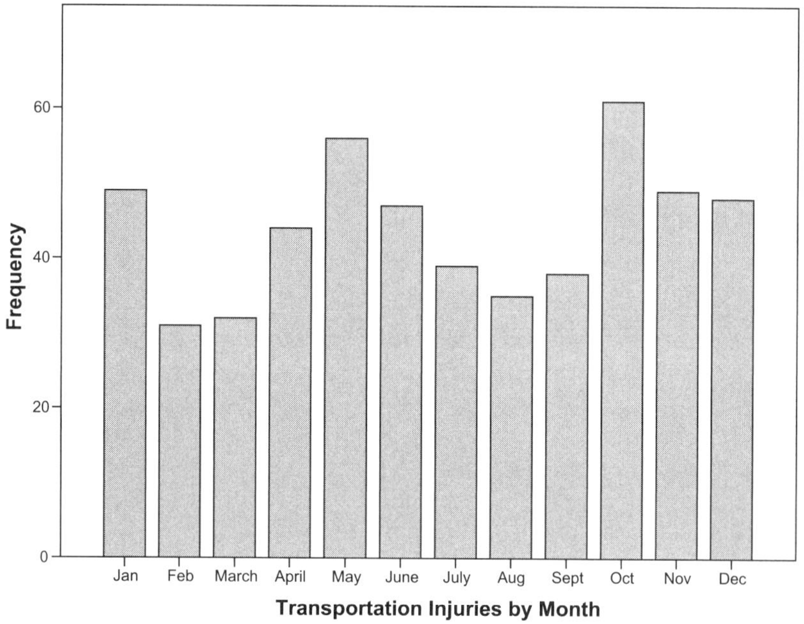

11.4. Admittance month of transportation-related injuries in the post–Civil War Seventh Cavalry. Note greatest frequency in October and least in February.

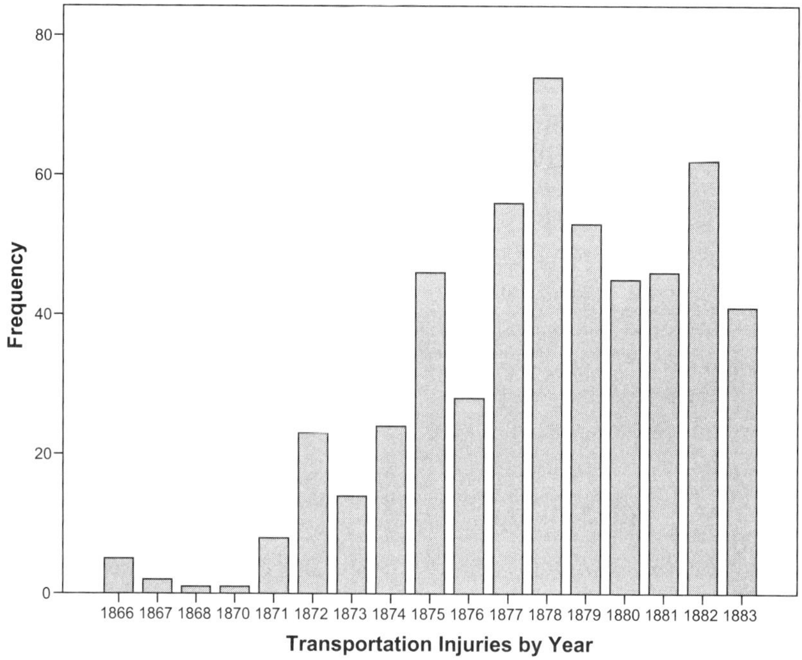

11.5. Admittance year of transportation-related injuries in the post–Civil War Seventh Cavalry. Note tendency for injuries to increase from the mid-1860s through the early 1880s.

Annual frequency of transportation-related injuries changed during the study period (table 11.4 and fig. 11.5). They increased from the 1860s into the early 1880s ($R^2 = 0.720$; injuries $= -7030.913 + [3.767 \times \text{year}]$), with 1878 and 1882 having particularly high numbers of transportation-related injuries.

This result is surprising. There should be little difference in Seventh Cavalry activities and mounts during the period. Perhaps the variation is related to changes in medical documentation rather than changes in injury frequencies.

GEOGRAPHIC REGIONS

Nearly 90% of the transportation-related injuries occurred in the northern plains. Fewer happened in the South, and fewest in the central plains.

AGE

The average age of the troopers suffering transportation-related injured differed from the age of those who were uninjured (t = 3.790, df = 462.89, p = 0.000; two-tailed, equal variances not assumed). The injured soldiers (25.40 years) averaged nearly a year older than the uninjured (24.46 years). Older soldiers may have had slowed response times and been more prone to conveyance-related injuries than their younger compatriots. This result also is surprising and contrasts with the frequency of present-day motor vehicle rates: today younger drivers are more accident-prone than older ones. Perhaps such a parallel does not extend to horse and wagon riders.

OTHER INTRINSIC VARIABLES

The other intrinsic variables showed no differences between injured and uninjured soldiers. Neither nativity (U.S.-born versus foreign-born; $\chi^2 = 0.32$, df = 1, $0.8 > p > 0.7$) nor height (t = 1.106, df = 6741, p = 0.269) reached statistical significance.

Internecine Violence, Skirmishes, and Injuries in the Plains and South

Images in movies and popular literature depict the nineteenth-century U.S. West as inhabited by an unruly, aggressive population. Whether the West of historians (such as Roger McGrath, Robert Utley, and Clare McKanna) or novelists (e.g., Louis L'Amour, Zane Grey, and—my favorite—Larry McMurtry), depictions of the frontier West ooze blood and violence. Bio-osteologists also tend to emphasize western skeletons involved in violent encounters (for example, Scott et al. 1998; Owsley and Bruwelheide 2008; Weathermon 2008).

The post–Civil War South is similarly depicted as an unsettled and violent-prone place. Both regions had frayed social fabrics and reputations as fostering cultures of violence, resulting in interpersonal flare-ups and fights. These reputations have taken on near mythical standing.

The Seventh Cavalry troopers' injuries included violent intramural and extramural interpersonal encounters in the West and South. In addition to conflict between Seventh Cavalry members and opposing forces, injuries were inflicted by fellow soldiers with fists and any other handy weapons. Injuries caused by comrades and citizens as well as those sustained in skirmishes are considered here. When honor, status, and poorly socialized young men were involved, fights were bound to happen within the group as well as between groups. Encounters with some civilians also resulted in conflicts.

Some areas in the post–Civil War United States were populated disproportionately by itinerant young adult males, many of whom had fought in the Civil War or experienced the war as children and adolescents. The Civil War "had an almost incalculable effect on the following decades" (Brown 1969:64). "The period from the Civil War to World War I was probably the most violent one in our history" (Brown 1970:3). When the armies mustered out men, they released fathers, farmers, clerks, and sociopaths alike into civil society.

Veterans had training and new attitudes toward violence as well as new lethal skills and experience. Violence in the post–Civil War period could be said to begin with the first assassination of a U.S. president, Abraham Lincoln, in April 1865 and continued for decades, including the second assassinated president, James A. Garfield, in July 1881. These decades spanned the core of our study period. Some authorities claim that the same violent trajectory continued from the past into today, with recent assassinations, mass murders, and serial murders representing perpetuation of the violent momentum established in the nineteenth century.

In addition to time, region, and experience, demographic distortions also occurred. Horace Greeley's popular edict "Go West, young man" was clearly directed at only one segment of the population. Either as a consequence of Greeley's directive or as a description of that demographic bulge, the frontier tended to be occupied in large part by young males. Few Euro-American females, few older males, few children, and few families inhabited the western frontier. Young adult males were well suited for the rigors of western life, with its freedom and economic opportunities that required hard labor, ready adaptability, and exposure to danger. Furthermore, many western migrants ascribed to a culture of swagger and violence. The frontier was summarized as being filled by "a self-conscious people, misfits, malcontents, folk who did not fit into the older, more established societies" (Roberts 1976:96). In addition to being brash, resenting authority, being quick to anger, and despising encroaching civilization (Roberts 1976), the demographic majority was an aberrant one.

Contemporary young men are often associated with being more violence-prone and more risk-taking than females and other age groups. Young men, it has been claimed, are "the heart of American violence" today as well as in the past (Courtwright 1996a:36). And because the western frontier had relatively few members of other demographic groups, poorly socialized young males dominated society, just as today young adult males dominate college bars on Saturday nights.

To this unstable mix of armed young men, add intoxication. Alcohol abuse lowered inhibitions and increased the probability of violence. Alcohol consumption served as an accelerant tossed on the fire.

So far this discussion has emphasized western frontier instability and the West as a clash location. But the frontier was not the only collision location in the late 1860s and 1870s. Recall that the South faced its own social and economic upheavals following the Civil War.

Southerners were stereotyped as prone to violence too. Even before the Civil War descriptions of the South included much violence among individuals and between groups. "Tales of duels, murder, and assault were stock items in scores of contemporary travel accounts, newspaper stories, and grand jury presentments" (Bodenhamer 1981:112–13). Modern historians have credited southerners with "a readiness to settle private disputes with fists, dirks, or even pistols" (Bodenhamer 1981:112–13). In part related to notions of honor, explosive encounters often occurred.

The Reconstruction South provided additional devastation wrought by the effects and aftereffects of war. The South suffered slow economic recovery, demographic perturbations in age and sex groups, and the psychosocial and political adjustments of the vanquished.

To evaluate these claims, this section examines indications of violent behavior in the Seventh Cavalry, during a period fifty years before establishment of the Federal Bureau of Investigation's Uniform Crime Reporting and a full century before the National Crime Victimization Survey was initiated. The Seventh Cavalry's medical records provide information on kinds of interpersonal violent injuries, perpetrators, actions causing injuries, anatomical parts involved, and extrinsic and intrinsic variables.

KINDS OF INJURIES

The most frequent injuries resulting from internecine interpersonal violence consisted of contusions ($n = 64$), gunshot wounds ($n = 37$), lacerations ($n = 33$), and incised wounds and fractures (both $n = 11$; table 11.1). Less frequent violent injuries resulted from bites, burns, concussions, dislocations, puncture wounds, and sprains.

The most frequent violence-related injuries were contusions. As an example, First Sergeant Edward Clyde received a contused left eye "in [a] personal affray" while stationed at Fort Buford in February 1883. Gunshot wounds constituted the next greatest number of interpersonal violent injuries.

Lacerations also occurred. As an example, John M. Marshall sustained a laceration when he was "hit on the head by a comrade in a brawl with an earthenware pitcher" at Fort Rice in January 1878. Because he was out of service until the next month, the pitcher was presumably not of the theatrical variety so often employed in classic western movies.

Fractures and incised wounds tied in frequency. Most fractures happened to recipients of violent action, but at least one person sustained a break resulting from his own aggressive act. John Schell broke his right fifth metacarpal (a bone in the palm of the hand near the little finger) while a prisoner fighting at Fort Yates in 1881. Such breaks, called boxer's fractures, are commonly sustained when punching someone with a fist.

Incised wounds constituted the second of the two tied types of injuries resulting from violence. As an example of such wounds, Micheal [*sic*] Daniels received "3 incised wounds with a knife by a comrade while both were drunk at a Negro dance" near Fort Yates in February 1879.

Less frequent violence-related injuries included sprains ($n = 9$), arrow wounds ($n = 7$), bites ($n = 4$), burns ($n = 3$), dislocations

(n = 2), and a concussion and a puncture wound (n = 1 for each). As an example of a sprain from an internecine encounter, Michael Pendergrass sprained his left shoulder when he was thrown on a box during a fight at Camp Hodgson in June 1880.

All arrow wounds occurred in 1867 near Fort Wallace. This incidence indicated transition from bow-driven to gunpowder-propelled projectiles in the late 1860s.

Bites among adversaries happened in fights too. All documented bites involved fingers and required amputations. To paraphrase modern-day physician Jeff Thomas of Chico, California, the human mouth is a cesspool of infectious agents. As an example, Allen Battle had "[a]n ulcer affecting the second and third phalanges of the right index finger. It resulted from a bite inflicted by an adversary in a fight" in Columbia, South Carolina, during July 1872. The subsequent infection necessitated the "[r]ight index finger [being] amputated at 1st phalangal [*sic*] articulation at Post of Spartunburg [*sic*] SC Aug. 15[,] 1872."

Some fights resulted in burns. John Mathasz's left second finger received a burn from a "comrade placing fire on finger." Nice comrade!

Both interpersonal violence-related dislocations involved left shoulder injuries received while wrestling a comrade.

The single violence-related concussion happened to August Schmidt. He sustained a brain concussion from being struck with a club during a brawl while in the field during August 1877.

A puncture wound was caused by a spear. J. T. Hamsted received an injury involving a "spear & G.S. [gunshot] wound" while near Fort Wallace in June 1867. And an apparent sharp force wound happened when a tomahawk struck Charles Clark's skull in June 1867 at Fort Wallace, causing his death.

PERPETUATORS: HOSTILES, CITIZENS, AND AMIGOS

Who caused these violence-related injuries? Documented perpetrators of such injuries included "friendly" citizens, officers and fellow troopers (89.6%), and Indian combatants (n = 19, 10.4%). All bites, burns, concussions, contusions, dislocations, incised wounds, and lacerations and most fractures and sprains were caused by citizens and fellow soldiers. All arrow wounds and many gunshot wounds were attributed to encounters with opposing Indians.

ACTIONS CAUSING VIOLENT INJURIES

Excluding for the moment the few who sustained injuries during skirmishes, intramural violent injuries occurred in brawls ($n = 67$), fights or personal affrays ($n = 46$), and other injurious activities (for example, being pushed, beaten, struck, kicked, and wrestled; $n = 36$).

ANATOMICAL LOCATIONS OF INJURIES

Violent interpersonal encounters impacted anatomical locations unequally. More than half of these injuries ($n = 86$, 52.1%) affected the head (scalp, face, lip, temple, brain, eyes, chin, and neck). Over one-fourth of the injuries involved an upper appendage ($n = 47$, 28.5%; arm, forearm, especially wrist, hand, and fingers). Approximately 8 percent of the injuries involved the torso ($n = 13$; breast, spine, thorax, back, lung, chest, rib, side, genitals, lumbar area). Other injuries affected the lower appendages ($n = 10$, 6.1%; thigh, leg, ankle, foot, toes), shoulder ($n = 8$, 4.8%), and hip ($n = 1$, 0.6%).

As the list shows, interpersonal aggression targeted the head—that most distinctive human and most vulnerable anatomical part. Such injuries demonstrated antagonists' desire to inflict damage and alter recognizable human features. These efforts seemed intent on dehumanizing and disfiguring the opponent.

The next most frequently affected region (the upper appendages, especially wrists, hands and fingers) sustained damage worthy of medical note. These injuries indicated mechanical failure when relatively small anatomical parts were hurled at rapid speeds and encountered larger, relatively immovable objects. When fragile anatomical structures were exposed to such forces, mechanical failure of tissues often followed.

The thorax (abdomen and lower limb anatomical regions, where few injuries happen) was not so susceptible to these physical forces. Considering the large surface areas and volumes of the thorax and abdomen relative to those of the head and upper limb, the small frequency of injuries in this area is remarkable. If injuries were simply a function of size or volume, the thorax and abdomen should have suffered the greatest number.

This distribution of internecine interpersonal violent injuries differed markedly from the distribution of transport-related injuries (presented in the previous section). Those transportation-related injuries involved lower appendages (55%), followed by upper appendages (15%), and the torso (12%). Interpersonal violent injuries, however, targeted the head, followed by upper appendages then lower appendages.

We now compare the violence-associated injuries by extrinsic and intrinsic variables.

TEMPORAL

Monthly internecine violence-related injuries varied but were not statistically significant ($p = 0.35$; table 11.2).

Seasonal violence-related injuries were similar in winter, summer, and fall, but plummeted in spring (table 11.3). The distribution was significant (one-sample $\chi^2 = p < 0.032$), with under-representation of injuries in spring contributing most to the relationship.

Violent injuries varied by year (table 11.4, fig. 11.6). The number of interpersonal internecine injuries rose during the late 1870s and early 1880s, when the Seventh Cavalry was posted on the northern plains. The fewest generally occurred in the late 1860s through the mid-1870s.

REGIONS

Because the Seventh Cavalry's shortest posting time occurred in the South, that region had the fewest violent-related injuries (n = 17; table 11.5). A few more occurred in the central plains (n = 20), probably in skirmishes with Indians. The greatest frequency was in the northern plains (n = 137, 78.7%), where the Seventh Cavalry spent of the most time. As demonstrated by the yearly distribution, the northern plains showed the greatest annual numbers of internecine injuries.

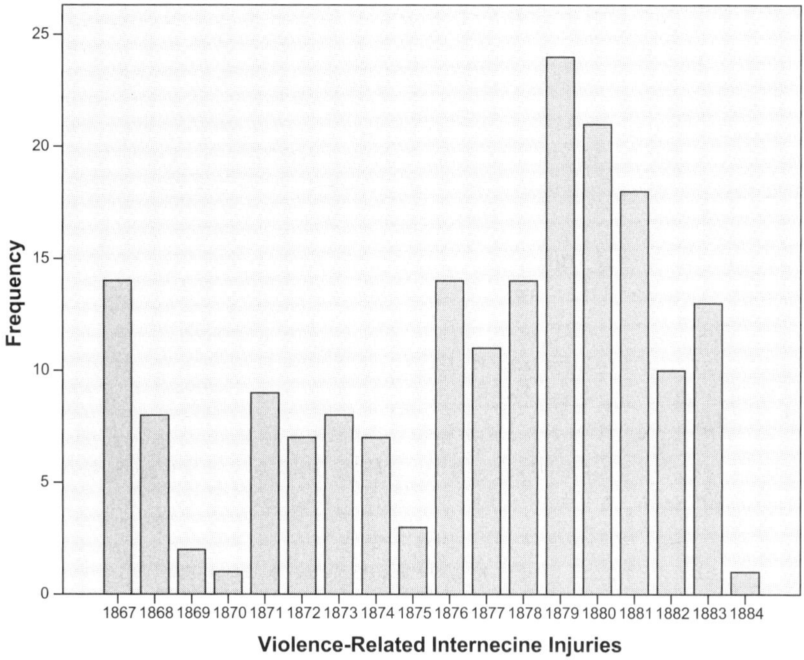

11.6. Admittance year of violence-related internecine injuries in the post–Civil War Seventh Cavalry. Note tendency for increased violence-related injuries in the late 1870s and early 1880s.

INTRINSIC VARIABLES

Some of the intrinsic variables showed differences in internecine violence-related injury frequencies (age and nativity). Others did not. A difference occurred between the ages of troopers suffering violence-induced injuries (mean 25.47 years) and the ages of the uninjured (mean 24.49 years; t = 2.367, df = 167.73, p = 0.019, equal variance not assumed). Injured troopers averaged a year older than the uninjured. Foreign-born troopers showed more frequent violence-related injuries than U.S.-born soldiers(χ^2 = 6.49, df = 1, $0.025 > p > 0.010$), although this difference did not achieve significance. Troopers suffering internecine violent injuries were on average shorter (67.49 inches) than the uninjured (69.13 inches), but no statistical relationship between height and violent injuries existed ($t = -0.183$, df = 6743, $p > 0.855$).

Battle-Related Injuries

The Seventh Cavalry's renown in large part resulted from the regiment's frontier battles. The Seventh Cavalry engaged in twenty-seven battles and skirmishes during the study period. Other regiments were engaged more frequently, but none suffered the combat deaths found in the Seventh Cavalry. This section considers battle-related injuries and the few deaths documented in the Carded Medical Records. Chapter 14 presents a more thorough assessment of deaths that occurred in the Seventh Cavalry and other regiments stationed in the post–Civil War West.

The Seventh Cavalry fought four major encounters, which are reviewed here (chapter 1 presents these battles in more detail). In chronological order, the first important fight occurred at the Washita River, now in Oklahoma, on November 27, 1868. The Seventh Cavalry surprised a Cheyenne village under the leadership of Black Kettle and fought a day-long battle before retreating. About three dozen Seventh Cavalry members were wounded or killed.

On August 4 and 11, 1873, while supporting the Northern Railroad Survey, the Seventh Cavalry fought running battles with northern Plains Indians along the Yellowstone River, now in eastern Montana. About a dozen Seventh Cavalry members were wounded or killed in these actions.

On June 25–26, 1876, the Seventh Cavalry's most famous encounter occurred: the Battle of the Little Bighorn. It was part of the Campaign of 1876, designed to force "hostiles" from roaming the northern plains onto reservations. The Seventh Cavalry discovered and attacked an enormous village of Lakotas, Cheyennes, and Arapahos. The battle continued for two days, ending when the Seventh Cavalry survivors were relieved by an advancing column. About 308 Seventh Cavalry members suffered wounds or death during the Battle of the Little Bighorn.

The last major encounter during our study period occurred the next year in September and October. As Chief Joseph and the Nez Perces progressed toward Canada, the Seventh Cavalry intercepted them on September 13, 1877, at Canyon Creek near the Yellowstone River in south-central Montana. The Seventh Cavalry lost twenty-two killed and forty wounded. The Nez Perces escaped that battle and continued north toward the U.S.-Canadian boundary. Later that month and in early October the Seventh Cavalry again fought the Nez Perces, this time in north-central Montana on Snake Creek (Bear Paw), less than fifty miles (eighty-two km) from Canada.

Analysis of this subset consisting of battle-related injuries requires a few methodological explanations. Dates of all injury Carded Medical Records were searched for those occurring near the times of these battles, indicating injuries that may have resulted from hostile encounters. Some Carded Medical Records indicated that the injuries were received in battle and a few that accidents caused them, while others required additional outside supporting information. Altogether 122 injuries could be attributed to battles (over 20 percent of all the injuries that the Carded Medical Records document).

KINDS AND LOCATIONS OF INJURIES

The causes and anatomical locations of the battle-related injuries (table 11.1) are presented first. Gunshot wounds caused most of the battle-related injuries. The Medical Record Cards indicated 99 gunshot wounds, the earliest ones at the Washita and continuing through the most recent Nez Perce encounters considered in our study. In addition, Carded Medical Records showed 4 arrow wounds received during battle, all suffered in the encounter at the Washita in 1868. That change from arrows to bullet wounds demonstrates a transition in Indian weapons from bows and arrows to firearms during the decades following the Civil War. The Carded Medical Records also documented 21 soldiers killed in action (KIA), all at the Washita. That documentation apparently indicates a change in record-keeping regulations from early records to late records related to deaths in battle. After the Washita battle, medical records fail to show KIAs from later encounters (a point revisited in chapter 14). Finally, a sprain to the left knee was sustained at Snake Creek.

Many but not all of the battle-related injury Carded Medical Records indicate the location injured, both by anatomical region and by side of the body. More right sides ($n = 51$) were injured in battle than left sides ($n = 41$), although that difference is not statistically significant (binomial $p = 0.348$).

About half of the battle-related injuries in the Carded Medical Records specified the body part involved, some indicating multiple locations for one trooper. For analytical purposes the anatomical regions were divided into six general areas: (1) head and face; (2) thorax and abdomen; (3) shoulder; (4) arm, forearm, wrist, and hand; (5) hip; and (6) thigh, knee, leg, ankle, and foot. Arm-forearm-wrist-hand tied with thigh-knee-leg-ankle-foot (both $n = 33$). Next most frequent, the shoulder and thorax-abdomen tied ($n = 15$), followed by head-neck ($n = 9$), and finally hip ($n = 6$). Note that among battle-related injuries limbs appear to have been more vulnerable than larger anatomical regions, such as the thorax-abdomen. Perhaps injuries to the thorax-abdomen and head-neck with their vital organs were more likely to be fatal than injuries to limbs. Thus surviving troopers with limb injuries would be more likely to come to the surgeons' attention, so their injuries made their way into the medical records. Parenthetically, it might have been possible to test this assertion using the Washita KIAs, but none of those medical records indicated the anatomical locations damaged in that battle.

Because the KIAs seem to be a special instance of battle-related injuries, documented only in the earliest Carded Medical Records and omitted from the more recent ones, they are excluded from further assessment in this section.

INTRINSIC VARIABLES

Perhaps as expected, individuals who suffered battle-related injuries had intrinsic parameters similar to those of individuals who escaped such injuries. Similarities between those injured and uninjured groups hold for birthplaces (U.S.-born versus foreign-born, $\chi^2 = 0.04$, df = 1, $0.90 > p > 0.80$), ages at enlistment ($t = -0.19$, df = 6741, $p > 0.985$), and stature ($t = -0.309$, df = 674, $p = 0.757$). Battle-related injuries affected troopers equally regardless of nativity, age, or height.

Summary

No U.S. military regiment lost more men in western frontier battles during the post–Civil War period than the Seventh Cavalry. Other regiments fought in more engagements but suffered far fewer casualties. The Seventh Cavalry fought in thirty-one battles and skirmishes in all, losing 328 men, nearly one-third of all combat deaths recorded for the period 1866 to 1891 (Johnson 2012). Those fights also resulted in about 166 injuries in the same period (Johnson 2012). Battle-related injuries accounted for many of the injuries documented in the Seventh Cavalry's medical records, but more injuries were derived from internecine fights than from encounters with hostiles. Regardless of cause, altogether injuries constituted nearly 20 percent of all ailments.

Considering all injuries together, contusions constituted the most numerous category, far more than double the number of sprains, the next most frequent injury. Incised wounds, lacerations, and gunshot wounds occurred less frequently. Temporal trends could be discerned. Injuries increased in January and during winter and decreased in August and during the summer. The annual distribution of all injuries varied, most likely due to changing exposure to trauma during the period.

Overall, most injuries happened in the northern plains, fewest in the South. Foreign-born soldiers reported more injuries than their U.S.-born counterparts, and older soldiers received more injuries than younger soldiers. No height differences existed between injured and uninjured soldiers.

The first focus on the subsets of these injuries was on those related to transportation. The majority of such injuries resulted from contact with horses and other ungulates, with fewer caused by vehicles. Most injuries in this category consisted of contusions, sprains, and lacerations. The lower appendage sustained the most injuries, followed by the upper appendage and then the torso. The greatest numbers of conveyance-related injuries happened in October and May, the fewest in February and March. Despite monthly differences, no seasonal differences emerged. But conveyance-related injuries increased from the 1860s into the early 1880s. Of the transportation-related injuries almost 90 percent happened on the northern plains. Greater mobility may have been required on the northern plains than in the Seventh Cavalry's previous assignments in other regions, leading to greater susceptibility.

Older troopers tended to have more transportation-related injuries than younger troopers, although the age difference between the groups was small. The other intrinsic variables (birthplace and height) showed no relationship.

The second focus was on internecine violent injuries. The post–Civil War West and Reconstruction South constituted two violent regions during an especially violent period. As the regiment's luck would have it, the Seventh Cavalry was stationed in both of those volatile regions during the mid-nineteenth century. The most frequent interpersonal injuries consisted of contusions, gunshot wounds, and lacerations. Perpetrators included intramural comrades (fellow troopers and civilians) and hostile forces. The most frequently reported injured parts resulting from these violent encounters were the head and neck, then the upper appendage, followed by the lower appendage.

The frequency of internecine violence-related injuries varied by time. Most violent injuries happened in June and December, the fewest in March and May. As might be expected from the monthly distribution, these kinds of injuries were lowest in spring.

The northern plains had greater numbers of internecine violent injuries than the central plains, with the least in the South. No intrinsic affects (nativity and height) achieved significance. Age differences approached significance but failed to achieve that threshold. Soldiers injured in violent encounters averaged about half a year older than uninjured soldiers.

The third focus involved injuries received from hostiles during major battles. The Seventh Cavalry fought twenty-seven battles and skirmishes during the study period. The Seventh Cavalry participated in four major encounters: Washita (1868), Yellowstone (1873), Little Bighorn (1876), and the Nez Perce Campaign (1877).

Gunshot wounds caused the vast majority of battle-related injuries, followed by KIAs (Washita only) and arrow wounds (Washita only). Some anatomical regions were more vulnerable than others. The upper and lower limbs came first, followed by the shoulder and thorax-abdomen, then the head-neck, and finally the hip. The two sides were injured equally. The presence and absence of battle-related injuries occurred randomly by nativity (U.S.-born versus foreign-born), age, and height.

CHAPTER 12

Post–Traumatic Stress Disorder and the Seventh Cavalry

P. Willey, Gary Plank, and Douglas D. Scott

Post-Traumatic Stress Disorder (PTSD) resulting from recent conflicts in southwest Asia has caught the attention of journalists and public alike (see, for instance, Goode 2009; National Institute of Health 2009; Finkel 2013; and Vogel 2013). PTSD has been defined as "a delayed stress syndrome caused by exposure to combat and can produce symptoms of rage, guilt, flashbacks, nightmares, depression, and emotional numbing, and can lead to a variety of grave and psychiatric problems—from unemployment to suicide" (Dean 1997:5). In addition to present-day expressions, anecdotal accounts indicate postwar stress syndromes affected soldiers thousands of years ago, raising the question of whether Seventh Cavalry troopers experienced similar impacts.

This chapter examines members of the post–Civil War Seventh Cavalry for indications of PTSD, using individual histories and an epidemiological approach and relating them to the Seventh Cavalry's three major encounters. But first background information on the history of postwar stress syndromes and modern definitions is presented.

History

Throughout history, troubling symptoms suffered by some war veterans have been reported. The behaviors had no readily identifiable medical or apparent physiological basis.

Ancient accounts suggested that postwar stress syndromes were not a new phenomenon (Battle of Marathon 2006; Persian Wars 2009). Herodotus related an account from the Battle of Marathon (490 BC). He described Epizelus, a Greek soldier. After the battle Epizelus recounted seeing a gigantic warrior with a huge beard who fought near him and killed his fellow soldier. Without apparent medical reason Epizelus was blind for the rest of his life.

During the Napoleonic Wars, soldiers reported tingling, twitching, and partial paralysis when they had been close to passing projectiles or explosions but dodged physical wounds. This condition was called "cerebro-spinal shock" or "wind contusions" (Jones 2006). During the U.S. Civil War, unexplained symptoms were reported, commonly called "soldier's heart" (Barton 2009). Eric Dean (1997) and Earl Hess (1997) reasoned that PTSD-like symptoms existed then, although the concepts and terms differ from those of today. They noted insanity (usually resulting in sequestration in an insane asylum and discharge from service), nostalgia (including depression and homesickness), irritable or soldier's heart (such as palpitations and "muscular exhaustion of heart"), and sunstroke (sometimes associated with nervousness and agitation). Additional symptoms included shortness of breath, chest pains, fatigue, headache, dizziness, diarrhea, and sleep disturbances.

During the South African Anglo-Boer War (1899–1902), British servicemen suffered "disordered action of the heart." This condition was believed to be caused by the constriction of the chest from the webbing of the heavy packs that the soldiers carried. Symptoms consisted of irritability, changes in personality, nightmares, fatigue, shortness of breath, back pain, rapid or irregular heartbeat, headaches, joint pains, and poor concentration (Jones 2006). Unfortunately, people at that time had few insights into the condition and minimal treatment.

Advances in psychology and understanding of human behavior since World War I have yielded more information about postwar stress syndromes, their causes, and their treatments. During World War I, for example, postwar stress symptoms were labeled "shell shock" (Grossman 2000). It was believed that its symptoms resulted from exposure to bomb and mortar shell explosions. Clinicians thought that exploding shells caused brain concussions, thereby producing the symptoms (Grossman 2000). That postwar stress syndrome was also called "combat stress reaction" and believed to develop in replacement soldiers sent to new units, where they perceived themselves as unwelcomed (Jones et al. 2002).

During World War II, the postwar stress syndrome was known as "battle fatigue" or "combat fatigue" (Marlowe 2000). The cause of the symptoms shifted from a biological basis to an experiential one (Marlowe 2000). These external factors included threat or danger, primitive living conditions, hunger and thirst, periods of intense fear and great boredom, disease and accident, grief from the loss of comrades, anxiety over domestic concerns, and unrest within the military unit (Marlowe 2000). Many of the World War II symptoms included gastrointestinal complaints (Jones 2006). Other symptoms were similar to those of World War I, such as sleep disturbance, trouble concentrating, diarrhea, fatigue, heart palpitations, and memory problems (Hyams et al. 1996).

In the Korean War psychological battle casualties were attributed to "operational exhaustion" (Barton 2009). Symptoms included fatigue, hyperventilation, and panic attacks (Hyams et al. 1996). The term "battle fatigue" was not used, but similar illnesses included manic-depression, anxiety neurosis, panic disorder, and chronic fatigue syndrome. These symptoms often appeared to be somatic. Combat stress reaction was a significant problem during this conflict, but only during the Vietnam War was the term "PTSD" applied. A distinction was made between Acute Combat Stress Reaction (ACSR) and PTSD. ACSR was the immediate result of psychological trauma, while PTSD referred to longer-term psychological trauma (Hyams et al. 1996).

During the Vietnam War, symptoms reported by soldiers included reexperiencing the traumatic event, increased arousal, feeling detached, anxiety, nightmares, difficulty sleeping, and irritability or outbursts of anger. Although symptoms varied, they often had long-lasting and debilitating effects. Until the post-Vietnam era treatment for PTSD involved removing the soldier from combat and little else (Grossman 1996).

Some similar and other dissimilar symptoms have been reported after the recent Persian Gulf, Iraq, and Afghanistan wars, including headache, joint and muscle pain, fatigue, shortness of breath, chest pain, diarrhea, skin rashes, forgetfulness, trouble concentrating, sleep disturbance, depression, and irritability. Such symptoms have been labeled the Gulf War Syndrome (Hyams et al. 1996).

Each war has different circumstances, so authorities are hesitant to label all postwar stress syndromes with the same title. As a further complication, symptoms are self-reported and interpreted by the examining physician. Many symptoms are similar, but some are specific to particular wars. For example, during World War I many symptoms concentrated around the heart, while during World War II symptoms centered on the abdominal area. As understanding and vocabulary have changed, so has the reporting and labeling of these symptoms (Hyams et al. 1996).

It is appropriate to consider the differing challenges that each war presented. During World War I, soldiers were exposed to more explosive ordnance than in earlier wars. During the Vietnam War, soldiers were exposed to Agent Orange as well as jungle conditions. That war introduced a new form of jungle warfare where the soldier was often unable to distinguish enemy combatants, allies, and civilians. During the Persian Gulf War, soldiers may have been exposed to chemical weapons and were subjected to desert conditions. Soldiers worried about enemy infiltration into secured areas, inability to distinguish between enemy combatants and civilians, and terrorist attacks, improvised explosive devices, and suicide bombings. Because of these differences clinicians have been reluctant to label all postwar stress syndromes with a single title. Despite these differences, however, many similarities in symptoms are reported. All symptoms appear to be related to patients' stress and anxiety.

Edgar Jones and Simon Wessely (2001) indicate that causes of postwar stress were related to similar stress-inducing situations. Work by the National Institute of Mental Health divided post–traumatic stress symptoms into three groups. The first category consisted of reexperiencing symptoms that included flashbacks, sweating, heart palpitations, nightmares, and intrusive thoughts. The second category included avoidance of places or circumstances, feeling numb emotionally, trouble with memory, loss of interest in previously enjoyable activities, and strong feelings of guilt or depression. The third category consisted of hyperarousal symptoms, including feeling tense or on edge, difficulty sleeping, angry outbursts, trouble concentrating, and being startled easily (National Institute of Mental Health n.d.).

Considering the prevalence of postwar stress syndromes following earlier wars, the question of the Seventh Cavalry's experience arises. Before examining those troopers' possible symptoms, PTSD symptoms in the twenty-first century are reviewed to place the Seventh Cavalry's experiences in context.

Current Definitions of PTSD

The *Diagnostic and Statistical Manual of Mental Disorders*, the bible of psychiatric clinicians, includes PTSD as an anxiety disorder (American Psychiatric Association [APA] 2013:271–80). It identifies PTSD as an expression of extreme terror or horror and disabling ineffectiveness following exposure to a traumatic event. PTSD may also result from the threat of a traumatic event or even hearing about such a traumatic event occurring to a close friend or relative. The trauma might be death, injury, or harm or threats that those events might occur.

The most common features associated with PTSD are terror, defenselessness, traumatization, an ongoing reliving of the traumatic experience (such as flashbacks), avoiding phenomena associated with the event (such as anniversaries, persons reminiscent of the event, or the location where an event occurred), psychological numbing (such as disinterest in previously pleasurable activities, detachment, or emotional remoteness), and heightened nervousness (such as anxiety, insomnia, or irritability). An increase in associated symptoms may also occur, such as depression, self-destructive or aggressive urges, substance abuse, and physical ailments.

PTSD symptoms usually begin within three months of the trauma. But onset may be delayed, with symptoms emerging six months or even longer after the event. In either acute or delayed expressions symptoms must persist for more than a month and must not have been present before exposure to the traumatic event. Resolution of PSTD symptoms occurs within three months in approximately one-half of the cases; the other half's symptoms persist more than a year (APA 2013:276–77). If the Seventh Cavalry shows PTSD-related conditions, we expect them to follow this chronological distribution.

Acute Stress Disorder (ASD), mentioned earlier under the older term, ACSR, is defined as "the development of characteristic symptoms lasting 3 days to 1 month following exposure to one or more traumatic events" (APA 2013:281). These symptoms happen close to the event and are short-lived, persisting a maximum of four weeks. Before a diagnosis of PTSD, the individual must have experienced symptoms for more than one month. Due to the diagnostic criteria of these disorders, they do not overlap, although a person with ASD may develop PTSD later (APA 2013:276).

The Seventh Cavalry was involved in three major encounters (table 12.1) and many lesser skirmishes. The earliest major

TABLE 12.1. Battles and battle-related stress periods involving the post–Civil War Seventh Cavalry

Battle name	*Date of battle*	*Prestress period*	*Acute stress disorder*	*Heightened PTSD*	*Continuing PTSD*
Battle of the Washita	November 28, 1868	November 1867–October 1868	December 1868	January–December 1869	January–December 1870
Battle of the Little Bighorn	June 25–27, 1876	June 1875–May 1876	July 1876	August 1876–July 1877*	August 1877–July 1878
Nez Perce Campaign	September 13 & September 30, October 5, 1877	September 1876–August 1877*	October 1877	November 1877–October 1878	November 1878–October 1879

*Note overlapping time interval of the Battle of the Little Bighorn's heightened PTSD period (August 1876–July 1877) and the Nez Perce Campaign's prestress period (September 1876–August 1877).

encounter happened in November 1868 on the Washita River against the Cheyennes. The second—the regiment's most famous battle—occurred in June 1876 on the Little Bighorn River. And the Seventh Cavalry engaged the Nez Perces at Canyon and Snake Creeks in Montana in September and October of 1877. All of these battles are treated more thoroughly in chapter 1 and in a plethora of scholarly books and articles.

The Seventh Cavalry medical records were examined for evidence of postwar stress symptoms. During the nineteenth century, little was known about the symptoms and their associated behaviors. Consequently, soldiers exhibiting stress-related symptoms were not identified or treated for those conditions. Seventh Cavalry Carded Medical Records and disciplinary documents, however, show examples of behaviors that might be associated with stress-induced symptoms. Here we present several individuals' postbattle experiences and provide an epidemiological assessment of violence, intoxication, and desertions.

Seventh Cavalry Troopers Possibly Displaying Symptoms of PTSD

On June 21, 1877, just a few days before the first anniversary of the Battle of the Little Bighorn, Private John J. Fay of the Seventh Cavalry's Company D appeared before a surgeon who diagnosed him as suffering from insanity. The previous year, during the Battle of the Little Bighorn, Fay had fought in both the Valley Fight and Hilltop Defense (Nichols 2000:99). He survived the three-day battle, apparently uninjured. After the winter at Fort Abraham Lincoln, Dakota Territory, his company and others left for the field in May 1877. They served as part of the effort to force the remaining recalcitrant Sioux and Cheyennes onto reservations and to intercept the fleeing Nez Perces and Chief Joseph. The correlation of Fay's insanity with the anniversary of the Little Bighorn suggests PTSD symptoms, involving both intrusive reexperiencing of the battle and an effort to avoid those recollections.

As defined in the mid- and late nineteenth century, insanity included a variety of mental derangements and was generally separated into three subdivisions: mania (mostly identified by agitation), melancholia (associated with depression, despondency, and lethargy), and dementia (indicated by impaired, distorted thought processes; Schroeder-Lein 2008:161). Insanity had recognized organic causes, such as head injuries and neurosyphilis, as well as psychological causes. The cause of Fay's insanity, unfortunately, went unrecorded in his military documents.

Two days after Fay's insanity diagnosis, on the eve of the Little Bighorn's anniversary, he was transferred from the field to Cantonment on Tongue River. Two months later he moved to more permanent installations. He went first to Fort Abraham Lincoln and later to Fort Rice, where, on September 15, 1877, he received a discharge from service for disability due to insanity. This discharge date occurred nearly three months after his initial diagnosis and a year before his official expiration of service (NARA RE M333, Rolls 31–43). Thus Fay left military life behind and became a civilian.

Whatever the intentions for his release from service, Fay's story did not end with his discharge. As a civilian he apparently recovered from insanity, flourishing and living a long life. In 1880 he was near Fort Meade, seemingly having followed the Seventh Cavalry from its Missouri River postings to that one near the Black Hills. There he had a wife and three children. Later he resided in Illinois. He lived to be eighty years old, dying in the U.S. Soldiers Home in Washington, D.C., the day after Christmas in 1932 (Nichols 2000:99), more than fifty years after his insanity diagnosis. The resolution of his insanity had been as successful as any modern therapist could hope for a patient.

In addition to insanity, other possible PTSD-related symptoms emerged from the Seventh Cavalry medical records. They include a Little Bighorn survivor, Private Ernest Wasmus, who experienced insomnia when he was about to engage the Nez Perces a year after that battle. Among the more than 20,000 medical records, only one other case of insomnia occurred.

As a final example, Private John R. Stewtker committed suicide with an overdose of opium. His death occurred while in company quarters at Fort Abraham Lincoln, five months after his involvement in the Little Bighorn (Nichols 2000:315).

As compelling as the individual stories are, another means of appraising PTSD in the Seventh Cavalry uses an epidemiological assessment.

Epidemiology and Epidemiological Expectations of PTSD

An epidemiological approach employs an overview of illness and health, searching for trends in groups and populations. Although based on individual health records, epidemiology does not focus on individuals. The records are summarized for a perspective on the group as a whole.

Our epidemiological predictions for PTSD in the nineteenth-century Seventh Cavalry are based on modern definitions (table 12.1; fig. 12.1). We expect symptoms associated with PTSD after combat at the Washita, at Little Bighorn, and in the Nez Perce Campaign. Three variables that may be associated with PTSD in the Seventh Cavalry records are examined: internecine violence, intoxication, and desertion.

These traits are analyzed by three PTSD-related periods. The year before the battles represents the normal baseline of those traits. Then PTSD symptoms should surge a month after the battles (the month-long non-PTSD ASD period). Heightened PTSD Period symptoms should occur during the first year after combat and a month of ASD. Continuing PTSD period symptoms should persist during the next year.

We employed two data sources to test those predictions: Regimental Returns and Carded Medical Records. More information concerning these sources is available in chapters 4 and 5. Three

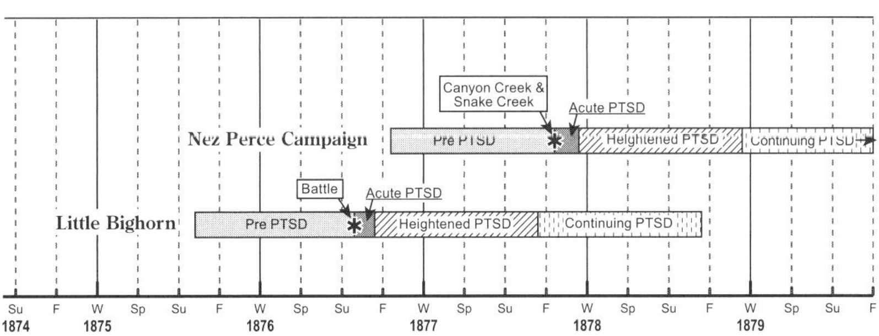

12.1. Time line of Seventh Cavalry encounters at the Battle of the Little Bighorn and Nez Perce Campaign correlated with Post–Traumatic Stress Disorder (PTSD). (Season abbreviations W = winter, Sp = spring, Su = summer, F = fall.) Chart drawn by Judy Stolen.

approaches are used. Modifying one of the approaches from chapter 11, we study aggression-produced injuries from internecine violence among the Seventh Cavalry members as well as with civilians and soldiers of other regiments. This analysis excludes physical trauma resulting from battles and skirmishes between the Seventh Cavalry and antagonistic groups. Those battle-related injuries resulted from institutional decisions, not from individual frustrations and volitions.

Second, alcohol was often available to Seventh Cavalry troopers and sometimes resulted in degrees of abuse, showing physical ailments. Indications of abuse noted in the medical records included inebriation, alcoholism, and delirium tremens. For our purposes the three alcohol symptoms were combined and analyzed together as intoxication.

In addition to violence and alcohol abuse, another PTSD symptom is avoidance of stimuli associated with the traumatic event. This can take many forms, but one means of avoiding military associations altogether is desertion, the unauthorized absence from military duty. Desertion is the ultimate means of dodging battle memories and occurred at amazingly high rates in the post–Civil War Seventh Cavalry (as described in chapter 5).

PTSD and Seventh Cavalry Brawls, Personal Affrays, and Internecine Violence

Temper flashes and violent behaviors may be among the most striking and blatant symptoms attributable to PTSD. If they occurred in the predicted fashion consistent with PTSD, the impact of violence among Seventh Cavalry members may indicate PTSD. For assessment of internecine violence by time, place, and intrinsic variables, see chapter 11.

Here we consider the relationship between internecine violent injuries and Seventh Cavalry battles and campaigns and the possibility that PTSD symptoms are expressed by increased internecine injuries.

The number of Seventh Cavalry violence-related injuries varies depending on the encounters and stress periods associated with them. We analyze the violence-related injury distributions for all three encounters combined then present the injury frequencies associated with each battle separately.

When all three battles are combined (Washita, Little Bighorn, and Nez Perce Campaign) and the internecine injury frequencies are compared with the number of unaffected enlisted men in the three periods (Prestress, Heightened Stress, and Continuing Stress), a statistically significant difference exists ($\chi^2 = 9.50$, df $= 2$, $p < 0.01$). Internecine injuries increase in the Continuing PTSD period. Injuries are under-represented in the Prestress and Heightened Stress periods, partially in keeping with expectations of our research hypothesis (fig. 12.2: injuries from skirmishes and small actions are omitted).

Considering each battle separately, unfortunately the internecine injury-related diagnoses associated with the Battle of the Washita in 1868 are too few to be amenable to statistical assessment.

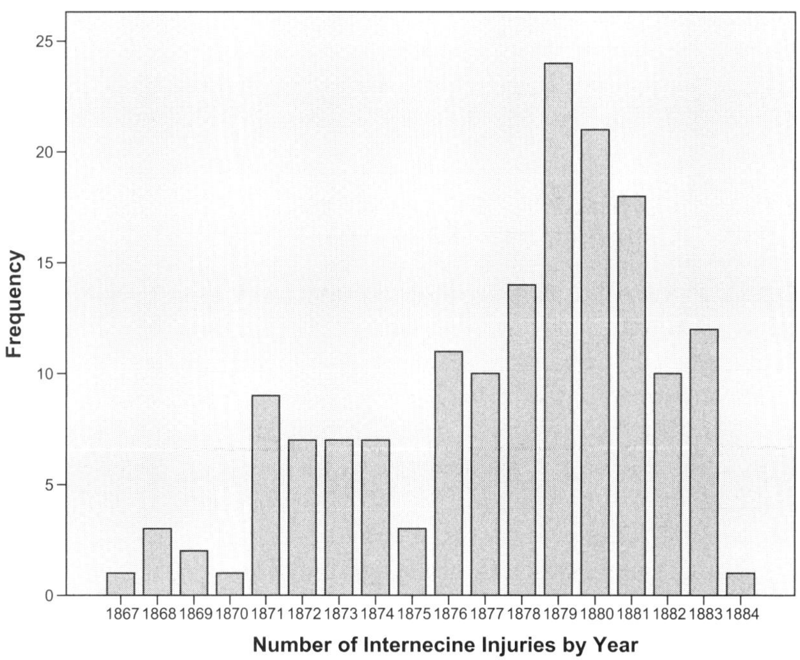

12.2. Number of Seventh Cavalry internecine injuries by year. Note increasing number of injuries, with greatest frequency in 1879, possibly associated with PTSD symptoms from the Little Bighorn and Nez Perce battles.

The Battle of the Little Bighorn in 1876 approaches but does not achieve significant differences ($\chi^2 = 4.35$, df = 2, $0.25 > p > 0.10$). And the 1877 Nez Perce Campaign shows statistically significant differences in the incidence of violence-related events ($\chi^2 = 10.18$, df = 2, $p < 0.01$). The greatest contributions to significance in the Nez Perce Campaign are the few Prestress period injuries and an increase in the Continuing PTSD period. The intermediate number of injuries in the Heightened PTSD period is approximately what would be expected under random circumstances. So, although the pattern shows complexity, internecine injuries generally rise as predicted in the period following exposure to stress, in keeping with PTSD predictions.

PTSD and the Drinking Seventh Cavalry

This section summarizes the second epidemiological parameter: intoxication. We start with temporal, geographic, and intrinsic variables, continuing with rank, and concluding with PTSD. All three intoxication diagnoses (inebriation, alcoholism, and delirium tremens) are lumped together for all analyses.

INTOXICATION BY TEMPORAL AND GEOGRAPHIC DISTRIBUTIONS

Intoxications peak in May, followed by the period of November through March. They are least frequent in June through August and in April. In the next larger temporal division intoxications show seasonal patterning ($\chi^2 = 9.22$, df = 1, $0.005 > p > 0.001$). Summer has fewer than expected intoxications and winter has more. Alcohol-related complaints change annually during the course of our study period. During the post–Civil War period, Seventh Cavalry alcohol-related diagnoses increase.

The posting locations were divided into the central plains, the South, and the northern plains. The number of intoxications while posted in the central plains ($n = 20$) is so small, however, that the region must be eliminated from statistical consideration. A difference exists between the intoxication numbers in the two remaining regions (South and northern plains) ($\chi^2 = 21.23$, df = 2, $p <$

0.001). Intoxication is under-represented in the South and over-represented in the northern plains.

INTOXICATION BY BIRTHPLACE, AGE, HEIGHT, AND RANK

This section examines intrinsic variables: birthplace, age, height, and rank. A significant difference exists between birthplaces (foreign-born vs. U.S.-born) and intoxication diagnoses (χ^2 = 13.86, df = 1, $p < 0.001$). Intoxication complaints rise among foreign-born soldiers and decrease among U.S.-born troopers.

What about the nineteenth-century images of the hard-drinking Germans and Irish? Comparing the Seventh Cavalry German-born troopers with U.S.-born by intoxications, no significant difference was found ($\chi^2 = 0.12$, df = 1, $p > 0.50$). Comparing the Irish-born sample with the U.S.-born, however, a difference does occur ($\chi^2 = 46.06$, df = 1, $p < 0.001$). The abundance of Irish intoxications and under-representation of U.S.-born intoxications produce the difference, in keeping with the nineteenth-century stereotype of the hard-drinking Irish (Wittke 1967:140–43).

The enlistment age of intoxicated troopers contrasts with the age of unintoxicated troopers ($t = 10.90$, df = 193.168, $p < 0.000$, two-tailed equal variances not assumed). Older troopers (average age 28.97 years) exhibit more frequent intoxications than younger ones (24.39 years).

No difference in stature occurs between intoxicated (mean 67.17 inches) and unintoxicated (mean 67.19 inches) soldiers. And no relationship exists between enlisted ranks and intoxications.

PTSD AND INTOXICATION

Now we examine the possibility that the Seventh Cavalry as a group may have used alcohol as a means of dealing with PTSD.

Considering all three encounters together (Washita, Little Bighorn, and Nez Perce Campaign), all intoxication diagnoses combined (inebriation, alcoholism, and delirium tremens) and three periods (Prestress, Heightened Stress, and Continuing Stress periods), the distribution approaches but does not achieve statistical significance ($\chi^2 = 4.246$, df = 2, $p > 0.10$).

Next we examine each encounter separately. Unfortunately, the alcohol-related diagnoses surrounding the Battle of the Washita are so infrequent that the distribution is not amenable to statistical assessment.

When the distribution of alcohol-related diagnoses associated with the Battle of the Little Bighorn are compared by three PTSD periods, differences occur ($\chi^2 = 8.81$, df = 2, $p < 0.005$). The greatest contributions to the results, however, are greater frequency of intoxications in the Prestress period and under-representation in the Heightened PTSD periods—the reverse of our expectations.

Finally, when the three stress periods involving the Nez Perce Campaign are considered, differences are found ($\chi^2 = 11.12$, df = 2, $p < 0.005$). The greatest contributions to this significance are the few Pre-PTSD period alcohol-related incidents and an increase in the Continuing PTSD period, as predicted.

PTSD and Desertions from the Seventh Cavalry

This section investigates the possibility that desertion rates reflect PTSD symptoms. Consideration of desertions by time, place, and intrinsic variables is presented in chapter 5.

Some Seventh Cavalry troopers may have expressed PTSD symptoms by deserting. When desertions and the three stress periods (Prestress, Heightened Stress, and Continuing PTSD) are compared for the three Seventh Cavalry encounters combined, the distribution approaches but does not achieve statistical significance ($\chi^2 = 5.95$, df = 2, $0.10 > p > 0.05$).

When desertion frequencies associated with the Washita are separated by PTSD periods and compared, they achieve significance ($\chi^2 = 23.91$, df = 2, $p < 0.001$). The most notable deviations from chance are a higher prebattle desertion rate and a lower desertion rate during the Heightened PTSD period. These results contradict our predictions.

There is something odd about desertions surrounding the Washita, however. While relatively low average monthly desertion rates are associated with the other two combats, a high average monthly desertion rate occurs around the time of the Battle of Washita. In fact the highest desertion rate of any one month in our entire study period occurred during the Prestress period before the Washita: 155 desertions occurred in March 1868—nearly 14 percent of the enlisted men. It is possible that desertions during this one aberrant month altered what was a distribution more in keeping with our predictions.

A statistically significant relation exists between the desertion frequencies associated with the Battle of the Little Bighorn and the three stress periods ($\chi^2 = 83.16$, df = 2, $p < 0.001$). Desertion rates before the Little Bighorn were low and later desertion rates increased, especially after the battle during the Heightened PTSD period.

When examining desertions by stress periods during the Nez Perce Campaign, the year after the Battle of the Little Bighorn, a statistically significant relationship emerges ($\chi^2 = 47.29$, df = 2, $p < 0.001$). Desertion rates before the Nez Perce Campaign were high, but desertion rates in the Heightened PTSD period were also high; only in the Continuing PTSD period did they fall. Other influences, such as the overlapping Little Bighorn postbattle period and the Nez Perce Campaign prebattle period, may confound these interpretations.

Summary

This chapter presents possible PTSD symptoms among the nineteenth-century Seventh Cavalry troopers from two perspectives: individual case histories and group epidemiological data. Individuals expressing possible PTSD symptoms include troopers suffering insanity, insomnia, and suicide. Individual case studies have an advantage of providing specific details, marshaled to suggest the presence of PTSD-like symptoms after a battle. Because of the lack of clinical details to support more exact diagnoses and the course of their ailments in the records, however, additional evidence is required.

Group epidemiological data have the advantage over case histories in considering all of the regiment's enlisted men together and possible symptoms that may be PTSD-related. Internecine injuries surrounding the Little Bighorn, although not statistically significant, are consistent. The Nez Perce Campaign supports our expectations, injuries being low before the campaign and increasing, especially in the second year following the campaign. Intoxication distributions surrounding the Battle of the Little Bighorn display the reverse of our predictions, while those associated with the Nez Perce Campaign are somewhat consistent: low in the Pre-PTSD period then increasing, especially as time continues after the conflict. Finally, desertion rates associated with the Little Bighorn fit our expectations, while those associated with the Nez Perce Campaign vary and only somewhat support our expectations.

Taken altogether, the three variables associated with the Seventh Cavalry's Little Bighorn and Nez Perce campaigns show mixed support for our PTSD hypothesis. Some of these symptoms and behaviors may involve PTSD-like responses, although a one-to-one relationship is neither possible to establish nor likely to exist.

Thus we argue that PTSD or PTSD-like symptoms existed in Seventh Cavalry troopers after the Little Bighorn and Nez Perce battles although those engagements involved different forms of combat than modern wars do. A pervasive set of long-lasting effects existed after exposure to horrific events, whenever they occurred, with or without the hallmarks of modern warfare. Not wishing to diminish present-day soldiers' sufferings resulting from combat in southwest Asia or elsewhere, we propose that in earlier periods many military combat veterans who served and suffered could be affected by PTSD-like symptoms. PTSD-like symptoms are not solely a modern affliction that results from new and terrifying conditions of warfare in the twentieth and twenty-first centuries. Using modern analytical techniques and the legacy of records left behind, we recognize and honor the sufferings and sacrifices of earlier generations of soldiers as well as present-day ones.

CHAPTER 13

Seventh Cavalry Medical Records Compared with Battle of the Little Bighorn Skeletons

P. Willey and Douglas D. Scott

How well do skeletons represent the illnesses that past individuals suffered? When an osteologist reconstructs the health and illness of dynastic Egyptians, prehistoric Indians, medieval French people, or casualties from the Battle of the Little Bighorn, how accurate are those assessments? How well do the Seventh Cavalry skeletal diseases reflect their living health?

The results of studies of skeletal samples are often presented as if they were living populations. Unfortunately, they are neither living nor populations. They consist of death assemblages and samples of populations. Although acknowledging the muteness and potential falseness of the human skeleton, human osteologists frequently proceed as if skeletons provide a definitive perspective on past populations' health and the diseases that they suffered.

As fortune would have it, some Seventh Cavalry troopers are represented and documented by both written medical records and skeletal remains. These two sources provide a means of comparing the differing perspectives that records and skeletons provide.

The post–Civil War Seventh Cavalry's Carded Medical Records offer a method of understanding diseases as they occurred and were diagnosed in the late nineteenth century. They identify many illnesses that we recognize today, including relatively minor ailments (such as acute diarrhea) as well as major life-threatening diseases (such as typhoid fever). These Seventh Cavalry medical records occur in a preantibiotic period. And the medical records precede application of modern clinical or laboratory tests. Acknowledging those technological limitations, they correspond with nearly all samples that bio-osteologists analyze. Skeletal samples usually predate antibiotic treatments and employ gross observations to make diagnoses.

For osteological comparisons with these historic medical records we use data from earlier studies of human bones of Seventh Cavalry casualties from the Battle of the Little Bighorn (June 1876). Bones of Seventh Cavalry members have emerged from the battleground and began being collected the year after the battle. Collection continued irregularly through the twentieth century. Recent osteological analyses and reports of those bones document the soldiers' illnesses and provide the osteological information required for comparisons with the Seventh Cavalry medical records.

By comparing the Seventh Cavalry's written medical histories with the Little Bighorn skeletal assessments we can determine how well these skeletons' alterations reflect ailments documented in medical records of that group during the mid-nineteenth century. We suggest comparability and divergences of other living groups' illnesses based on information gained from bio-osteological studies. This chapter presents the bio-osteologists' reflective assessments of skeletal limitations and describes the methods employed. A brief results section and more extensive discussion follow, ending with a summary and conclusions.

Background

At its simplest level paleopathology has three general goals, each posing many skeletal challenges: (1) diagnosis of a specific individual's diseases, (2) assessment of a group's diseases, and (3) interpretation of a population's co-evolutionary adjustment with diseases. Each goal requires accurate identification of diseases, which necessitates hurdling skeletal challenges.

Identifying diseases from skeletons poses four major challenges. First, skeletons available for study are often incomplete, and elements present are frequently fragmentary.

Second, skeletal series typically consist of small sample sizes, contrasted with large numbers of people present in living groups.

Third, bone lesions are often ambiguous, in part because bone can change only by increasing, decreasing, or both increasing and decreasing simultaneously. So bone reaction is limited, making a diagnosis of a specific disease difficult.

Fourth, bones often fail to document brief, nontraumatic events, registering only some major or persistent insults.

Unless these hurdles can be overcome—or at least understood—paleopathology's goals are jeopardized. Seventh Cavalry medical records and Little Bighorn skeletons provide a means of assessing these challenges.

Materials and Methods

Materials employed for this comparison derive from skeletons recovered from the Little Bighorn Battlefield, Montana, and Seventh Cavalry Carded Medical Records.

Seventh Cavalry's Carded Medical Records were the same ones used elsewhere in this work with a few additional modifications. In some instances the primary diagnoses were worded differently than the nineteenth-century nosology categories. But those diagnoses showed similarities such that those terms could be correlated with the established categories. Unlike some other assessments in this volume, the present analysis omitted less certain diagnoses, such as "others of this category" and "those with less exact diagnoses" as well as blank, unidentified, and vague diagnoses. The remaining medical cards, consisting of 18,945 diagnoses, constituted the data set (table 13.1).

In addition to the medical records, the other data set consisted of bones from the Battle of the Little Bighorn. Discoverers and battle survivors returned to the field and collected skeletal remains. Most available skeletons were discovered after the grand exhumation of enlisted men's remains and their reburial in 1881. Some bones were overlooked by the reburial parties, however, and were subsequently found on the battlefield by park staff and visitors. Archaeological investigations also recovered human remains (Scott et al. 1998), which were part of our analytical data set. Scott et al.

TABLE 13.1 Modified number and percentage of post–Civil War Seventh Cavalry diagnoses using a nineteenth-century military disease classification system

Order (numbers) and likelihood of skeletal involvement (letters)	*Disease*	*Number*	*Percentage within order*
	CLASS I. ZYMOTIC DISEASES, n = 6598 (34.8%)		
1. Miasmatic Diseases			
A*	Typhoid fever	78	1.5
A	Typhus fever	4	0.1
A	Typho-malarial fever	17	0.3
A	Remittent fever	231	4.3
A	Quotidian intermittent fever	959	17.8
A	Tertian intermittent fever	693	12.9
A	Quartan intermittent fever	8	0.1
A	Acute diarrhea	2418	45.0
A	Chronic diarrhea	37	0.7
A	Acute dysentery	133	2.5
A	Chronic dysentery	11	0.2
A	Epidemic cholera	31	0.6
A	Erysipelas	50	0.9
A	Pyemia	1	0.0
A	Smallpox	1	0.0
A	Varioloid	6	0.1
A	Chicken pox	1	0.0
A	Measles	18	0.3
A	Mumps	23	0.4
A	Tonsillitis (quinsy)—Woodward's "Inflammation of Tonsils"?	602	11.2
A	Diphtheria	1	0.0

**Note:* A = No or highly improbable skeletal involvement, B = Might involve skeleton, might be skeletally diagnosed, C = Skeletal involvement likely, certain. Categories without instances in the Seventh Cavalry medical records were omitted from this table.

TABLE 13.1 *(continued)*

Order (numbers) and likelihood of skeletal involvement (letters)	*Disease*	*Number*	*Percentage within order*
A	Epidemic catarrh (influenza)	29	0.5
A	9. Congestive intermittent fever	3	0.1
B	19. Debility	23	0.4
	Total	**5378**	**99.9**
2. Enthetic Diseases			
A	Primary syphilis	269	31.1
B	Constitutional syphilis	204	23.6
A	Gonorrhea	317	36.6
A	Gonorrhea orchitis	58	6.7
A	Gonorrhea ophthalmia	1	0.1
A	Stricture of urethra (gonorrhea)	13	1.5
A	Bite of serpents	3	0.3
	Total	**865**	**99.9**
3. Dietic Diseases			
B	Starvation	2	0.6
B	Scurvy	32	9.0
A	Inebriation	221	62.3
A	Delirium tremens	23	6.5
A	Chronic alcoholism	77	21.7
	Total	**355**	**100.1**
CLASS II. CONSTITUTIONAL DISEASES, n = 996 (5.3%)			
1. Diathetic Diseases			
B	Gout	1	0.1
A	Acute rheumatism	541	58.5
B	Chronic rheumatism	337	36.5
B	Anemia	18	2.0

(continued)

TABLE 13.1 *(continued)*

Order (numbers) and likelihood of skeletal involvement (letters)	*Disease*	*Number*	*Percentage within order*
A	Dropsy (when not a mere symptom of disease of heart, liver, or kidneys)	8	0.9
B	Tumor	19	2.1
	Total	**924**	**100.1**
2. Tubercular Diseases			
B	Consumption	68	94.4
A	Scrofula	4	5.6
	Total	**72**	**100.0**
	CLASS III. PARASITIC DISEASES, *n* = 50 (0.3%)		
A	Itch	27	54.0
A	Tape worms	23	46.0
	Total	**50**	**100.0**
	CLASS IV. LOCAL DISEASES, *n* = 6740 (35.6%)		
1. Diseases of the Nervous System			
A	Apoplexy	0	0
A	Convulsions	5	0.5
A	Epilepsy	40	4.3
A	Headache	312	33.8
A	Insanity	20	2.2
A	Inflammation of the brain	5	0.5
A	Inflammation of the spinal cord	1	0.1
A	Nostalgia	3	0.3
A	Neuralgia	469	50.9
B	Paralysis	12	1.3
A	Sunstroke	13	1.4
C	50. Toothache	42	4.6
	Total	**922**	**99.9**

TABLE 13.1 *(continued)*

Order (numbers) and likelihood of skeletal involvement (letters)	*Disease*	*Number*	*Percentage within order*
2. Diseases of the Eye			
A	Conjunctivitis	313	90.7
A	Iritis	14	4.1
A	Cataract	3	0.9
A	Night blindness	10	2.9
A	57. Ophthalmia	5	1.4
	Total	**345**	**100.0**
3. Diseases of the Ear			
B	Otorhoea (Otorrhea)	70	57.4
A	Inflammation of the internal ear	21	17.2
B	Deafness	22	18.0
A	59. Earache	9	7.4
	Total	**122**	**100.0**
4. Diseases of the Organs of Circulation			
A	Inflammation of pericardium	11	13.3
A	Inflammation of endocardium	1	1.2
A	Hypertrophy of heart	5	6.0
A	Valvular disease of heart	51	61.4
A	Varicose veins	15	18.1
	Total	**83**	**100.0**
5. Diseases of the Respiratory Organs			
A	Asthma	13	0.6
A	Catarrh	1379	61.7
A	Acute bronchitis	513	23.0
A	Chronic bronchitis	40	1.8
A	Epistaxis (Same as 76. Hemorrhage from nose)	5	0.2

(continued)

TABLE 13.1 *(continued)*

Order (numbers) and likelihood of skeletal involvement (letters)	*Disease*	*Number*	*Percentage within order*
A	Inflammation of larynx	19	0.9
A	Inflammation of lungs	104	4.7
B	Inflammation of pleura	153	6.8
A	Dropsy of chest	1	0.0
A	77. Hemorrhage from lungs	7	0.3
	Total	**2234**	**100.0**
6. Diseases of the Digestive Organs			
A	Colic	219	19.3
A	Constipation	397	34.9
A	Cholera morbus	35	3.1
A	Dyspepsia	129	11.3
A	Inflammation of stomach	15	1.3
A	Inflammation of bowels	7	0.6
A	Inflammation of peritoneum	1	0.1
A	Hemorrhage from stomach	3	0.3
A	Hemorrhage from bowels	1	0.1
A	Fistula in ano	14	1.2
A	Piles	221	19.4
A	Prolapsus ani	3	0.3
A	Femoral hernia	4	0.4
A	Inguinal hernia	44	3.9
A	Acute inflammation of liver	15	1.3
A	Dropsy from hepatic disease	1	0.1
A	Jaundice	21	1.8
A	Inflammation of the spleen	2	0.2
A	Enlarged spleen	5	0.4
	Total	**1137**	**100.0**

TABLE 13.1 *(continued)*

Order (numbers) and likelihood of skeletal involvement (letters)	*Disease*	*Number*	*Percentage within order*
7. Diseases of Urinary and Genital Organs			
A	Inflammation of kidneys	11	5.0
B	Diabetes	3	1.4
C	Gravel and stone	3	1.4
C	Calculus	5	2.3
A	Inflammation of bladder	16	7.3
A	Incontinence of urine	24	11.0
A	Inflammation of testicle (not gonorrheal)	118	53.9
A	Hydrocele	1	0.5
A	Varicocele Woodward's IV, 4, no. 69	26	11.9
A	106. Difficulty of urination	12	5.5
	Total	**219**	**100.2**
8. Diseases of the Bones and Joints			
C	Inflammation of periosteum	2	5.1
C	Inflammation of bones	1	2.6
C	Caries	1	2.6
C	Necrosis	6	15.4
C	Inflammation of [j]oints	24	61.5
C	Anchylosis	5	12.8
	Total	**39**	**100.0**
9. Diseases of the Integumentary System			
A	Abscess	238	14.5
A	Boil	973	59.4
A	Carbuncle	13	0.8
A	Ulcers	164	10.0

(continued)

TABLE 13.1 (*continued*)

Order (numbers) and likelihood of skeletal involvement (letters)	*Disease*	*Number*	*Percentage within order*
A	Whitlow	164	10.0
A	Skin diseases (not including [illegible] or affections or itch)	87	5.3
	Total	**1639**	**100.0**
	CLASS V. VIOLENT DISEASE AND DEATH, *n* = 4561 (24.1%)		
1. Wounds, Injuries, and ["Accidents"?]			
A	Burns and scalds	97	2.1
B	Contusion	2004	44.0
B	Concussion of the brain	12	0.3
B	Sprains	802	17.6
B	Dislocations	51	1.1
B	Frostbite	301	6.6
C	Simple fractures (not gunshot)	142	3.1
C	Compound fractures (not gunshot)	8	0.2
B	Gunshot wounds	394	8.6
B	Incised wounds	330	7.2
A	Lacerated wounds	278	6.1
B	Punctured wounds	80	1.8
A	Poisoning by [name your poison!]	59	1.3
B	2. Homicide	1	0.0
B	3. Suicide	2	0.0
	Total	**4558**	**100.0**
	TOTAL (5 classes excluding inexact and blank/vague diagnoses) *n* = 18,945 (100.1%)		

Source: Based on U.S. Army Regulations (1881); Woodward's (1870) illness categories added, with his numbers preceding the illness.

(1998:133–227) summarized analyses of these skeletal remains, including original analyses (Snow and Fitzpatrick 1989; Scott and Snow 1991; Scott and Owsley 1991; Willey et al. 1996; and Willey 1997). Skeletal lesions were placed into standard paleopathological groups, including congenital/developmental (hereditary or acquired during growth), infectious (caused by micro- or macro-organisms), traumatic (caused by physical forces), and degenerative (caused by wearing during long-term use) alterations. For the present comparisons we ignored battle-related perimortem, fresh-bone alterations. Only antemortem skeletal ailments that may have come to the attention of surgeons and entered into medical records were included. Altogether some 1,305 skeletal elements or element portions representing at least 44 individuals have been reported (Scott et al. 1998:233, table 29).

Finally, the diseases' likelihood of being expressed skeletally was assessed. The first category included those ailments in which no skeletal involvement was possible or at least likely to appear. The second category involved antemortem diseases that may have produced skeletal lesions, some of which might have been identified from the bones. And the third category consisted of diagnoses that would likely or certainly have caused skeletal alterations. These probabilities of skeletal expressions were based on general osteological summaries (Aufderheide and Rodríguez-Martín 1998; Ortner 2003)

Results

SKELETONS FROM THE LITTLE BIGHORN BATTLE

Table 13.2 lists diseases noted in publications describing skeletons from the Battle of the Little Bighorn. Congenital/developmental, infectious, traumatic, and degenerative ailments dominate the list.

Congenital alterations of Little Bighorn skeletons mostly involved axial skeletal elements, from the skull through thorax and vertebral column. An example of congenital alteration was a two-headed, bicipital left rib (CNC Grave 455, unassigned; fig. 13.1). Developmental alterations, sometimes associated with habitual or "occupational" behaviors, mostly affected the periarticular surfaces of the lower limbs.

TABLE 13.2. Antemortem alterations of skeletons from the Little Bighorn Battlefield by disease categories

Disease category	*Skeletal lesion*	*Little Bighorn skeleton affected*
Congenital diseases and developmental defects		
	Asymmetrical occipital condyles	CNC Burial 4
	Possible slight wry neck	CNC Burial 4
	Bicipital rib	CNC Grave 455 (burial unassigned)
	Lumbar 5 neural arch absent	Marker 128
	Sacral-coccygeal fusion	CNC Burial 8B
	Shortened mandibular ramus—microsomia? (or possibly degenerative)	CNC Burial 8B
	Lytic lesion adjacent to head of femora	CNC Burials 3 and 5
	Poirier facets	CNC Burials 1, 2, 3, 4, 5, 6B, and 7
	Possible bipartite patella	Markers 86–87
	"Squatting" facets	CNC Burials 1, 2, 3, and 5
Infectious diseases		
	Slight periostitis both tibiae	CNC Burials 5 and 6B
Traumatic diseases		
	Compressed vertebral body	Markers 67–68
	Shoulder separations?	CNC Burial 1
	Cowboy "thumb"—phalanx	CNC Burial 7
	Fractured frontal	CNC Burial 2
	Fractured? clavicles	CNC Burial 3
	Fractured radius	CNC Burial 4
	Fractured ribs	CNC Burial 8B
	Fractured third cuneiform	CNC Burial 1
	Fractured metatarsal V	CNC Burial 4
	Fracture of foot	Marker 105

TABLE 13.2. *(continued)*

Disease category	*Skeletal lesion*	*Little Bighorn skeleton affected*
Degenerative changes		
	Degenerative changes of temporomandibular joint	CNC Burials 2 and 8B
	Osteoarthritis	CNC Burials 1 and 4.
	Osteophytosis	Reno Crossing, Markers 33–34, 67–68, CNC Burials 1, 2, 4, and 8B
	Osteophytosis	Markers 9–10, 33–34, 67–68, and 105, CNC Burials 1, 7, and 8B
	Ossified ligamentum flava	CNC Burials 1, 2, 3, 4, 5, 7, and 8A
	Depressions for Schmorl nodes	CNC Burials 1, 2, 3, 4, 5, 7, 8A, and 8B
	Shoulder	CNC Burials 3 and 7
	Elbow	Markers 9–10, Reno Crossing, CNC Burials 3 and 7
	Wrist	CNC Burial 8B
	Metacarpal	CNC Grave 453 (unassigned)
	Hips	CNC Burials 1, 3, and 4
	Knees	CNC Burials 1 and 7
	Talocrural joint	CNC Burial 1
	Toes	Markers 112 and 113

Note: CNC = Custer National Cemetery.

Degenerative changes resulted from long-term use of joints and articulations and involved almost all joints. The most severe degenerative joint changes attacked the spine, affecting the intervertebral bodies (depressions for Schmorl's nodes; fig. 13.2). And antemortem traumatic alterations mostly affected the appendicular skeletal elements.

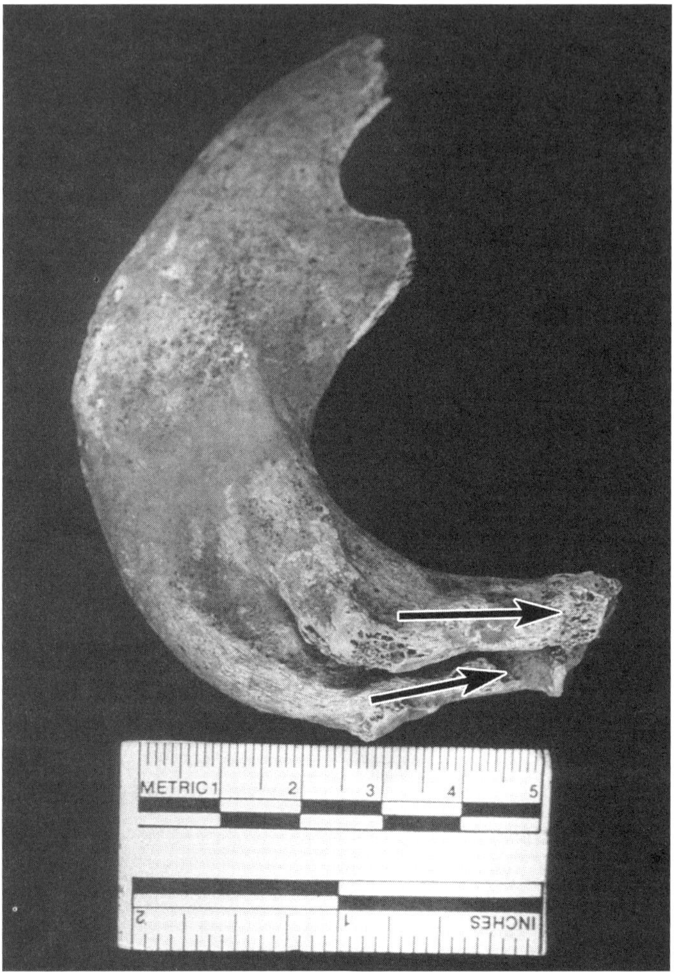

13.1. Fused left rib with two heads (*arrows*) from Little Bighorn. Custer National Cemetery Grave 455 (burial unassigned). Photo PW362.

Although less frequent than the other ailments, a few inflammatory alterations emerged too. Periostitis affected tibiae of two skeletons (fig. 13.3), suggesting moderate but persistent infections.

Altogether, diseases from the Little Bighorn Battlefield skeletons were few, especially when contrasted with illnesses documented in the Seventh Cavalry's medical records.

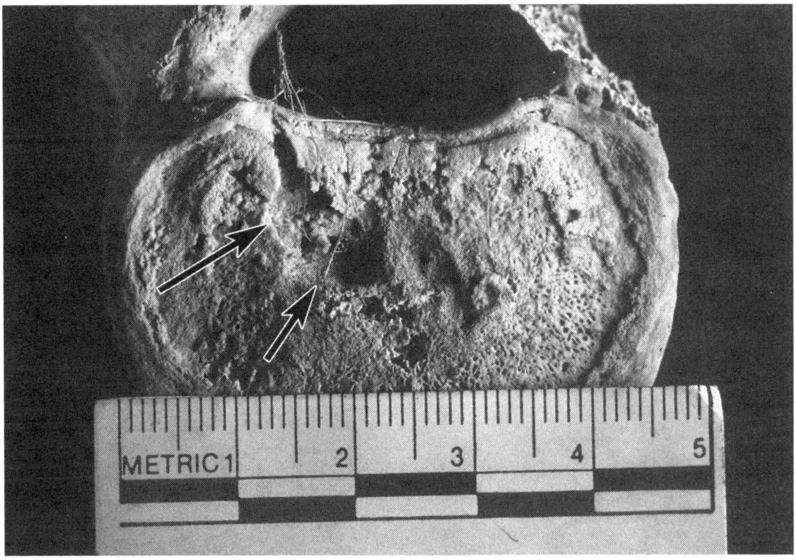

13.2. Lumbar vertebral body displaying degenerative depressions (*arrows*) associated with Schmorl nodes from Little Bighorn. Anterior is down. Custer National Cemetery Burial 8B. Photo PW522.

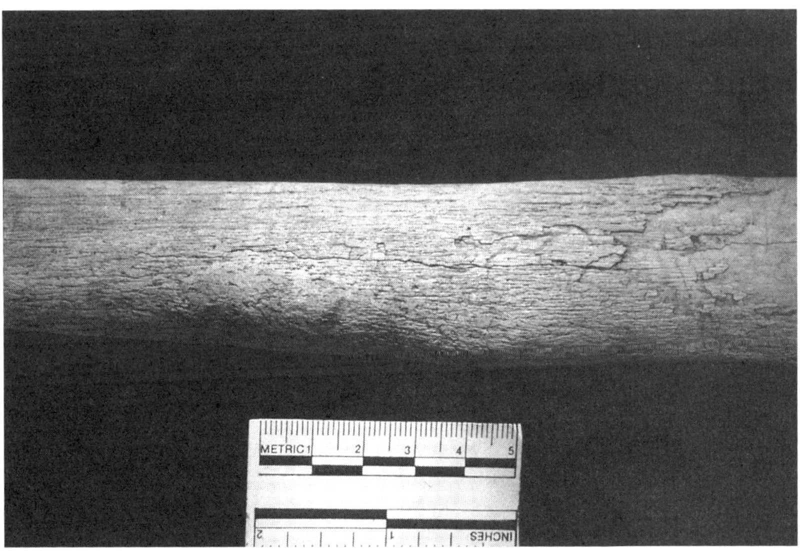

13.3. Medial surface of left tibia showing inflammatory response from Little Bighorn. Note plaque-like bone on most of surface and unaffected bone to right. Superior is right. Custer National Cemetery Burial 6B. Photo PW439.

SEVENTH CAVALRY MEDICAL RECORDS

Table 13.1 presents illnesses noted in Seventh Cavalry medical records. Beginning with the smallest nosology unit, the most frequent specific disease diagnoses consisted of acute diarrhea (n = 2,418), contusion (n = 2,004), catarrh (n = 1,379), boils (n = 973), quotidian intermittent fever (n = 959), tertian intermittent fever (n = 693), tonsillitis (n = 602), acute rheumatism (n = 541), and acute bronchitis (n = 513).

Next in the structural hierarchy, the best-represented disease orders consisted of miasmatic diseases (n = 5,378, mostly acute diarrhea), wounds and injuries (n = 4,558, mostly contusions), respiratory diseases (n = 2,234, mostly catarrh), integumentary system ailments (n = 1,639, mostly boils), and digestive organ complaints (n = 1,137, mostly constipation).

The greatest numbers in the largest category, class, showed local diseases (n = 6,740, mostly involving respiratory organs), zymotic disease (n = 6,598, mostly miasmatic diseases), and violent disease (n = 4,561, mostly wounds and injuries).

DISEASES LIKELY TO CAUSE SKELETAL INVOLVEMENT

A minority of these illnesses that the medical records documented would have been expressed skeletally. To assess the quantities involved, we divided the records' illnesses into three groups (table 13.3, fig. 13.4). Nearly three-quarters of the Seventh Cavalry

TABLE 13.3. Distribution of post–Civil War Seventh Cavalry medical records by likelihood of expressing skeletal lesions

	No skeletal involvement	*Possible skeletal involvement*	*Likely or certain skeletal involvement*	*Total*
Number	13,789	4941	215	18,945
Percentage	72.8	26.1	1.1	100.0

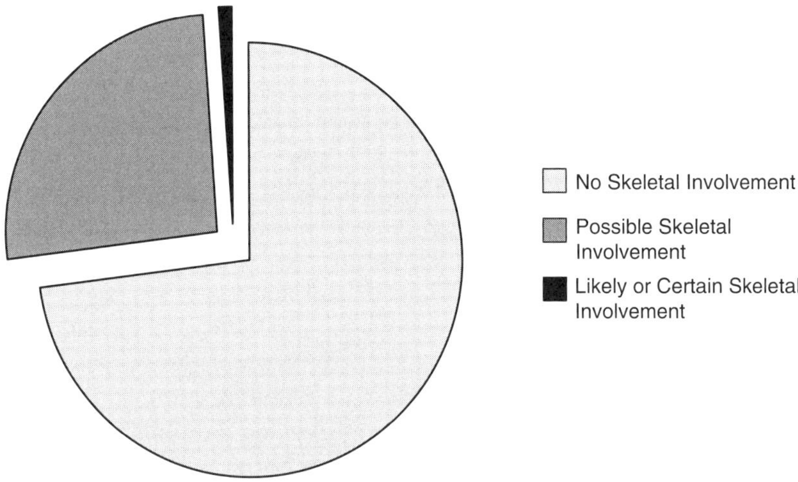

13.4. Illnesses in Seventh Cavalry medical records and their likelihood to be displayed skeletally. Note that the majority of illnesses in the records were unlikely to produce skeletal lesions and only 1 percent were likely to produce discernible lesions.

records (72.8%) fell into the category of no skeletal involvement. Almost all of the remaining illnesses (26.1%) showed possible skeletal involvement. And the last few records (only 1.1%) constituted diseases that were likely or certain to have altered skeletons. Based on these results, few of the Seventh Cavalry's medical record illnesses would have shown in the troopers' skeletons.

SKELETAL AND RECORD COMPARISONS

Skeletons from the Little Bighorn displayed various kinds of illnesses. The greatest number fell in the congenital or developmental category. Despite this, none of these illnesses probably came to the surgeons' attention. Some medical records, however, suggested congenital or developmental defects. Medical records likely associated with congenital/developmental defects included fistula in ano (n = 14), and femoral and inguinal hernias (n = 4 and 44, respectively). All of these documented congenital/developmental defects involved soft tissue, however, not bones. These record numbers represented less than 0.2 percent of all the medical records—a frequency overshadowed by skeletal evidence for congenital or developmental alterations.

Degenerative changes were the next most frequent category of alterations in the skeletons. With the possible exception of a few alterations, most of them were unlikely to be noted by nineteenth-century military surgeons. This is not true for changes to the spine, some of which were severe. Surgeons may have recorded those complaints as neuralgia or perhaps rheumatism.

Antemortem traumatic changes happened next most frequently in the Little Bighorn skeletons. Most of the injuries that the skeletons showed were notable and probably came to the surgeons' attentions. They included fractures and a possible shoulder separation. In the final category, Little Bighorn skeletons indicated few infections, which also might have been noted by surgeons.

Little Bighorn skeletal remains showed some ailments and conditions, however, that the Seventh Cavalry medical records appeared to have under-represented. They demonstrated high frequencies of dental problems. Using the Seventh Cavalry dentitions from the Custer National Cemetery as a subset of the skeletons' oral health (Willey et al. 1996), three major dental conditions occurred: active carious lesions, abscesses, and antemortem tooth loss. Carious lesions active at the time of death happened in more than a quarter (27.4%) of the teeth present (fig. 13.5), and active abscesses were present in 0.5% of the sockets; 11.4% of the teeth were lost antemortem. Altogether, those figures involved nearly 40% of the teeth or sockets—a remarkably high proportion of dental illness for such a young adult group.

In contrast, the medical records documented few dental problems. Only 42 toothaches were listed among all of the medical complaints—less than 0.25% of the records. It is possible that other diagnoses indicated but masked dental issues that the skeletons manifested. Those other diagnoses may have included otherwise unspecified rheumatism, abscess, and neuralgia. In addition, barbers and blacksmiths rather than surgeons probably dealt with many oral illnesses. These alternative "dental practitioners," however, left no written records of their extracurricular handiwork.

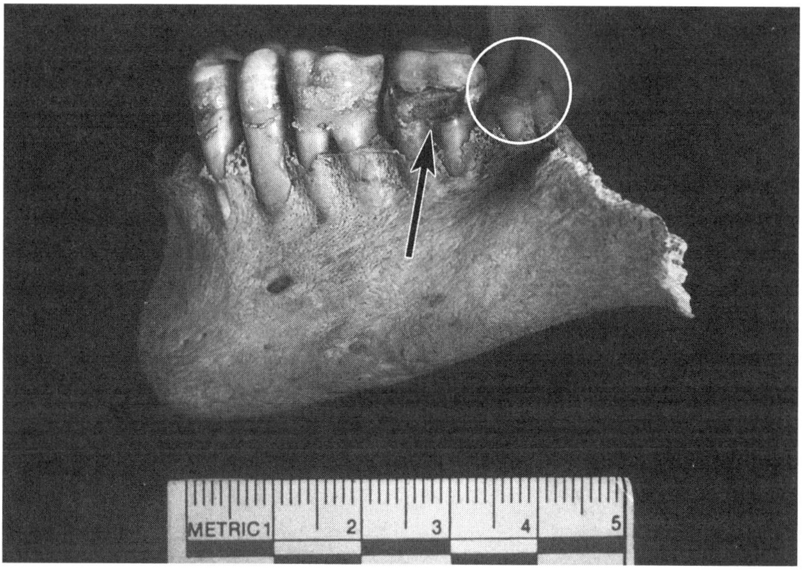

13.5. Left mandible showing carious lesions active at the time of death. Second molar with large caries at cement-enamel juncture (*arrow*) and third molar missing crown due to caries (*circle*). Custer National Cemetery Burial 8B. Photo PW514.

IDENTIFIED TROOPERS' SKELETAL LESIONS AND THEIR MEDICAL RECORDS

Another approach involves comparing identified skeletons and their osseous lesions with those individuals' medical records. Three troopers' skeletons have been identified with confidence (Scott et al. 1998:320–24, table 47). Another two previously identified skeletons must be eliminated from consideration here. Mitch Boyer (identified from remains at Markers 33–34) was an interpreter and thus fell outside military medical documentation. And the skeleton in CNC Burial 2 once identified as Corporal George Lell has subsequently been shown not to be his (Willey et al. 2003, 2004). So the three remaining identified skeletons are those of Sergeant Edward Botzer, Farrier Vincent Charley, and Sergeant Miles O'Hara.

Sergeant Botzer's remains have been identified as those discovered at the Reno Crossing in 1988 (Scott and Snow 1991).

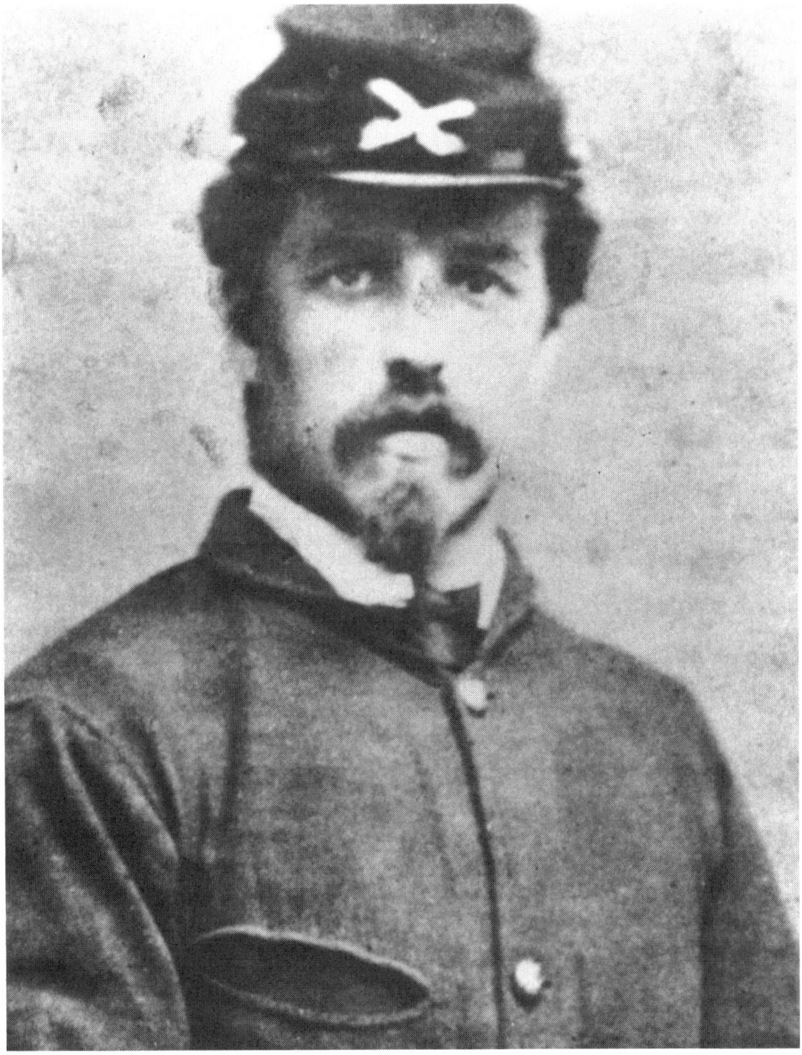

13.6. Portrait of Sergeant Edward Botzer, whose remains were discovered in the Reno Retreat Crossing. Courtesy Little Bighorn Battlefield National Monument, public domain image.

The remains consisted of only the skull, clavicle, and humerus. Medical records for Botzer (fig. 13.6) documented eleven events in his tenure with the Seventh Cavalry. He suffered four bouts of intermittent fevers and two remittent fevers while serving in the South. While in the South he complained of constipation (1875) and diarrhea (1876). Two other illnesses were nearly back-to-back complaints of chronic rheumatism in 1874 while stationed at Fort Abraham Lincoln. Although it is possible that Botzer's rheumatism may have involved the skeleton, that association could not be established without more specific document information. The only other recorded ailment possibly leaving a skeletal lesion was a contusion suffered in November 1872 at Laurensville, South Carolina. The medical record omitted the anatomical location. No comparable skeletal lesion occurred, but so few bones were recovered that the possibility remains that skeletal elements were involved. Other than perimortem injuries, Sergeant Botzer's skeleton showed periodontal disease and antemortem tooth loss, neither having corresponding medical records.

Farrier Vincent Charley was identified as being CNC Burial 4 (Scott and Willey 1996; Willey 1997). The remains constituted a nearly complete skeleton. Charley's medical history consisted of three complaints. Two of them were unlikely to show skeletal lesions (diarrhea and boil). But in February 1872, while in Chester, South Carolina, Charley reported a contusion and abrasion. Although the anatomical location of that wound or wounds went unstated, the record may have corresponded to the skeletons' fractured right fifth metatarsal. Lacking additional specific details, however, this association is unlikely. The skeleton also displayed a healed fracture of the right radius midshaft, an injury that most likely would have come to the surgeon's attention if it occurred while Charley was in service. Charley's mandible demonstrated third molars that had been extracted or lost within a year or two of his death, during the period when he was in the Seventh Cavalry (his first enlistment began in March 1871). But none of Charley's medical records mentioned toothaches or extractions. The skeleton also displayed lesser conditions, such as degenerative joint disease and an extra-articular facet.

Sergeant Miles O'Hara's remains have been identified as those found in the Hilltop Defense, L-Entrenchment, Burial 1 (Scott

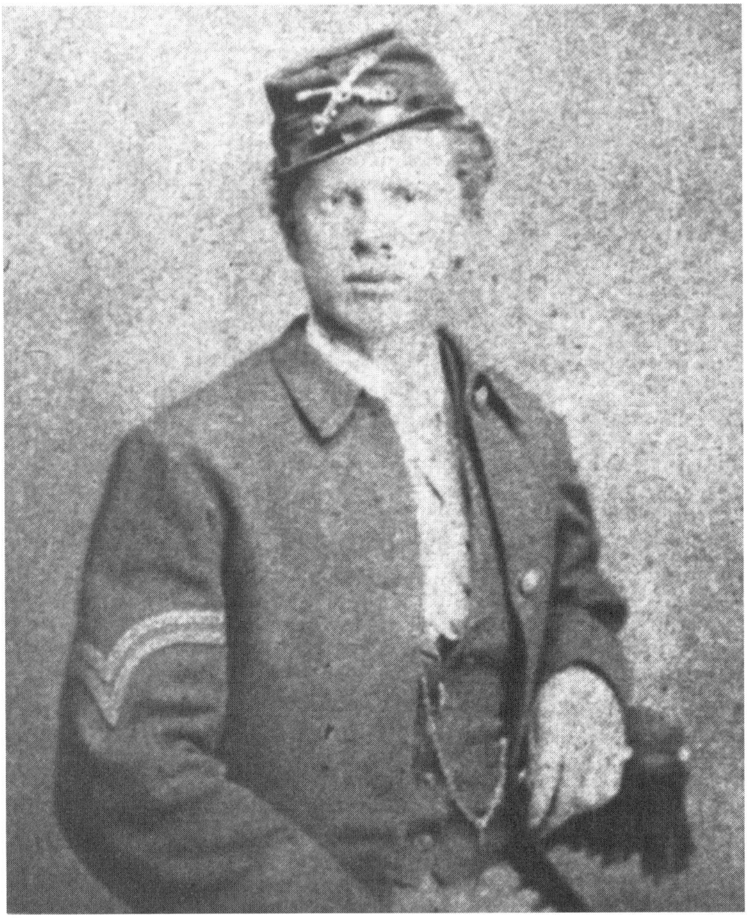

13.7. Portrait of Sergeant Miles O'Hara, whose remains were found in a rifle pit at the Reno-Benteen defense site. Courtesy Little Bighorn Battlefield National Monument, public domain image.

et al. 1988; fig. 13.7). The major bones present consisted of the skull, hyoid, cervical vertebra, coccyx, left scapula, left humerus, left radius, left ulna, left femur, and several ribs. Other than antemortem tooth loss and a carious lesion, no skeletal lesions were noted. Sergeant O'Hara's medical records showed no ailments whatsoever, although he had been in the Seventh Cavalry almost four years when he died. Perhaps he was in excellent health, a claim that the skeleton may support.

In summary, no definitive relation exists between the identified skeletons and those troopers' medical records. A number of explanations may in part explain those absences.

Challenges and Limitations

In some ways this assessment of a skeletal sample's efficacy to reflect illness in a living group forms a particularly stringent one because of five challenges. First, many of the Little Bighorn skeletal elements were fragmentary and most skeletons were partial. The recovered skeletal series represented only a small portion of the approximately 268 U.S. casualties from the battle. The skeletal remains embodied only 17 percent of the number of U.S. casualties from the battle (Scott et al. 1998:230). When considering the bones separately, the skeletal element count amounted to a mere 2.4 percent of the total from those casualties (Scott et al. 1998:233–34). But it must be noted that both fragmentation and small sample size create common challenges in many bio-osteological studies, not only for skeletons from the Little Bighorn.

Second, the present study employed a relatively healthy young adult male sample. Before enlistment, they had survived the throes of childhood growth, rapid bone remodeling, and the most devastating childhood diseases. Enlistment requirements screened potential troopers and eliminated those whose premilitary ill health disqualified them from service, thus excluding potential enlistees with major congenital defects and debilitating injuries. The recruits who were accepted were males, thus evading diseases that predominate among females. And the troopers were in prime adulthood when killed, too young to display many of the degenerative effects and long-term infections found in middle-aged and old people. Consequently, the relatively good health of the skeletons might in part reflect those advantages, which are not often seen in other skeletal series.

Third, some ailments documented in the medical records were those of recidivists. For example, as noted in chapter 8, intermittent fevers often persisted with ongoing symptoms, not a single event. And the skeletal alterations generally showed one-time and lengthy episodes. So medical records may have overcounted and over-represented some diseases, while skeletons indicated only the end result of diseases as a single osteological manifestation.

Fourth, medical records consisted of diseases that happened only during the enlistment period. In general, few pre-enlistment ailments found their way into the medical records. Exceptions may have included persistent infections (such as malarias and some STIs) and other diseases with recurring symptoms. Skeletal lesions, however, such as healed fractures, may have occurred years or decades before enlistment. They would not have been recorded by surgeons if the event happened before enlistment but would been noted by human osteologists.

Finally, differences in understanding and interpreting etiologies and pathogenesis occur between the nineteenth-century medical records and twentieth-century skeletal assessments. Seventh Cavalry surgeons were tasked with treating and returning troopers to service. Twentieth-century osteologists attempted to document all skeletal lesions, whether they impacted service or not.

Summary

Osteologists study skeletons to make inferences about past individuals and the populations they represent, including the diseases they suffered. Unfortunately, the skeletal system, when it does respond to disease, reacts in a limited, frequently confounding manner, often making reliable diagnoses of specific diseases challenging. The impact of those limitations is largely unknown.

This chapter attempts to rectify that deficiency by comparing diseases of the skeletons from the Battle of the Little Bighorn with illnesses documented in the Seventh Cavalry's medical records. The comparison reveals a number of principles.

Among the few Little Bighorn skeletons studied, diseases consisted mostly of congenital/developmental defects and degenerative and traumatic lesions. The Seventh Cavalry's medical records, in contrast, most frequently documented diarrhea, contusions, catarrh, boils, and fevers—few of which likely affected the skeleton.

Nearly 75 percent of the medical record illnesses would not have been expressed skeletally. About 25 percent of the medical records might have resulted in skeletal lesions. And only about 1 percent of the medical record illnesses would likely or certainly have altered the skeleton. This hypothetical compartmentalization of the Seventh Cavalry's medical records demonstrates under-representation of medically documented diseases in the Little Bighorn skeletons.

Skeletons from the Little Bighorn grossly under-represented some of the largest categories of medical record diseases, including infectious diseases and ailments of the integumentary system. But the Little Bighorn skeletons displayed more congenital/developmental defects, antemortem trauma, and dental disease than the medical records documented.

Another means of comparing skeletons and medical records involved several skeletons from the Little Bighorn who had been identified. Little if any correlation between skeletal and medical records was found by comparing identified skeletons with those same troopers' medical records. The disjunction between skeletal and medical record diseases persisted in this comparison.

Some of these discrepancies may be explained by the differences between the two data sets. The Little Bighorn skeletal sample was small and fragmentary, as most skeletal samples are. The troopers were an unusually healthy young adult male group, who probably displayed few diseases suffered by the very young or old or females of any ages. Some of the diseases that the Seventh Cavalry troopers documented were ongoing ailments, especially some of the infectious diseases. Their medical records may have contained multiple accounts of a single developing disease, while the skeletons showed the disease once. Another issue was that the medical records only included those ailments that happened during the enlistment period, while the skeletons carried with them all osteological insults that occurred before enlistment as well as those that occurred during service. Finally, nineteenth-century surgeons' understanding and documentation of disease differed from twentieth-century osteologists' approaches. The two groups' goals diverged, and so did their results.

The Little Bighorn skeletons tell one story while Seventh Cavalry medical records tell another, with little overlap between the two sources. Each approach is useful but largely discordant. But there is hope for some resolution of these polar perspectives.

Overspecificity in skeletal disease identification has been criticized by paleopathologists. Some authorities recommend using broader categories to identify skeletal diseases to avoid misdiagnosis (Waldron 1994:28–41; Ortner 2003). The potential for DNA to identify specific diseases from skeletal remains has emerged recently (Ortner 2003:111). Thus greater disease specificity may be possible and greater comparability between the two approaches may be achieved.

CHAPTER 14

Frontier Post–Civil War Military Enlisted Men's Deaths and Those in the Seventh Cavalry

Billy Markland, Douglas D. Scott, and P. Willey

The preceding chapters involve morbidity of the post–Civil War Seventh Cavalry, but not specifically mortality. The two are broadly related, of course; disease and injury may result in death. But the two processes are not necessarily the same. Many diseases are moderate. A boil, for instance, is unlikely to cause death. So mortality provides another means of understanding the Seventh Cavalry's most severe illnesses. If a trooper's death preceded attention from the surgeon, then the demise was unlikely to be reported, at least in the medical records. Consequently, deaths often went undocumented in the medical records (see chapter 11 for twenty-one examples of soldiers killed in action).

In part that under-reporting of deaths represented application of the nineteenth-century military nosology. Deaths appeared on the official list of ailments only in the cases of homicide, suicide, and execution. The more than twenty thousand Seventh Cavalry medical records included only one homicide and two suicides. Death by itself was not an official diagnostic category.

Nonetheless, two additional Seventh Cavalry medical records presented death as the primary diagnosis. While en route to Fort Dodge in December 1868, Private William McManus, an Irish immigrant, died after serving a year with the Seventh Cavalry. The medical record did not indicate the cause of his death, only that he was "admitted for burial."

The second death diagnosis in the Seventh Cavalry medical records was that of Private Markus Weiss, who emigrated from Hungary to the United States. He was in his second enlistment when he died in November 1879 at Fort Meade. He suffered "[c]ompound fracture of skull—simple fracture of neck right femur and left humerus. . . . Buried under a gravel bank while on fatigue duty, and instantly killed."

So the Seventh Cavalry's medical records documented only a few deaths. Did that absence indicate a sickly but vital regiment? Other records (described below) indicate that at least 451 Seventh Cavalry enlisted men died between 1866 and 1883 in the West alone. In addition to these deaths twenty-one Seventh Cavalry soldiers died while stationed in the South. To understand military mortality we must turn to a record set other than the medical records. Using that data set, we compare the Seventh Cavalry's deaths with those of the other regiments in the West, supplemented with deaths in the South.

Materials and Methods

Military records documenting military deaths differed from those depicting medical histories. Frontier deaths were abstracted from the National Archives and Records Administration (NARA) microfilms of Enlistment Registers and Monthly Regimental Returns (M233). Southern deaths were transcribed from NARA RG 94 Records of the Adjutant General's Office, 1780s–1917, Register of Deaths, volume 4, July 1869 to June 1872, and volume 5, July 1872 to June 1874, Entry 642. In addition to other information, the records included the enlisted man's name, regiment and branch of service, cause and manner of death, when and where death occurred, and the enlisted man's birthplace, age at enlistment, height, and terminal rank. Markland transcribed frontier records into an Excel file (his March 13, 2012, revision was used in this assessment). Dates for officers' deaths were derived from two primary sources. Officers of line regiments (infantry, cavalry, and artillery) were obtained from the regimental returns of those regiments. Staff officers' deaths were acquired from the annual Army Registers.

The overall database includes information from 1848 through 1891, for a grand total of 11,766 frontier military deaths. The analyses presented here, however, are limited to the period comparable to the Seventh Cavalry medical records. These enlistments began in August 1866 and continued through the end of 1882. Two methodological steps were required to compare the Seventh Cavalry deaths with those of other regiments. For this purpose we omitted frontier deaths in 1871 and 1872, when most of the Seventh Cavalry was stationed in the South, not the West, and terminated this analysis with 1882, after which few Seventh Cavalry deaths occurred. The entire western regular military deaths totaled 4,747 in this analytical database. Some entries lacked information, necessitating their omission from analysis. Because of the absence of comparable overall Reconstruction data, Seventh Cavalry deaths in the South are presented in the discussion section only.

Statistics consisted of hand-calculated chi-square tests as well as SPSS Statistics 20.0 (SPSS 2011) calculated descriptive statistics and *t* tests.

Results and Comparisons with the Seventh Cavalry

In this section we compare the frontier military deaths and the Seventh Cavalry deaths. The results are divided into deaths by regimental branch, cause and category, time, place, rank, and intrinsic information, including birthplace, enlistment age, and height as well as rank.

BRANCHES OF THE ARMY

Not surprisingly, the greatest number of frontier military deaths occurred in the two military branches with the greatest number of enlisted men: cavalry and infantry (table 14.1). Deaths in the cavalry roughly equaled those in the infantry. Fewer deaths occurred in the artillery, ordnance, and medical departments. Other branches had even fewer deaths.

TABLE 14.1. Distribution of post–Civil War frontier military deaths by branch of service

Service branch	*Frequency*	*Percent*
Unknown	1	.0
Artillery	151	3.2
Cavalry	2208	46.5
Commissary Dept.	4	.1
Dept. of the Pacific	2	.0
District of New Mexico	2	.0
Engineers	6	.1
General Services	20	.4
HQ Dept. CA	1	.0
Infantry	2236	47.1
Medical Department	38	.8
Ordnance Department	46	1.0
Provost Marshal	7	.1
Signal Corps	17	.4
Subsistence Department	5	.1
Total	4745	100.0

Note: Notice that the greatest number of mortalities occurred in the cavalry and infantry, the two branches with the greatest number of soldiers.

CAUSES AND CATEGORIES OF DEATHS

This section deals with two aspects of death. Cause of death indicates the specific illness or injury producing the soldier's demise. As examples, the death records note cholera and gunshot wounds as causes of death. Category of death clusters those specific fatal illnesses and injuries into broad groups. For example, accidents and diseases constitute two such broad categories.

The causes of death were distributed widely, falling into more than 450 different terminal events. Examples of the most numerous causes of deaths included Indians (n = 693), gunshot wounds (n = 550), drowning (n = 346), typhoid fever (n = 237), cholera

(n = 221, excluding 11 cholera morbus), consumption (n = 201), and many deaths from unknown causes (n = 235). Some of these causes were ambiguous. Deaths attributed to Indians, for example, might have been caused by gunshot or arrow wounds or by a number of other more specific actions.

Category of deaths clustered those hundreds of causes of death into a nine broad groups: death from accidents, disease, died of wounds received (DOWR), execution, killed in action (KIA) or in the line of duty (KILD), missing, presumed dead (MPD), murdered, and suicide (table 14.2 and fig. 14.1).

The majority of military frontier deaths occurred in the disease category, followed by accidental deaths. Together they encompassed over 70 percent of the frontier military deaths. Accidental

TABLE 14.2. Distribution of post–Civil War frontier military deaths by category and regiments

	SEVENTH CAVALRY		ALL REGIMENTS	
	Frequency	*Percent*	*Frequency*	*Percent*
Accident	33	7.3	781	16.5
Disease	83	18.4	2587	54.5
DOWR–in action	14	3.1	76	1.6
DOWR–in line of duty	0		5	.1
DOWR–other	11	2.4	248	5.2
DOWR–performing duty	0		1	.0
DOWR–unknown	5	1.1	70	1.5
Executed	0		1	.0
Killed in action (KIA)	280	62.1	597	12.6
Killed in the line of duty (KILD)	0		17	.4
Missing, presumed dead (MPD)	5	1.1	30	.6
Murdered	5	1.1	74	1.6
Suicide	3	0.7	175	3.7
Unknown	12	2.7	83	1.7
Total	451	100.0	4745	100.0

Note: DOWR = died of wounds received.

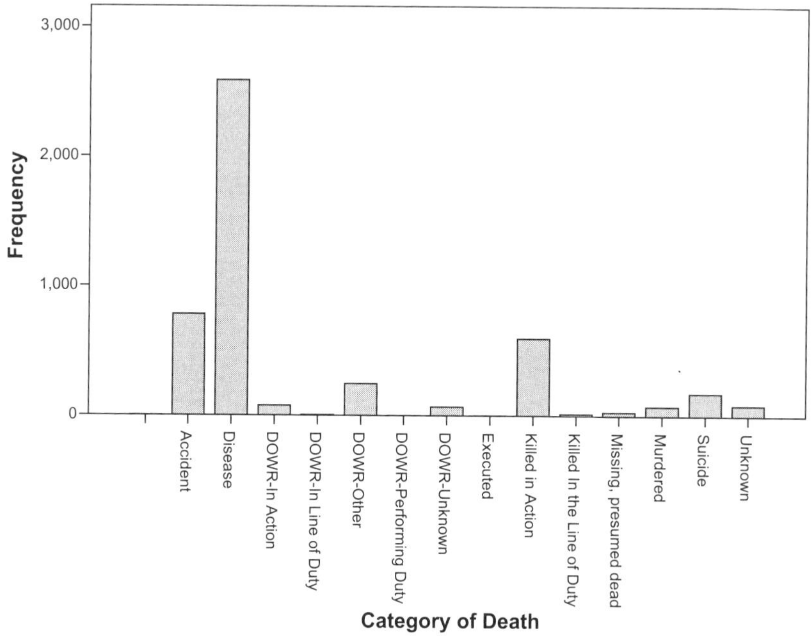

14.1. Categories of post–Civil War military frontier deaths. Note that most deaths resulted from disease, not from antagonistic encounters. Even deaths from accidents outnumber those killed in action. DOWR = died of wounds received.

deaths alone outnumbered killed in action (KIA), the third most frequent category of death.

All of the battle- and encounter-related violent deaths added together (DOWR, KIA, KILD, MPD, and murdered) totaled less than one-quarter of the total deaths. So soldiers in the post–Civil War West were three times more likely to die of causes other than those involved in interpersonal encounters. Although proportionally few, suicides were the next most frequent category of deaths.

Statistically significant differences emerged between overall frontier military death categories and Seventh Cavalry death categories ($\chi^2 = 1140.64$, df $= 5$, $p < 0.001$). The greatest contributors to this significance were the Seventh Cavalry's under-representation of deaths from accidents and disease and over-representation of KIAs. This conclusion might have been anticipated. Many of the

Seventh Cavalry's KIAs resulted from major engagements in the Washita, Little Bighorn, and Nez Perce encounters.

TIME OF DEATH: MONTH, SEASON, AND YEAR

The time when deaths occurred was patterned. The month of death deviated from random (one-sample χ^2, $p < 0.000$; table 14.3 and fig. 14.2). Greatest frequencies of deaths were from June through October. The fewest deaths happened in November through May. If death failed to take a holiday during the cooler months, at least he took some time off during the holiday season. These distributions were probably not due to troop strength, at least if the other western frontier's regiments follow the Seventh Cavalry's enlistment pattern. More likely the frequency of deaths was based on activities and exposures during the warmer months of June through October.

TABLE 14.3. Post–Civil War military frontier deaths by month

Month of death	*Frequency*	*Percent*
January	359	7.6
February	267	5.6
March	331	7.0
April	285	6.0
May	353	7.4
June	615	13.0
July	550	11.6
August	444	9.4
September	454	9.6
October	381	8.0
November	357	7.5
December	348	7.3
Total	4744	100.0

Note: Notice higher frequencies in June through October, lower ones in November through May.

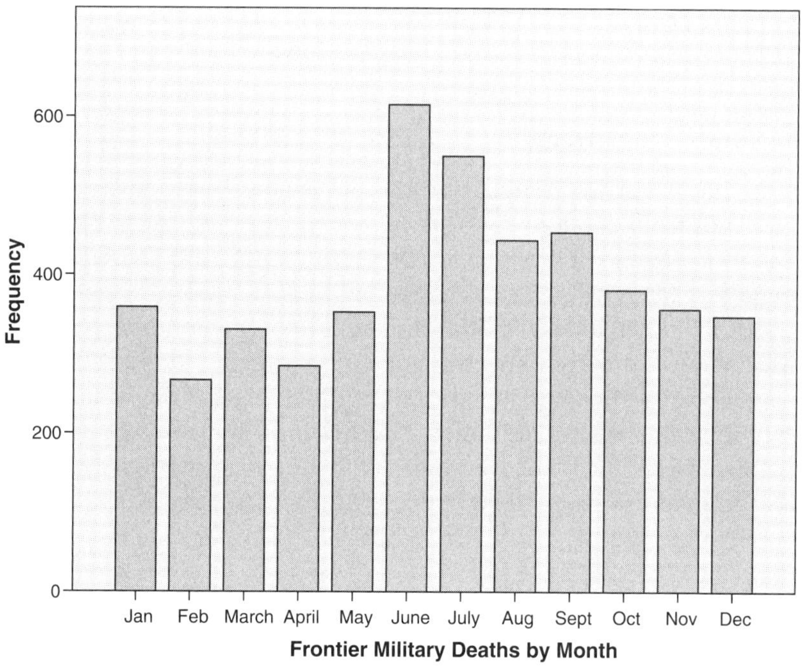

14.2. Monthly post–Civil War military frontier deaths. Note that the deaths peak in June through October and fall in November through May.

The Seventh Cavalry's deaths followed those distributions, largely from battles in June, September, and November.

Overall, western military deaths also differed by season (one-sample χ^2, $p < 0.000$; table 14.4 and fig. 14.3). The greatest frequencies of deaths were in summer and fall. Fewest deaths occurred in winter and spring. Like the monthly tallies, these seasonal distributions were probably not due to troop strength alone. Frequency of deaths was most likely based on activities and exposures during the hot summer and continuing into fall.

The Seventh Cavalry western deaths showed a similar pattern, with exaggerated seasonal peaks and valleys ($\chi^2 = 273.13$, df $= 3$, $p < 0.001$). The greatest Seventh Cavalry exaggerations were summer highs and spring lows.

The number of military frontier deaths annually fluctuated wildly (table 14.5 and fig. 14.4). The greatest numbers of annual deaths generally happened in the late 1860s (1867–70) and

TABLE 14.4. Post–Civil War military frontier deaths in the Seventh Cavalry and other regiments by season

Season	*Seventh Cavalry*	*Other regiments*	*Total frequency*	*Percent of total*
Winter	34	940	974	20.5
Spring	16	953	969	20.4
Summer	302	1307	1609	33.9
Fall	100	1092	1192	25.1
Total	452	4292	4744	100.0

Note: Notice higher death frequencies in summer and fall, lower ones in winter and spring.

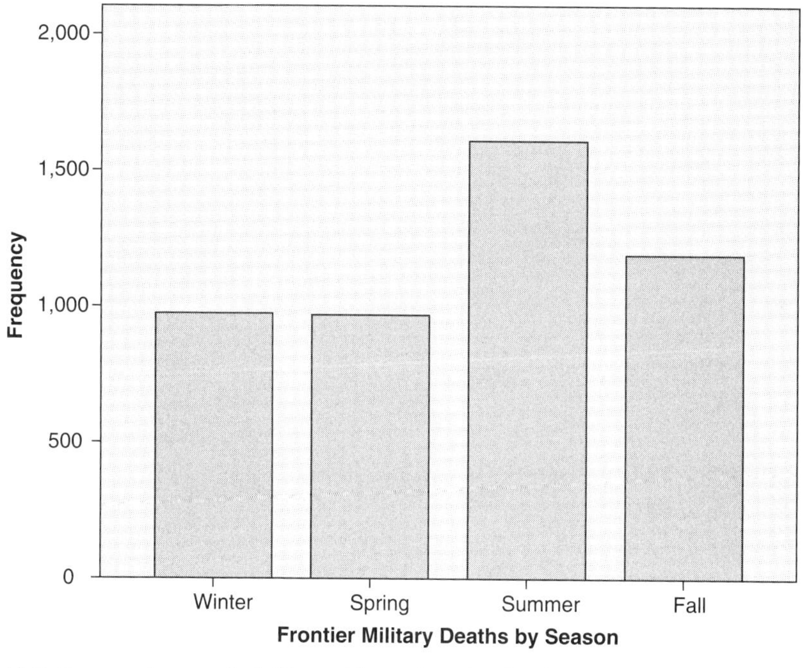

14.3. Seasonal post–Civil War military frontier deaths. Note that the deaths peak in summer and fall and plummet in winter and spring.

TABLE 14.5. Annual military frontier deaths in post–Civil War Seventh Cavalry and other regiments

Year	*Seventh Cavalry*	*Other regiments*	*Total frequency*	*Percent of total*
1866	26	55	81	1.7
1867	42	530	572	12.0
1868	30	314	344	7.2
1869	11	291	302	6.4
1870	17	337	354	7.5
1871	3	278	281	5.9
1872	0	281	281	5.9
1873	10	260	270	5.7
1874	8	217	225	4.7
1875	3	146	149	3.1
1876	249	183	432	9.1
1877	27	271	298	6.3
1878	6	205	211	4.4
1879	4	208	212	4.5
1880	3	194	197	4.1
1881	4	187	191	4.0
1882	3	159	162	3.4
1883	5	130	135	2.8
1884	0	22	22	.5
1885	0	13	13	.3
1886	0	8	8	.2
1887	0	5	5	.1
Total	451	4294	4745	100.0
Missing			2	.0
Total			4747	100.0

Note: Notice high frequencies in late 1860s and mid-1870s and lows in 1880s. Seventh Cavalry deaths in the South (1871: $n = 9$, 1872: $n = 8$, and 1873: $n = 4$) are omitted here.

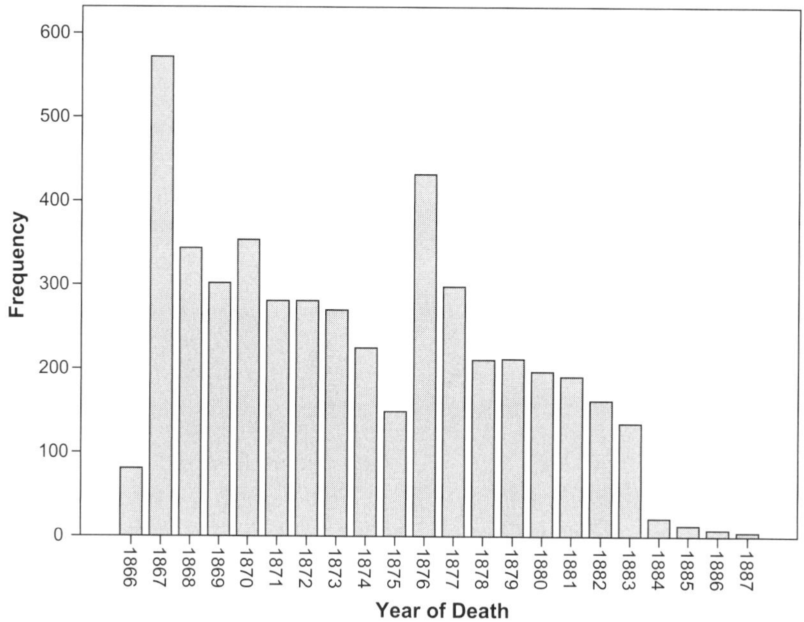

14.4. Annual post–Civil War military frontier deaths. Note that the deaths peak in the late 1860s and mid-1870s.

mid-1870s (1876 and 1877). The fewest deaths occurred in the early 1880s. Deaths tended to decline after 1870, with the exception of the mid-1870s rise.

Much of the variation in these death numbers can probably be explained by the number of susceptible soldiers. In 1866, for instance, at the end of the Civil War, few regulars occupied the West. But as troop strength increased the number of men exposed to western rigors increased. Thus the number of deaths rose in subsequent years.

The number of troops in the West explains some of the increased deaths in 1866–68, but not all of them. Surely troop strength remained high in the following decades, but the number of deaths generally decreased. There was an increased emphasis on hygiene after the cholera epidemics of the mid-1860s. In addition, better transportation increased availability of antiscorbutic foods and medical care. The dramatic increase in deaths in the years following the end of the Civil War may have involved two cholera epidemics and one yellow fever epidemic as well as an upsurge in

TABLE 14.6. Early post–Civil War military frontier deaths by year and the three most frequent categories of death

Year	*Accident*	*Disease*	*KIA*	*Total*
1866	2 (2.9)	66 (97.1)	0	68 (100.0)
1867	75 (13.9)	432 (80.0)	33 (6.1)	540 (100.0)
1868	48 (16.6)	211 (73.0)	30 (10.4)	289 (100.0)
1869	54 (22.9)	160 (67.8)	22 (9.3)	236 (100.0)
1870	76 (26.1)	200 (68.7)	15 (5.2)	291 (100.0)

Note: Percentages by row in parentheses.

Indian hostilities. The 1867 increases are as dramatic as they are perplexing (table 14.6).

Death from disease reigned as the majority category for every year, varying from more than two-thirds of deaths to almost all of them. The high frequency of deaths from disease was probably due to groups of men who were new to service and were exposed to diseases that they had not been subjected to before enlistment. Accidental deaths came next in numbers, varying from less than one-tenth to one-fourth of the total. KIAs were the least frequent of the three major categories of death, fluctuating widely from none to about 10 percent of the annual total.

Seventh Cavalry western deaths differed significantly from the other frontier regular deaths by year ($\chi^2 = 1123.83$, df $= 14$, $p < 0.001$). The Seventh Cavalry had fewer deaths than expected in 1869–70, 1873–75, and 1878–82 (recall that a 1871–72 gap occurred during the Seventh Cavalry's deployment outside the West, in the South). Only in 1876, the year of the Little Bighorn Battle, did the Seventh Cavalry's deaths exceed those found in other regiments. Part of that under-representation of Seventh Cavalry deaths may be explained by the next topic: where the Seventh Cavalry was posted in the West.

DEATHS BY STATE AND TERRITORY

Military frontier deaths did not happen randomly by geographic location either (table 14.7). The greatest number of army deaths

TABLE 14.7. Locations of post–Civil War military frontier deaths

Location	*Frequency*	*Percent*
Unclear	2	.0
Alaska Territory	18	.4
Arizona Territory and Arizona	382	8.0
At sea	8	.1
British Columbia	1	.0
California	263	5.5
Colorado Territory and Colorado	124	2.6
Dakota Territory	303	6.4
Idaho Territory and Idaho	92	1.9
Illinois	1	.0
Indian Territory (Oklahoma)	233	4.9
Kansas	548	11.5
Mexico	7	.1
Missouri	112	2.4
Montana Territory	495	10.4
Nebraska Territory and Nebraska	158	3.3
Nevada Territory and Nevada	31	.6
New Mexico Territory and New Mexico	306	6.5
Nicaragua	35	.7
North Dakota	1	.0
Oregon Territory and Oregon	48	1.0
South Dakota	1	.0
Texas	1175	24.8
Unknown	7	.1
Utah Territory and Utah	51	1.0
Washington Territory and Washington	80	1.7
Wyoming Territory and Wyoming	265	5.5
Total	4747	100.0

Note: Notice greatest frequencies in Arizona, Dakota, Kansas, Montana, and especially Texas.

occurred in Texas (n = 1,175), Kansas (n = 548), Montana Territory (n = 495), Arizona Territory (n = 382), and Dakota Territory (n = 305). Although the Seventh Cavalry was posted in several of these death-ridden states and contributed its fair share of the mortalities there, it was not posted in Texas, where the greatest number of deaths happened.

Contrasted with the locations with the greater numbers of deaths, the fewest military frontier deaths happened in areas marginal to the West proper, such as Illinois (n = 1) and Alaska Territory (n = 18), and in places outside U.S. boundaries, such as at sea (n = 8), in British Columbia (n = 1), in Mexico (n = 7), and in Nicaragua (n = 35) (almost all Nicaragua deaths happened in 1866 and 1867 from cholera when troops were transported to the west coast via the isthmus of Panama).

Troop strength probably served as the major determiner of death frequencies. In addition, the nature of assignments and presence of infectious agents and violence probably influenced these frequencies. And time had a synergistic effect.

Intrinsic variables such as birthplace, age, and stature as well as rank also impacted death frequencies.

BIRTHPLACE

Birthplaces of military frontier casualties were not random (table 14.8). The majority of deaths were among U.S.-born soldiers (55.9%), although foreign-born deaths followed closely (44.1%). Among foreign-born mortalities, the greatest numbers hailed from Ireland (n = 912), Germany (n = 631: excludes Bohemia [n = 1]), England (n = 185), and Canada (n = 112). These numbers probably parallel troop strength from each of those countries and reflect migration patterns during the mid-nineteenth century.

No statistical difference was found between the proportion of U.S.-born and foreign-born deaths in the Seventh Cavalry and in the other regiments ($\chi^2 = 0.50$, df = 1, $0.30 > p > 0.50$). Comparable to the general trend mentioned above, slightly more U.S.-born than foreign-born Seventh Cavalry soldiers died on the frontier.

TABLE 14.8. Birthplaces of post–Civil War soldiers who died on the frontier

Location	*Frequency*	*Percent*
Uncertain	3	.1
At sea	3	.1
Austria	11	.2
Belgium	4	.1
Bohemia	1	.0
Canada	112	2.4
Cuba	1	.0
Czechoslovakia	2	.0
Denmark	26	.5
England	185	3.9
France	37	.8
Germany	631	13.3
Greece	2	.0
Haiti	1	.0
Holland	6	.1
Hungary	6	.1
Ireland	912	19.2
Italy	1	.0
Jamaica	1	.0
Luxemburg	1	.0
Mexico	3	.1
Netherlands	3	.1
New Zealand	1	.0
Norway	6	.1
Russia	5	.1
Scotland	60	1.3
South Africa	1	.0
South America	1	.0
Spain	3	.1
Sweden	10	.2
Switzerland	42	.9
United States	2653	55.9
Wales	9	.2
West Indies	4	.1
Total	4747	100.0

ENLISTMENT AGE

The enlistment ages of survivors and frontier casualties were similar (table 14.9). About three-fourths of first enlistment deaths occurred between the ages of 21 and 30, with a spike at 21, the youngest official enlistment age. Probably because of a greater

TABLE 14.9. Age at enlistment of soldiers who died on the post–Civil War frontier

*Age (Years)**	*Frequency*	*Percent*
16	5	.1
17	8	.2
18	49	1.0
19	62	1.3
20	57	1.2
21	1061	22.4
22	559	11.8
23	349	7.4
24	280	5.9
25	272	5.7
26	255	5.4
27	258	5.4
28	218	4.6
29	168	3.5
30	155	3.3
31	129	2.7
32	126	2.7
33	110	2.3
34	124	2.6
35	90	1.9
36	58	1.2
37	56	1.2
38	45	.9

TABLE 14.9. *(continued)*

*Age (Years)**	*Frequency*	*Percent*
39	42	.8
40	48	1.0
41	25	.5
42	21	.4
43	27	.6
44	12	.3
45	12	.3
46	8	.2
47	9	.2
48	8	.2
49	6	.1
50	4	.1
51	3	.1
52	2	.0
53	3	.1
54	3	.1
55	2	.0
56	1	.0
57	1	.0
59	1	.0
62	2	.0
65	1	.0
Total	4735	99.7
Missing	12	.3
Total	4747	100.0

*Age rounded to the most recently completed whole year.

number of deaths among older soldiers, however, the mean enlistment age of all western frontier regular deaths was 26.2 years.

These ages follow standard enlistment rules. During most of the post–Civil War period, minimum enlistment age stood at 21 years, with some exceptions. Musicians and youths 18 to 21 with parental consent could enlist (Ewing 1894:174). The "too young" enlistees (under 21) who died on the western frontier totaled 181 (3.8% of our sample), a tragic count but a small proportion of the overall deaths.

Regulations established 35 years or 30 years (for the cavalry) as the upper age limit (Ewing 1894:179). Among the frontier regular deaths, 1,134 (23.9%) enlisted at 30 or older. Possibly these older soldiers were permitted to reenlist, although other such oldsters could not enlist for a first time. Older soldiers likely proved more vulnerable to severe illnesses and injuries terminating in death than younger soldiers in the prime of life.

The Seventh Cavalry frontier deaths differed from those of other regiments (t = 3.868, df = 620.573, p = 0.000, two-tailed test, equal variances not assumed). Seventh Cavalry mortalities averaged about a year younger than those in the other regiments (Seventh Cavalry 25.38 years versus others 26.33 years). Other regiments' deaths may possibly have been skewed by some older individuals who suffered terminal diseases. Many of the Seventh Cavalry's deaths occurred from battle injuries, before the soldiers aged or reenlisted.

Height

Enlistment heights of the frontier regular deaths formed a relatively normal, "bell curve" distribution (fig. 14.5). The mean was 67.1 inches, average for post–Civil War soldiers. Some distortions happened at the extremes, however, most likely based on enlistment regulations.

Although enlistment regulations for stature varied considerably during the post–Civil War period, the minimum height generally stood at about 65 inches, give or take an inch (Ewing 1894:179–80). Among the frontier military mortalities, however,

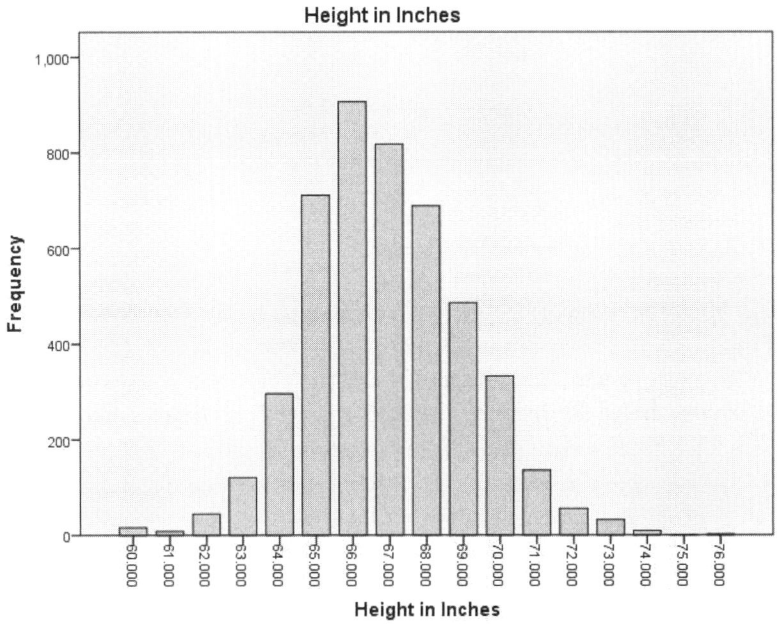

14.5. Enlistment statures of soldiers who died on the frontier. The distribution generally follows a normal distribution but is shifted (skewed) to the right, suggesting implementation of enlistment regulations barring shorter potential enlistees. Statures rounded to nearest inch.

the shortest stature fell to a mere 58.375 inches—nearly 7 inches below the regulation minimum. And that soldier was not alone. The proportion of deceased western soldiers with less than the regulation minimum height of 65 inches amounted to 11.5% (n = 537) of the military frontier deaths. This frequency was striking, but it might have been even greater. The distribution (fig. 14.5) appears slightly asymmetrical, with a steeper slope on the shorter side and a more gradual slope on the taller side. This distribution probably indicates some enforcement of regulations, excluding shorter men from enlistment.

At the other stature extreme, the regulations established 76 inches as the maximum stature for cavalry, but no maximum existed for other branches. Only two of the military frontier casualties were that tall; none was taller.

Statures of Seventh Cavalry western deaths compared well with those from other frontier regiments, showing no difference ($t = -1.694$, df = 4662, $p = 0.090$, two-tailed test, equal variances assumed).

RANK

Most of the military frontier deaths involved lower ranks (table 14.10). Privates constituted three-fourths of the deaths, corporals 5%, all sergeants combined 8.9%. Recruits in the few weeks before they achieved a formal rank appeared to be at high risk, constituting 4.8% of all mortalities. Recruits' deaths most likely demonstrated failure to thrive in military life and exposure to new diseases associated with crowding many men together in close quarters.

To compare the ranks of other western regiments' mortalities with those of the Seventh Cavalry, the ranks were lumped together as elsewhere in this volume (senior and junior noncommissioned officers versus rankers). The ranks of the Seventh Cavalry's deaths differed from those in other regiments ($\chi^2 = 15.74$, df = 2, $p < 0.001$). The major (no pun intended) difference was the over-representation of Seventh Cavalry junior noncommissioned officers. If commissioned officers were included in this assessment, Seventh Cavalry officers probably would have been over-represented among the dead when contrasted with other military frontier west regiments too. Battle-related catastrophic mortalities were independent of rank, so the Seventh Cavalry suffered proportionally more officer deaths by combat than any other regiment.

Discussion

Death constitutes the arbiter of morbidity and terminator of life. So this chapter deals with the ultimate impact of diseases and injuries, not the lesser, survivable ailments often documented in Seventh Cavalry medical records. The soldiers, for the most part, survived almost all of those ailments. This chapter also expands the scope of study beyond the Seventh Cavalry to infantry and all other

TABLE 14.10. Distribution of post–Civil War military frontier regular deaths by rank

Rank	*Frequency*	*Percent*
Valid	2	.0
Unknown	1	.0
Drillmaster	1	.0
1st class private	5	.1
1st sergeant	64	1.3
2d class private	17	.4
3d class private	1	.0
Artificer	14	.3
Blacksmith	32	.7
Bugler	9	.2
Chief musician	3	.1
Chief trumpeter	1	.0
Commissary sgt.	10	.2
Corporal	255	5.4
Discharged soldier	1	.0
Drummer	1	.0
Farrier	23	.5
Fifer	1	.0
Hospital steward	35	.7
Lance sergeant	1	.0
Musician	39	.8
Ordnance sergeant	15	.3
Principal musician	10	.2
Private	3564	75.1
Quartermaster sergeant	18	.3
Recruit	228	4.8
Saddler	23	.5
Saddler sergeant	2	.0
Sergeant	308	6.5
Sgt. major	4	.1
Subcook	2	.0
Trumpeter	35	.7
Unknown	3	.1
Wagoner	19	.4
Total	4747	100.0

regiments serving on the post–Civil War frontier. Despite this difference, the data and our interpretations had inherent limitations.

The mortality data, like the medical records, omitted officers, civilian contractors, women, and children. So in that sense the death records paralleled the limitations of the medical records, omitting the same groups. Both sources presented only enlisted men.

The military frontier regular deaths also omitted a portion of the post–Civil War Seventh Cavalry deaths. For a little over two years (1871–73), the Seventh was posted in the South, not in the West. Hence deaths occurring during those years were excluded from these comparisons, thus presenting an incomplete perspective. It behooves us to examine those Seventh Cavalry deaths that happened in the South.

During the Seventh Cavalry's posting in the South, 21 deaths occurred. Thus the years in the South showed reduced mortality (1871: $n = 9$, 1872: $n = 8$, and 1873: $n = 4$). Only the later years on the northern plains had comparably few deaths. Most of the southern deaths happened in South Carolina ($n = 13$) with fewer mortalities in Tennessee, North Carolina, Alabama, Kentucky, and Mississippi. Southern deaths struck privates ($n = 17$) more than all of the other ranks combined. The principal cause of deaths was lung ailments ($n = 7$), followed by typhoid and other fevers ($n = 4$ and 3, respectively), and injuries ($n = 3$), as well as less frequent causes.

Finally, our statistics involve mortality counts, not ratio of deaths to survivors. So we may be presenting a distorted perspective by excluding information related to entire regimental strength. It would be laborious and complex to count troop strength of those serving on the frontier, but a laudable task. We are uncertain how dead/survivor proportions may differ among regiments and alter the results presented here.

Summary

This chapter describes western frontier military regular casualties from 1866 through 1882. During those years, 4,747 soldiers died in that region. In addition it compares Seventh Cavalry deaths to those in other regiments.

Among the western frontier regulars, death struck the infantry and cavalry about equally. Other branches with fewer enlisted men showed fewer deaths. Most deaths were caused by violent or accidental events, encounters with Indians and gunshot wounds being the two most frequent. The records documented many other causes, most providing specific details of the causes of death.

The disease category produced the majority of deaths, followed by accidents. KIA and other interpersonal violence categories amounted to less than a quarter of all deaths.

By month most deaths happened from June through October, when exposure to disease, accident, and violence rose. The fewest deaths happened from November through May. Seasonal deaths reflected this same pattern. The greatest number of deaths happened in summer and fall, dropping in winter and spring. The number of annual deaths changed during the two decades studied. The early years produced the greatest number of deaths, which dropped slowly through the period, with the exception of a mid-1870s spike.

Deaths also showed geographic patterning. The most dangerous state of all by far was Texas. Kansas, Montana Territory, and Arizona and Dakota Territories trailed the Lone Star State in mortality. A combination of troop strength and vulnerabilities to disease and violence probably influenced these patterns.

Deaths of U.S.-born enlisted men outnumbered those of foreign-born soldiers. This pattern probably reflected the numbers of enlistees. Most enlistments of soldiers who died happened at 21 years, the earliest "regular" enlistment age. Less than 4% of those who died enlisted at an age younger than 21. Enlistment age of soldiers who died averaged about 26. Regulars who died on the frontier averaged 67 inches tall. Approximately 11% of the soldiers who died there were shorter than the official regulation stature of 65 inches.

Most of the western frontier regular deaths occurred among the lower ranks. Their deaths were likely due to their overwhelming numbers. Perhaps surprisingly, recruits constituted nearly 5% of all deaths, suggesting heightened vulnerability in the first weeks of military service.

How did Seventh Cavalry deaths reflect these overall western frontier military mortalities? They showed similarities in nativity (U.S.-born versus foreign-born) and stature.

But we also found differences. The Seventh Cavalry displayed greater proportions of KIAs, doubtless from the regiment's several major campaign encounters. Conversely, the Seventh Cavalry's deaths from accidents and diseases constituted smaller proportions than in other regiments.

In addition, the Seventh Cavalry's seasonal death numbers displayed an exaggerated western mortality pattern: summer deaths were especially high and spring deaths particularly low. The Seventh Cavalry showed heightened mortality during one year: 1876, when the Battle of the Little Bighorn occurred. In other years the Seventh Cavalry's deaths fell below those of other regiments.

Finally, the Seventh Cavalry displayed an unusual pattern of deaths by ranks. Seventh Cavalry junior noncommissioned officers died in greater proportions than similar ranks of the other regiments in the West, probably due to the catastrophic nature of the regiment's battle-related fatalities.

CHAPTER 15

Health of Urban American Civilians, Children, Women, and Old Men in the Late Nineteenth and Early Twentieth Centuries

Colleen Milligan

This chapter embraces a different perspective than preceding chapters, most of which provide data-oriented health assessments of one small demographic sliver. They deal with post–Civil War Seventh Cavalry soldiers, who were all white males, mostly between twenty-one and thirty years old. In addition, almost all of the soldiers spent their enlistments serving on the western frontier or in the Reconstruction South. Few of them were stationed in urban areas.

Consequently, earlier chapters exclude children, women, and older white males as well as all other heritages. In addition, they mostly omit urbanites. Although of course some similarities exist between the illnesses of the troopers and those of these others, we expect marked differences in the ailments that they experienced.

To provide a broader perspective on U.S. health, we turn to a midwestern urban group of the late nineteenth and early twentieth century that represents both sexes, all age groups, and "others." This study examines groups not eligible for military service—or military health care. Instead they fell under the purview of an emerging public health movement.

This chapter reviews nineteenth-century illnesses, the rise of urban areas, the emergence of public health movements, and change in disease and mortality into the early twentieth century.

Illnesses documented in Milwaukee are compared with those of the Seventh Cavalry.

Nineteenth-Century Health

The impact of communicable diseases was a major health concern in nineteenth-century America. They affected many members of society, regardless of social standing, sex, age, or ethnicity. Throughout much of the century the prominent view concerning the spread of disease was the miasmatic theory. According to that approach, malarias were associated with marshy lands, choleras with contaminated water supplies, and fevers with crowded housing, army camps, jails, and other institutions where the dirt and filth abounded. Individuals concerned with public health in the United States first approached the topic as a war against contagions and later initiated a prevention movement (Duffy 1990). Although diseases presented major challenges in all regions, urban centers produced particular hurdles because they concentrated peoples and contagious diseases in close proximity. State and municipal agencies pondered improving the urban environment and combating the epidemic and endemic diseases that arose (Duffy 1978).

The Rise of Urban Centers and the Public Health Movement

Industrialization of America's cities shifted people from the countryside into urban centers. This change altered environments where people lived and produced new cultural dynamics. The mortality and fertility trends associated with the change were often interpreted as evidence of a biological response to new cultural stressors (Omran 1977). These stressors included overcrowding in urban centers and insufficient urban infrastructure, especially related to public sanitation.

Eighteenth-century America saw major disruptions in cities from virulent epidemics (Leavitt 1978). At the dawn of a new century the first permanent board of health was established in Boston in 1799, after a series of outbreaks of yellow fever, a common infectious disease in the late eighteenth and early nineteenth centuries. The city board managed quarantine and sanitation in the city (Duffy 1990). These projects increased awareness of America's public health problems.

Temporary city boards of health were established in other cities when an epidemic threatened, only to be disbanded after the crisis. Between 1800 and 1830, despite rising concern over public health, few steps were taken to establish permanent organizations (Duffy 1990). At the same time, the connection between government assistance and community efforts weakened. As the nation's cities grew, largely from the influx of immigrants, the community responsibility for the indigent and infirm decreased (Duffy 1990).

By the mid-nineteenth century people residing in or near urban areas outnumbered those living in rural communities. Rapid population growth and overcrowding from increased immigration overwhelmed sanitation systems in cities. Hence disease in urban populations often resulted in epidemic outbreaks. Diseases such as malaria persisted endemically in all regions of the United States. Infectious disease was a major threat to all segments of society, but most deaths occurred among infants, children, adolescents, and young adults. High rates of infant mortality in particular were a primary concern of public health officials during the pre–Civil War period (Duffy 1990). Infectious diseases struck every city, town, and community and were an ever-present concern to groups across the United States.

An unintended result of the abolition movement and Civil War was diminished support for public health initiatives (Duffy 1990). Most support for public health occurred in urban areas. Urban initiatives emphasized quality of water, disposal of waste and sewage, sanitation (such as street cleaning), and indigent institutionalization (Leavitt 1978). The Civil War resulted in immense social changes, including increasing numbers of indigents in the cities. Because epidemics normally struck the poorest neighborhoods hardest, poverty was linked with public health concerns.

The impression that poverty spread disease meant that cities needed to address the issue of institutional care for the indigent and incapacitated when slow progress was made with public health initiatives. At the beginning of the nineteenth century almshouses and a sense of community responsibility for the poor corresponded with the creation of boards of health when epidemics threatened. As the nineteenth century progressed, the almshouse began to be replaced with larger institutional structures. *The State and Public Welfare in Nineteenth-Century America* (Anonymous 1976) looked at five reports concerning the establishment of institutions for the care and detainment of America's paupers in the nineteenth century. The reports, written between 1833 and 1877, addressed the issue of responsibility for maintenance and upkeep of state-run institutions. They also noted that laws dictating the pauper system were heavily intertwined with other laws concerning public welfare. Despite the efforts of city-level health initiatives and state-run institutions, vital statistics gathered after 1830 showed a steady decline in health across America as the nineteenth century progressed (Duffy 1990). Urban growth and the problems that came with that increase were addressed inadequately at the city level.

During the years surrounding the Civil War, little national support for public health movements existed, despite the lessons learned from sanitation associated with war and military encampments. Civilians were introduced to the concept that human waste disposal was related to enteric diseases, the need for fresh produce to avoid vitamin deficiencies, and the value of quarantine measures to control the spread of disease. Starting in 1865, permanent city health departments were established in American cities (Duffy 1990). Support for public health at the state and national levels followed by the end of the 1860s.

Like city boards of health, state boards of health started in Massachusetts in 1869 (Milwaukee Health Department [MHD] 1876–77). When the American Health Department formed in 1872, only three states and the District of Columbia had similar organizations. The American Public Health Association arose concurrently when the role of pathogens began to be publicized by Louis Pasteur, Joseph Lister, and Robert Koch (Bernstein 1972). Medical knowledge concerning pathogens and the importance of sanitation played a major role in shaping public health policies during the late nineteenth century. Vaccination campaigns and regulation of food and milk quality were added to public health efforts. The advocacy of public health movements spread from the east coast to the Midwest then to the South in the second half of the nineteenth century. By the beginning of the twentieth century the movement had reached the west coast (Duffy 1990). During this time, all regions showed a slow decline in infant mortality and modest increase in life expectancy.

This chapter examines one city in the midwestern region: Milwaukee. Wisconsin's State Board of Health was the eleventh established, in 1876 (MHD 1876–77). It was one of a swell of new organizations within the United States and set a foundation for the current Wisconsin Department of Health Services. Milwaukee, however, began its own public health initiatives even earlier, in 1867, when the city was granted permission by the state legislature to create a city board of health (Leavitt 1982; Gurda 2006). The city's efforts, starting in the mid- to late nineteenth century, highlighted the struggle to control infectious diseases targeting segments of Milwaukee's population.

Milwaukee

Milwaukee's history showed a city dedicated to public health innovations and reforms. Early efforts by Milwaukee's Board of Health were dominated by sanitation efforts, such as monitoring the condition of Milwaukee's slaughterhouses, the quality of the city's water and ice, and the disposal of garbage and sewage (Still 1948). To thwart the spread of disease, Milwaukee dealt first with the deplorable condition of the city's various wards and city streets. Densely populated neighborhoods, open sewers, manure in the streets, and industrial waste created an environment conducive for pathogens to develop and disseminate (Leavitt 1982). In addition to poor sanitation, contaminated food and milk spread contagions across Milwaukee.

Efforts to improve the condition of the city began with the creation of the Board of Health in 1867. The following year Milwaukee faced a smallpox epidemic. The city's response, led by the board, included vaccination campaigns and school closings, thus limiting the spread of the disease (Leavitt 1982). Epidemics such as this one increased support for the newly formed board. Like all major American cities, however, Milwaukee struggled to find a balance between politics and the need for reform. Economics complicated issues, such as regulation of the city's slaughterhouses and the city's water system. Milwaukee's focus on manufacturing and commerce attracted thousands of immigrants to the city, drawn by industrial labor opportunities. But the stress encountered in the urban environment and crowded living spaces increased the severity of epidemics in the city (Leavitt 1982). The municipal government balanced expansion of Milwaukee's manufacturing interests with the need to regulate the wastes that these industries produced (Leavitt 1982).

Infectious diseases, particularly airborne and waterborne ones, were a constant threat in American cities during the nineteenth century. Board activity focusing on infectious disease centered on isolating Milwaukee's sick. Milwaukee suffered from periodic epidemics, including smallpox, diphtheria, influenza, cholera, and typhoid fever. Rapid growth and overcrowding increased the city's mortality rates from infectious diseases. From 1860 through 1930 respiratory and gastrointestinal infections caused most deaths (Leavitt 1982). Public health concerns associated with these diseases drew the attention of politicians, businesses, schools, and residents. Lack of medical knowledge about the contagions present in the city led to the use of a variety of patent medicines. Elixirs and homeopathic remedies became popular consumer products, with private individuals and businesses advertising their products in an unregulated pharmaceutical market (Lipsky and Sharp 2001).

Despite the impact of illnesses on the city and its history of public health reform, enacting reactive measures was not always smooth. The *11th Annual Report of the Board of Health of the City of Milwaukee* (MHD 1877–78) details the city's efforts to combat smallpox and frustration with the populace's lack of understanding concerning the importance of preventive measures such as vaccination. Resistance to smallpox vaccination concentrated on the nature of the vaccine, which produced scarring. The vesicle created by the vaccine becomes a pus-filled blister, which eventually scabs and creates a small scar. Despite repeated epidemics, resistance to preventive measures was common in the nineteenth century.

Infant mortality continued to be a leading problem ten years after the creation of the Milwaukee Board of Health. In addition, children and adults were susceptible to infectious disease. Table 15.1 displays the mortality pattern for 1877 (MHD 1877–78).

TABLE 15.1. Milwaukee deaths by age groups and sex for 1877

Age	*Male percent*	*Female percent*	*Total percent*	*Number of deaths*
Under 1 year	18.0	15.8	33.8	757
1 to 5 years	11.3	10.4	21.7	487
5 to 20 years	5.3	6.5	11.8	265
20 to 30 years	3.5	4.2	7.7	172
30 to 40 years	3.1	2.2	5.3	118
40 to 50 years	2.3	1.9	4.3	97
50 to 60 years	3.9	2.2	6.1	137
60 to 70 years	2.7	1.7	4.4	99
70 to 80 years	1.9	1.6	3.5	79
Over 80 years	0.6	0.7	1.4	32
Totals	52.8	47.2	100.0	2243

Milwaukee Health Department 1877–78.

Considering all age cohorts, leading causes of death in 1877 were associated mostly with contagions. From the tenth to the first most frequent, deaths were caused by cholera infantum, violence, meningitis, diarrhea, diphtheria, stillborn and premature births, scarlet fever, consumption, infantile convulsions, and smallpox. Although present throughout the United States during the nineteenth century, these diseases were particularly lethal in larger cities because the pathogens spread rapidly in those densely populated areas. Infant mortality primarily involved cholera infantum, diarrhea, stillborn and premature births, and infantile convulsions. Infant deaths from gastrointestinal infections in particular remained the greatest problem facing the city, highlighting the relationship between infectious disease and contaminated food and water (MHD 1877–78).

During the subsequent two decades (1880–1899), the city's efforts to control disease concentrated on vaccination campaigns and city sanitation. Milwaukee also increased institutionalization of the sick, disabled, and indigent. By 1882 the county had established separate institutions to house children, the poor, people with a chronic debilitating illness or physical disability, and the mentally disabled (Richards and Kastell 1993).

The impact on the leading causes of death can be seen in the *16th Annual Report of the Commissioner of Health of the City of Milwaukee* (MHD 1892–93). Tuberculosis (known as consumption), diphtheria, diarrheal diseases, marasmus (severe malnutrition, usually associated with infant deaths), pneumonia, convulsions, bronchitis, heart disease, senility, and accidents accounted for the majority of deaths. The city's efforts reduced deaths from some pathogens. One of the most notable differences in the leading causes of death is the absence of smallpox and the rise of heart disease and senility. When Milwaukee suffered another smallpox epidemic, the impact was mitigated by the city's vaccination campaigns. The vaccination programs enacted in Milwaukee's schools were often more successful than community measures. Starting in 1873, the city school board required smallpox vaccination for all students beginning the public schools (Leavitt 1982).

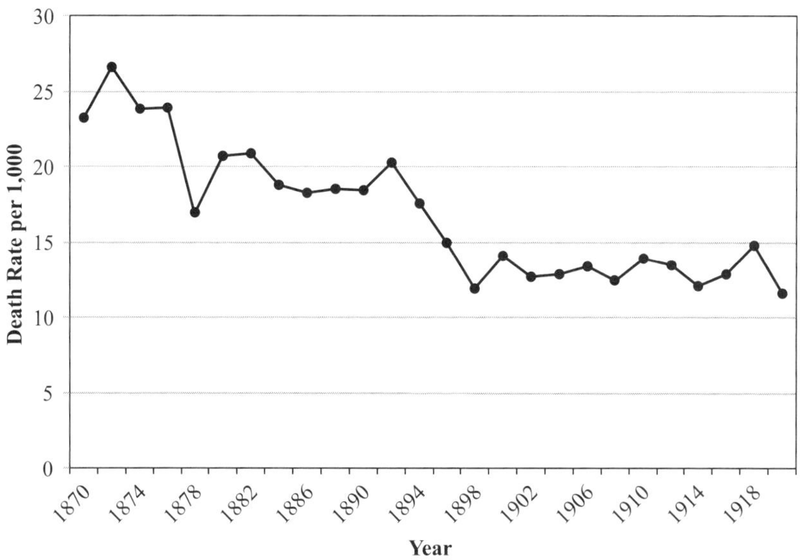

15.1. Death rate per 1,000 for Milwaukee from 1870 to 1920. (Data abstracted from Leavitt 1982.)

Efforts to combat epidemics often exceeded the attention given to more endemic problems, such as tuberculosis. Figure 15.1 shows the death rate for the city of Milwaukee between 1870 and 1920. It demonstrates an overall declining death rate but shows Milwaukee's continued struggle with epidemics. The marked decline after 1878 followed a smallpox epidemic in 1876, one of several smallpox epidemics that hit the city before 1900. Although minor by nineteenth-century standards, the last peak involved the impact of the 1918 influenza outbreak on the city's death rate.

By the beginning of the twentieth century death rates had fallen in American cities, including Milwaukee. Table 15.2 presents the mortality pattern from the 1899–1900 *Annual Report of the Commissioner of Health of the City of Milwaukee*. The infant mortality rate remained greatest among all age cohorts. But the percentage of total deaths was lower for those between the ages of one and

TABLE 15.2. Milwaukee deaths by age groups and sex for 1900

Age	*Male percent*	*Female percent*	*Total percent*	*Number of deaths*
Under 1 year	18.0	12.9	30.9	1,247
1 to 5 years	6.2	5.8	12.0	484
5 to 10 years	1.9	1.7	3.6	143
10 to 20 years	2.1	2.3	4.4	177
20 to 30 years	3.0	4.0	7.0	282
30 to 40 years	3.8	3.4	7.2	288
40 to 50 years	4.5	3.4	7.9	319
50 to 60 years	3.2	3.0	6.2	251
60 to 70 years	3.7	3.9	7.6	304
70 to 80 years	4.0	4.9	8.9	357
80 to 90 years	1.9	1.9	3.8	152
90 to 100 years	0.1	0.4	0.5	21
Over 100 years	0.0	0.02	0.02	1
Totals	52.4	47.6	100.0	4026

Source: Milwaukee Health Department 1899–1900.

five as well as those under the age of thirty than earlier. The table also shows a dramatic increase in the percentage of total deaths for those over the age of sixty, reflecting an increasing life span.

Changes in the Twentieth Century

Using historical records and archival research, mortality trends can be examined for cause-of-death information and cause-specific mortality (Gage 2005). Degenerative diseases replaced infectious diseases as the leading causes of death during the twentieth century, indicating an epidemiological transition (Omran 1977; Barrett et al. 1998; Gage 2005). Figure 15.2 shows a 1921 summary of the major causes of death in Boston, New York City, Philadelphia, and New Orleans between 1815 and 1914 (Anonymous 1921). The bar chart (Balance of Mortality) shows a decrease in infectious diseases and an increase in degenerative diseases. Most noticeably, the death rate rises for both heart disease and cancers and declines for all infectious diseases except pneumonia.

The figure summarizes the patterns of mortality found throughout the United States during the nineteenth century. The early part of the century reflected a struggle to control periodic epidemics, with little attention to preventing reoccurrences. The increased death rate between 1840 and 1864 is attributable to growing American urban

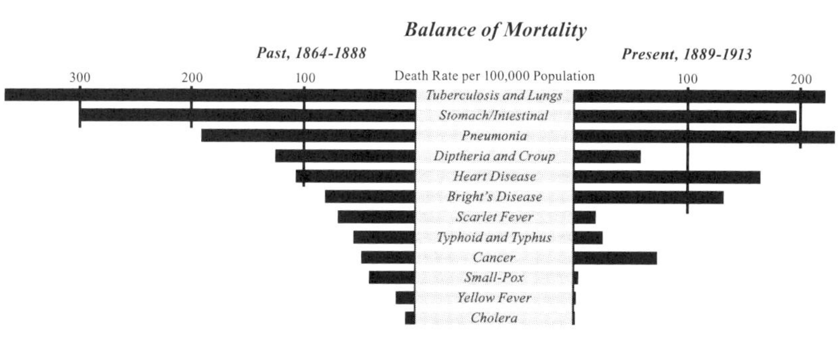

15.2. Decline in infectious diseases, particularly tuberculosis and diphtheria, and increase in degenerative and neoplastic diseases, notably heart problems and cancer, during the nineteenth and early twentieth centuries. (Modified from Anonymous 1921:102.)

areas with immigrants increasing the population (Anonymous 1921). In contrast, the post–Civil War period displays evidence of continued epidemics but also demonstrates a declining number of deaths despite a growing population. Most noticeably, the advent of the twentieth century is associated with a drop in the death rate.

Unlike the earlier theory concerning the role of a "miasmic" environment, medical science advanced the ideas of curative medicine and the promotion of germ theory between 1870 and 1930 (Leavitt 1982). Despite this change, the preantibiotic era showed little development in the ability of medicine to treat and cure either acute or chronic illnesses. With the exception of the development of vaccines for illnesses such as diphtheria and smallpox, medicine's contributions to public health for the most part simply explained how contagions were passed and what measures improved urban environments to mitigate the impact of these contagions (Leavitt 1982).

The annual reports from Milwaukee's Heath Department presented causes of death. Six diseases (typhoid fever, diphtheria, tuberculosis, pneumonia, cancer, and heart disease) emerged as the leading causes of death in Milwaukee during the nineteenth century and early twentieth century. Figure 15.3 shows the frequency of each of these six diseases in five-year intervals starting in 1895 and ending in 1905 (MHD 1907). The frequencies of typhoid fever and diphtheria declined. The frequencies of cancer and heart disease (both degenerative diseases), in contrast, showed a general increase during those years. Although a slight decrease in tuberculosis occurred, historic information highlighted the steady impact that both tuberculosis and pneumonia had on the mortality rates in Milwaukee. The city's efforts to combat tuberculosis were minimal before 1912, the year when the health department added a division for tuberculosis (MHD 1912).

The decrease of infectious diseases and the increase of degenerative diseases, both in Milwaukee and nationally, were trends that continued throughout the twentieth century. The nineteenth century in the United States was impacted by the presence of contagions in the general populace, so that every region, city, and community was affected. The first substantial efforts to improve the nation's health were enacted during this time, however, many of which still play roles in public health concerns today.

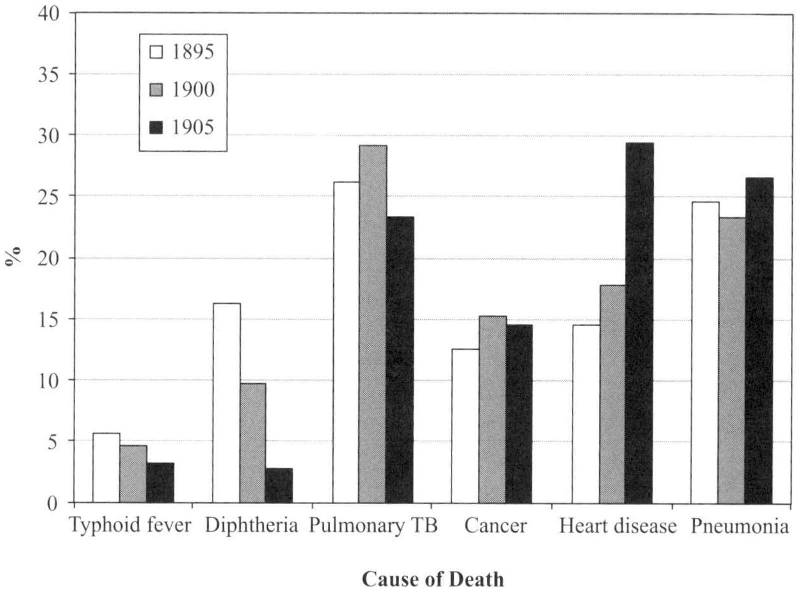

15.3. Changes in cause of death in Milwaukee: 1895, 1900, and 1905. Percentage determined by the number of deaths by cause divided by the total number of deaths from these six major death causes in the year intervals. (Data abstracted from Milwaukee Health Department 1907.)

Summary and Comparisons

This chapter takes a broad perspective on illness, beyond the post–Civil War Seventh Cavalry that earlier chapters have emphasized. It encompasses archival and other historical records from the late nineteenth and early twentieth centuries documenting mortality in urban areas, with an emphasis on Milwaukee, Wisconsin.

Differences between the two data sets emerged. The Seventh Cavalry's military illnesses and medicine contrasted with Milwaukee's public health movement and the city's overall mortality.

Positioned in the frontier West and Reconstruction South, the Seventh Cavalry stations differed from Milwaukee, a large midwestern city. The Seventh Cavalry records were limited to the two decades immediately following the Civil War, while the Milwaukee data included that period, continuing into the early twentieth century. The Seventh Cavalry enlistments consisted almost solely of young adult males, versus the presence of all ages (including children and the elderly) and both sexes in Milwaukee. And the Seventh Cavalry represented a relatively healthy group (at least healthy enough to pass enlistment requirements), contrasted with individuals of all health backgrounds that an urban area could assemble.

Cause of deaths highlighted the differences between Milwaukee and the Seventh Cavalry. Early in the period (1868), smallpox, diphtheria, influenza, cholera, and typhoid fever dominated Milwaukee's death records. In the next decade (1877), smallpox, consumption, scarlet fever, diphtheria, meningitis, and violence contributed most to deaths in Milwaukee. And from 1880 through 1899 tuberculosis, diphtheria, diarrheal diseases, pneumonia, convulsions, bronchitis, heart disease, senility, and accidents caused most of Milwaukee's deaths. Despite this plethora of diseases, accidents, and lethal potentials, Milwaukee death rates declined from 1870 through 1920.

The Seventh Cavalry showed few similarities to and many differences from Milwaukee moralities. In one of the few similarities, the Seventh Cavalry demonstrated a general decline in the number of deaths from 1867 through the mid-1880s.

The majority of deaths in the post–Civil War Seventh Cavalry resulted from violence, injuries, or accidents (totaling nearly 75 percent of all deaths), many of them battle- or skirmish-related. As an example, deaths at the hands of "Indians" amounted to approximately 63 percent of the total number of deaths. Infectious diseases came next, with cholera (about 5 percent of all deaths), consumption and other lung-related distresses (nearly 4 percent), and typhoid fevers (about 2 percent) being the most frequent infection-caused deaths in the Seventh Cavalry.

But the Seventh Cavalry had no cases of the other dominant infections that impacted Milwaukee: no deaths from influenza, smallpox, scarlet fever, or diphtheria. Meningitis and convulsions, frequent urban killers, caused only a few Seventh Cavalry deaths. Finally, as might be expected in a relatively youthful military sample, the Seventh Cavalry had few cases of degenerative disease deaths (such as heart diseases and cancers), while Milwaukee suffered an increasing number of degenerative deaths over time.

In some ways this comparison between the Seventh Cavalry and Milwaukee deaths reflects changes that continue to be made today. It reveals a rural-to-urban migration and includes a demographic contrast between a more youthful group with a group including older individuals as well as subadults. The study shows epidemic diseases diminishing and chronic and degenerative diseases increasing as causes of deaths. So the comparison serves as a stark, if somewhat artificial, example of mortality changes from a nineteenth-century pattern to a more contemporary one.

CHAPTER 16 Summary and Discussion

P. Willey and Douglas D. Scott

The Seventh Cavalry served as the iconic regiment in the post–Civil War U.S Army. Its charismatic leader, George Custer, and high-profile encounters with Plains Indians, including the Battle of the Little Bighorn, led to this image. Although the regiment stood out in many ways, the Seventh Cavalry and its troopers reflected characteristics of other regiments during the period. To expand these comparisons, this work describes the health and illness of the Seventh Cavalry and explores similarities and differences with other groups.

Building on previous work related to the military in the frontier West and in the Reconstruction South, this book assesses the Seventh Cavalry's health and illness, beginning with the regiment's inception in 1866 and continuing into the early 1880s. This interdisciplinary work rests at the intersection of many fields and disciplines, particularly western expansion, military history, illness, history of medicine, medical anthropology, human biology, epidemiology, demography, osteology, and anthropometry. The study takes an ecumenical, anthropological approach.

This book has four sections: foundations and background to Seventh Cavalry medical studies, materials and methods, health results, and comparative studies. Here we examine the studies for broader trends and themes. This concluding chapter surveys temporal, regional, and biological parameters for indications of broader trends and themes.

Seasonal differences in diseases emerge from some of our studies. Winter was a desperate time, showing increased numbers of ear, nose, and throat (ENT) and respiratory diseases, including influenza, catarrh, bronchitis, and pneumonia. Such increases in ENT and respiratory diseases in the nineteenth century anticipated similar seasonal distributions of those same diseases today.

All injuries also rose in winter, not just frostbite. This increase is surprising, because injuries involving recent soldiers in U.S. Army Basic Combat Training show the opposite result (Knapik et al. 2002). In that study, trainees showed higher injury incidence during summer than in fall.

Some of the post–Civil War injuries stemmed from fights with comrades and citizens, which also increased in winter. This distribution is also somewhat surprising based on present-day results. At least compared to property crimes, violent crimes now are generally greatest in summer, not winter (McDowall et al. 2012).

Some of the post–Civil War injuries were probably fueled by alcohol. As might be expected, intoxication also soared in winter.

Seasons other than winter presented challenges. Seventh Cavalry desertions peaked in spring, as they did in other post–Civil War regiments (Rickey 1963:147; Coffman 1986:672). Reasons given for desertion often included inadequate housing, poor diet, egotistical officers, and low pay. But deserters also included opportunistic men, enlisting at the end of summer, remaining in service through the winter, then seeking better opportunities outside military service in spring.

Summer and fall showed other hazards, particularly malaria, reflecting the seasonal pattern recognized earlier during the Civil War. The recent U.S. pattern for distribution of malaria demonstrates a similar summer-fall peak, although probably for different reasons. The current distribution largely involves summer travelers returning from malarial countries to the United States who are infected with malaria (Cullen and Arguin 2013).

Annual decreases, fluctuations, and increases also occurred. Malaria generally decreased over the decades of study, as did desertions. Other diseases periodically spiked and then fell to previous low levels. Influenza peaked in 1867 then dropped. Other illnesses showed similar periodic crests, such as sexually transmitted infections (STIs) (1871–72) and general injuries (1868 and 1878).

Finally, transportation-related and internecine injuries increased during the two decades of this study. Some of these annual differences may have been time-related, but others may have been caused by changes in posting locations.

Turning to geographic differences, the Seventh Cavalry's first posting region—the central plains—had high frequencies of malaria and desertions. While stationed in the South, the Seventh Cavalry's incidences of STIs soared. That increase probably resulted from greater sexual opportunities there than in the more remote, less populated central and northern plains. Finally, in the northern plains the Seventh Cavalry showed high incidences of ENT ailments, bronchitis, frostbite, and other physical injuries in the northern plains, including those caused by conveyances and interpersonal trauma.

In addition to temporal and geographic variables, biological parameters influenced disease susceptibility. Those physical parameters included nativity, age, stature, and rank.

Immigrants were at greater risk, with more vulnerability to many diseases than their native-born counterparts. Foreign-born troopers suffered more infectious diseases, including tuberculosis, malaria, and STIs.

Foreign-born troopers also showed greater frequencies of general injuries as well as injuries from internecine fights when intermural skirmishes were excluded. In addition, foreign-born troopers were more frequently intoxicated, especially the Irish-born soldiers. And foreign-born troopers deserted more frequently, particularly the German-born. None of the parameters studied showed greater susceptibilities or proportions among U.S.-born than among foreign-born soldiers.

Among the many challenges that immigrants faced, disease was a prime one. It is claimed that youngsters rapidly adjust physiologically to the environment where they were born (Kaplan 1988). But when such people moved or were even in the midst of moving, those adjustments to their native lands did not necessary suit them well for their new homes. They proved susceptible. Newly arrived European immigrants usually landed in major eastern port cities. Often crowded into substandard housing, eating new foods, and hit by acculturation, they were ripe for infectious disease.

Under such circumstances, an illness gradient developed. It was greatest immediately on arrival and became less so with time, exposure, and adjustment to the new environment (Little and Baker 1988:168). This change also had parallels among newly enlisted U.S.-born recruits, who probably experienced a similar illness gradient when freshly enlisted in the army.

Possible explanations for the behaviorally related vulnerabilities of immigrants included foreign-born troopers taking greater risks than U.S.-born ones, living isolated from paternal cultural norms and expectations, and acculturating slowly to the customs of a new nation.

Among personal parameters, height mattered. Shorter troopers suffered a few more internecine injuries than taller ones, although the distribution failed to achieve statistical significance. Surprisingly, taller soldiers reported more cold injuries than shorter ones.

Age demonstrated a few differences in illnesses. Younger troopers proved more vulnerable to some dangers. For example, they reported more STIs than older ones. Perhaps Venus called more loudly to the more youthful men with increased hormone levels and less sense than to the older ones.

In addition, desertions occurred more frequently among younger soldiers, possibly due to the impulsiveness and ambiguity associated with some youths. Perhaps they believed that better opportunities existed elsewhere and rashly left military service. Young adults have been characterized as lacking experience, taking risks, seeking thrills, being impulsive, and abusing alcohol (Robertson 1998:119). Maybe these characteristics explain some of the age-related impacts on younger troopers.

Older soldiers, however, sustained more injuries (including internecine and conveyance-related ones) than younger ones. This increase perhaps resulted from slower reflexes and decreasing strength-to-weight ratios among the older troopers. Older soldiers also exhibited greater frequencies of intoxication.

We should put "young" and "old" into a nineteenth-century perspective. Life expectancy for a white male born in 1850 (about the average birth year of our Seventh Cavalry cohort) was only 39.5 years, about half of the life expectancy for white males born in 1990 (Haines 2000:308, table 8.2). And the average age of husbands at first marriage used to be 27.0 years, with the wife's age being several years younger (1880 census in Haines 2000:319). On average, by the time troopers in the post-Civil War Seventh Cavalry enlisted they had lived more than half of their lives. If they conformed to the marriage patterns of the day, they would need to consider wedding at the time when their second five-year enlistment began.

Disease incidences showed relatively few differences by rank. Only cold injuries approached statistical significance, with rankers reporting more episodes of frostbite than junior noncommissioned officers.

Finally, five major challenges require discussion. First, Seventh Cavalry medical records present the mere tip of the illness iceberg. Many of the regiment's ailments doubtless went unreported, were tolerated, or were self-treated, self-medicated, or ignored by the sufferer. As one example, skeletal evidence demonstrated widespread dental ill-health contrasted with the few dental complaints documented in the records (chapter 13). Surgeons in the post–Civil War period generally did not treat dental ailments, so the poor dental health of the period went unrecorded. Many other ailments undoubtedly also went unreported or under-reported in the medical records.

Second, some illnesses remained asymptomatic. One example is syphilis, which may infect individuals without showing symptoms (chapter 9). Many other illnesses may have lacked symptoms. Without symptoms, no self-respecting trooper would report for sick call, let alone be diagnosed with the illness.

Third, medical records were maintained irregularly, at least sometimes. For instance, medical records were poorly kept while on march or in transit. When the Seventh Cavalry moved onto northern plains in April 1873, as an example, "Custer's Blizzard" welcomed them (chapters 1 and 10). Despite personal accounts to the contrary, medical records documented no cold injuries during that month, although frostbite must have occurred. Elizabeth Custer and others described this situation. Other marches no doubt were not so well chronicled. Written narratives indicated that snow blindness happened at the Battle of the Washita (Chandler 1960:20–25), although no cases appeared in the medical records. Seventy-five men suffered scurvy in May 1867 (Barnitz in Utley 1977:51), but the medical records showed only a dozen for the entire year. Similar issues may dog mortality records, with six troopers said to have died near Bon Homme, Dakota Territory, in 1873 (Chandler 1960:39), but none appearing in the death records.

So in several ways the ailments that the medical records noted are only the tip of the iceberg. Similar under-reporting has been noted in the twentieth-century general practice too (Last 1963). Such under-reporting must have been even more distorted in the nineteenth century.

This point leads to a recommendation. Medical records should be supplemented with other documents for a fuller understanding of events and health impacts. Medical records may be complemented by personal narratives (chapter 10), other military publications (for example, Otis 1871), and skeletal remains (chapter 13) for a more complete health perspective. We encourage researchers tackling this or a similar subject to employ a holistic research and investigation paradigm.

Fourth, in most cases we have failed to identify the severity of injuries or disease. Some events were minor and transitory, while others constituted substantial threats to life and persisted for months, even resulting in a medical discharge or death. Today, for instance, injuries are rated on a Trauma Score or Injury Severity Score. Some evaluation of severity is available indirectly on the Carded Medical Records by using time out of service (the difference between the admission and release dates). Chapters 7, 8, and 10 provide such assessments, which could be extended to other studies as proxies for severity.

Fifth, nineteenth-century diagnoses may have confused and confounded ailments in terms of their modern diagnoses and distinctions. Surgeons worked within organizational and cognitive structures that situated diseases in a framework different from those of today (see chapter 3). The military medical records often provided specific observations and symptoms that could have been caused by several different agents if assessed by today's standards. Lacking the understanding that germ theory provided and without recourse to laboratory tests, more definitive diagnoses were unimaginable at the time. Consequently, the Carded Medical Records recognized only some of the major illnesses that were identifiable at the time and recorded them.

Recidivism complicated these assessments in the opposite direction. Persistent ailments may have amplified the numbers beyond reality.

Following the initial illness episode, this reasoning goes, some infection and injury symptoms persisted and continued appearing in the medical records. Examples of infectious disease persistence may have included pulmonary ailments (chapter 7), malaria (chapter 8), and syphilis (chapter 9). In some cases the records may have indicated an initial infection, followed by sequellae resulting from the original event. In other instances, however, the person may have been infected and reinfected many times following the initial infection. It was unclear if one or more infections occurred. In either case the impact of chronic diseases stretched over months and years, affecting troop strength and readiness each time, whether they were newly acquired infections or not.

Conclusions

This work demonstrates the value of analyzing multiple lines of evidence, various primary records, and archaeologically recovered human remains. All of those sources are placed within the context of the history and development of the fields of illness and medical science. These seemingly disparate sources, when analyzed in concert, provide new insights into the health of a single unit of the U.S. Army for two decades following the Civil War. This study illuminates many details of the lives and deaths of those who served in the U.S. Seventh Cavalry from 1866 to 1884. The details garnered from the medical records, both on an individual level and at the epidemiological group level, enlarge and enrich the picture of the men who served in the Seventh Cavalry in that period.

They were neither the unsoiled, healthy heroes represented by Errol Flynn in *They Died with Their Boots On* nor the maniacal one-dimensional soldiers portrayed in *Little Big Man* or *Dances with Wolves*. They were men with characteristics of all humans, facets of both heroes and heels.

Documenting that reality, we have analyzed and interpreted a vast data set. The results provide a proxy model of illness, injury, and medical practice for the post–Civil War army as a whole. In some respects the Seventh Cavalry appears to have been a cross section of the U.S. Army during that period. By extension the present information can be used to make inferences about soldiers in other units as well as young adult white civilians. Thus the data and interpretations of the medical history of the Seventh Cavalry presented here serve as a model for studies of other units, other periods, and even soldiers of other countries. But the Seventh Cavalry's history included some notable exceptions, particularly involving mortalities.

The men of the Seventh Cavalry were not an inordinately sickly lot, but they shouldered their share of illnesses and injuries. Their medical records reflected their roles as "peacetime" soldiers doing arduous and sometimes hazardous and stressful duty. They suffered the spectrum of ailments that young males were all too susceptible to when placed in close company. They likewise fell prey to the lure of alcohol and sexual contact, which sometimes led to unfortunate results. The medical treatment that these men received was first rate by the standards of the time, but it was constrained by the medical knowledge of the day and the practitioners available to treat them. Medical science advanced rapidly during the study period, but that knowledge had little impact on the treatments available to the men of the Seventh Cavalry. The epidemiological transition from infection-dominated illnesses to degenerative-derived ones happened in the decades that followed. The medical records and this anthropological study of the men of the Seventh Cavalry sketch missing pieces of their lives, giving us a new sense of their medical trials and tribulations.

Appendix

List of Surgeons Associated with the Seventh Cavalry

Douglas D. Scott and Patrick J. Collison

Some proper name spellings are questionable because they were deciphered from the records of various clerks with a wide variety of handwriting styles. Where possible the spellings were verified in other sources, but not all acting assistant surgeons are listed in other sources.

For simplicity, this appendix omits states in the first section (Alphabetical List of Surgeons Associated with the Seventh Cavalry). The second section (Posts Affiliated with the Seventh Cavalry and Surgeons Stationed There) includes modern state names rather than the names of the territories when the Seventh Cavalry was stationed there.

Alphabetical List of Surgeons Associated with the Seventh Cavalry, 1866 to 1884

Abbreviations: AAS acting assistant surgeon; AS assistant surgeon; NPRR Northern Pacific Railroad.

Alden, Charles, AS, Jan.–Dec. 1883, Jan.–Sept. 1884, Fort Yates
Allen, S. J., AAS, NPRR, 1873; Sept.–Dec. 1873, Jan.–April 1874, Fort Rice; Black Hills Expedition 1874
Barlow, William, AAS, Feb.–Dec. 1882, Jan.–Dec. 1883, Jan.–Dec. 1884, Fort Leavenworth

Barnette, J. B., AAS, Mar.–June 1872, Opelika
Bartholf, J. K., AAS, June, Sept.–Oct. 1871, Columbia
Beach, S. S., AAS, July–Dec. 1872, Opelika; Oct.–Nov. 1874, Greensboro; Oct.–Dec. 1874, Jan.–April 1875, Livingston
Beechemin, Louis, AS, Aug.–Dec. 1878, Jan.–Dec. 1879, Jan.–April 1878, July–Oct. 1880, Jan.–April 1881, Fort Meade
Bell, Ralph, AAS, Nov. 1878, Fort A. Lincoln; Mar.–Oct. 1879, Fort Meade
Benham, R. B., AS, Jan.–April 1881, Fort A. Lincoln
Bergen, Andrew C., AAS, Black Hills Expedition 1874
Biart, Victor, Surgeon, Nov. 1881–May 1883, Fort Leavenworth
Boughton, J. Frazer, AAS, Sept. 1873, Fort A. Lincoln
Brown, J. Morris, AS, Nov.–Dec. 1866, Jan.–May 1867, Fort Morgan; July–Nov. 1867, Fort Reynolds
Bryan, B. J., AAS, Dec. 1872, Jan.–Feb. 1873, Oxford
Burkwell, M. C., AAS, NPRR 1873
Bushnell, George, AS, Mar.–Dec. 1881, Jan.–Sept. 1882, Fort Yates
Byrne, C. C., AS, July–Sept. 1875, Fort A. Lincoln
Byrnes, J. C., AAS, July–Sept. 1875, Fort Randall
Chase, V. B., AAS, Oct. 1866, Fort Ellsworth
Cinker(?), Augustus, AAS, Dec. 1866, Fort Larned
Coates, Isaac, AAS, Hancock Expedition 1867
Collins, H. C., AAS, July–Oct. 1871, Meridian
Crandall, James B., AAS, Nov. 1866, Fort Dodge; Jan.–Feb. 1867, Fort Larned
Crayton, Louis W., AS, Oct.–Dec. 1880, Jan.–Dec. 1881, Jan.–Oct. 1882, Fort Buford
Cronkhite, H. M., AS, Feb.–Dec. 1872, Jan.–Feb. 1873, Spartanburg
Davis, F. A. (H.?), AAS, assigned to Cavalry Barracks, Dec. 1873, Jan.–Mar. 1874, Fort A. Lincoln; June–Dec. 1874, Jan.–April 1875, Fort Rice
Davis, Thomas B. AAS, Oct.–Dec. 1876, Fort Rice; Jan.–Mar. 1877, Fort Abercrombie
Davis, William B. AS, in field with Seventh Cavalry, Nov. 1877; Jan.–Mar., June–Dec. 1878, Jan.–June, Aug.–Dec. 1879, at Fort Buford; July 1879, Jan.–May, July–Dec. 1880, detached service; June 1880, Jan.–Oct. 1881, June–Dec. 1882, Jan.–Dec. 1883, Jan.–Dec. 1884, Fort Totten
Deeble, H. M., AAS, Aug.–Dec. 1881, Jan.–Mar., July–Dec. 1882, Jan.–Dec. 1883, Jan.–April, June–Dec. 1884, Fort Yates

DeGraw, C. S., AS, Jan.–Dec. 1867, Jan.–Feb., June 1868, May 1869, Fort Dodge

Delany, Alfred, AS, Jan.–April 1871, Fort Hays

De Wolf, James, AAS, Nov.–Dec. 1875, Jan.–Mar. 1876, Fort A. Lincoln; Little Bighorn (KIA)

Du Bose, E. W., AAS, Black Hills Expedition 1874; June 1875–Aug. 1875, April, June 1878, Fort A. Lincoln

Ferguson, James L., AAS, Oct.–Dec. 1873, Jan.–Mar., Nov.–Dec. 1874, Jan.–April, Aug.–Dec. 1875, Jan.–Mar. 1876, Fort Totten; Nov.–Dec. 1877, Jan.–Mar., May–Aug., Oct.–Dec. 1878, detached service; April and Sept. 1878, Jan.–June 1879, Fort Yates

Fitch, A. F., AAS, Nov.–Dec. 1866, Jan.–Mar. 1867, Fort Hays; Sept.–Dec. 1867, Jan.–April 1868, April, 1869, Fort Dodge

Fitzgerald, A., AS, Mar. 1869, Fort Leavenworth; Nez Perce Campaign Aug.–Oct. 1877

Fitzgerald, J. W., AAS, Sept.–Dec. 1867, Jan.–April 1868, Fort Lyon

Forwood, W. H., AS, Sept., Dec. 1866, Jan.–Mar. 1867, Fort Larned; Dec. 1867, Jan.–1868, Fort Dodge; July–Sept. 1868, Fort Larned

Freeman, J. W., AAS, Oct.–Dec. 1881, Jan.–Dec. 1882 (detached service with Seventh Cavalry, June–July 1882), Jan.–May 1883, Fort Meade

Fryer, Benjamin, Surgeon, Nov.–Dec. 1881, Jan.–Dec. 1882, Jan.–Dec. 1883, Jan.–July 1884, Fort Leavenworth

Frynham, John F., AAS, Aug.–Dec. 1872, Laurenville

Gardner, Edwin F., AS, July 1877, Fort A. Lincoln; Nez Perce Campaign Aug.–Oct. 1877

Gibson, Joseph, AS, Dec. 1872, Jan.–May 1872, Yorkville

Goddard, C. E., AS, Nov.–Dec. 1884, Fort Yates

Hartsuff, A., Surgeon, Dec. 1884, Fort Larned

Harvard Valery, AS, May–Oct. 1877, in field with Seventh Cavalry; Nov.–Dec. 1877, Fort A. Lincoln

Harvey, John, AAS, May–Nov. 1871, Unionville; Dec. 1872, Jan.–Feb. 1872, Yorkville; April–Sept. 1872, Lincolnton; Dec. 1872, Jan.–Feb. 1873, Charlotte; NPRR 1873; Sept.–Oct. 1873, Fort A. Lincoln

Hatch, C. W., AAS, Nov.–Dec. 1876, Fort Abercrombie

Heger, Anthony, Surgeon, April–Dec. 1873, Jan.–Sept. 1874, Fort Snelling

Hilliard, E. D., AAS, Nov.–Dec. 1867, Fort Reynolds

Hoffman, W. J., AAS, NPRR 1873
Howard, W. King, AS, Oct.–Dec. 1870, Jan.–April 1871, Fort Wallace
Hubbard, V. Buren, AS, Dec. 1872, Jan.–Feb. 1873, Jackson Barracks
Irwin, Bernard D. J., AS, May 1880, Fort Meade
Johnson, R. W., AS, Nov.–Dec. 1882, Jan.–Dec. 1883, Jan.–Dec. 1884, Fort Buford
Kimball, J. A., AS, NPRR 1873; June 1875, Fort Randall; July 1875 on detached service with Seventh Cavalry
Kinoblauch, L. F., AAS, Oct.–Dec. 1874, Jan.–Dec. 1875, Jan.–April 1876, Shreveport
Kinsman, J. H., AS, Aug.–Oct. 1876, Fort A. Lincoln
Krine, T. C., AAS, June–Sept. 1871, Winsboro; Nov. 1871, Yorkville
La Bare, John, AAS, NPRR 1873; Oct.–Dec. 1873, Jan.–Oct. 1874, Fort A. Lincoln
Lippincott, Henry, AS, Hancock Expedition 1867; Nov.–Dec. 1867, Oct.–Dec. 1869, Jan.–April, Nov.–Dec. 1870, Jan.–Feb. 1871, Fort Leavenworth; Washita 1868
Lloyd, Frederick, AAS, Sept.–Dec. 1879, Mar. 1880, Feb. 1882, Fort A. Lincoln
Lord, George E., AAS, Black Hills Expedition May–July 1875; Little Bighorn (KIA)
Loring, Frederick, AAS, Sept. 1880, Fort Meade
Lytton, J. F., AAS, May, Nov.–Dec. 1871, Jan.–Feb. 1872, Chester; Dec. 1872, Jan.–Feb. 1873, Newberry
Magruder, Daniel or David, Surgeon, Nov.–Dec. 1867, Jan.–Aug., 1868, Mar.–May, Oct.–Nov. 1869, Jan.–Aug. 1870, Fort Leavenworth
Manderville, William B., AAS, Feb. 1873, Jackson Barracks; Oct.–Dec. 1874, Jan.–Mar. 1875, New Orleans; May 1875, Fort Randall
Mann, A. H., AAS, Jan.–Feb. 1873, Opelika
Marselis, N. H., AAS, Nov.–Dec. 1874, Jan.–Feb. 1875, Fort A. Lincoln
Maus, Louis M., AS, Nov.–Dec. 1877, Jan.–Dec. 1878, Jan.–Oct., Nov. 1879, Jan.–Dec. 1880, Jan.–April 1881, Fort Yates
McCall, W. P., AAS, July–Aug. 1884, Fort Leavenworth
McQuerry, George, AS, Oct.–Dec. 1884, Fort Meade
Meacham, Abel, AS, Oct.–Dec. 1870, Fort Hays
Meyer, George D., AAS, Dec. 1872, Jan. 1873, Jackson Barracks

Middleton, J. V. D., AS, Oct.–Dec. 1875, Jan.–Sept. 1876, Fort A. Lincoln; Oct. 1876, detached service to Standing Rock; Nov.–Dec. 1876, Jan.–Mar. 1877, Fort A. Lincoln; Surgeon, Sept.–Dec. 1883, Jan.–Dec. 1884, Fort Leavenworth

Middleton, Passemore, AS, April–May, July 1871, Elizabethtown; Surgeon, Sept.–Dec. 1884, Fort Leavenworth

Milham, John J., AS, Feb.–Dec. 1871, Jan.–Dec. 1872, Jan.–Mar. 1873, Taylor Barracks

Miller, George M., AAS, Jan.–July 1868, Fort Reynolds

O'dell, R. William, AAS, Mar.–Aug. 1871, Bagdad; Oct.–Dec. 1874, Jan.–Dec. 1875, Colfax

Owsley, W. T., AAS, Jan.–April 1875, Opelika

Paulding, Holmes O., AS, July–Nov. 1877, in field with Seventh Cavalry; Dec. 1877, May–June 1878, Fort A. Lincoln; July–Sept. 1878, in field with Seventh Cavalry; Nov. 1878, Fort A. Lincoln

Perin(?), Glover, Surgeon, Sept.–Dec. 1870, Jan.–Feb. 1871, Fort Leavenworth

Pleasant, Thomas H., AAS, May–Nov. 1880, Fort A. Lincoln

Pope, Benjamin F., AS, Aug.–Dec. 1871, Jan.–Feb. 1873, Elizabethtown

Price, C. E., AAS, Nov.–Dec. 1872, Jan.–Feb. 1873, Lebanon

Rector, Pierson, AAS, June–Dec. 1871, Jan.–Feb. 1872, Rutherfordton; Feb. 1873, Charlotte

Redd, Robert G., AAS, April, July–Aug. 1871, Mt. Vernon; June–Dec. 1872, Jan.–Feb. 1873, Yorkville; Sept.–Dec. 1875, Jan.–Sept., Nov.–Dec. 1876, Jan.–July 1877, Fort A. Lincoln

Renick, William, AAS, Dec. 1867, Jan.–Mar. 1868, Fort Leavenworth; Washita 1868; Nov.–Dec. 1869, Jan.–May 1870, Fort Lyon

Roberts, T. N., AAS, Sept.–Oct. 1871, Columbia

Ruger, H. H., AAS, May–Dec. 1871, Jan. 1872, Spartanburg; Jan. 1872, Mar.–Dec. 1872, Jan.–Feb. 1873, Unionville; NPRR 1873; Nov.–Dec. 1876, Jan.–July, Nov.–Dec. 1877, Jan.–Mar., June–Oct., Dec. 1878, Fort Totten; July–Sept. and Nov. 1878, detached service in the field; Jan.–Dec. 1879, Jan.–Dec. 1880, Jan.–Dec. 1881, Jan.–June, Aug.–Dec. 1882, Jan.–Mar. 1883, Fort Totten

Russell, W. T., AAS, Mar.–April 1871, Spartanburg

Sabin, W. E., AAS, Feb.–Dec. 1884 (at wood camp July 1884), Fort Meade

Sanderson, J. L., AAS, Nov.–Dec. 1882, Jan.–Dec. 1883, Jan.–Dec. 1884, Fort Meade

Shaw, James, AAS, Sept.–Oct. 1874, Fort Totten
Sheaver, M. M., AAS, Nov.–Dec. 1869, Jan.–Dec. 1870, Jan.–April 1871, Fort Wallace
Shiffmen, B., AAS, May–June 1867, Fort Lyon
Simons, J. A., AAS, Sept.–Dec. 1880, Jan.–Aug. 1881, Fort Meade
Skinner, F. C., AAS, April 1871, Chester
Smith, Andrew K., Surgeon, Aug. 1871, Atlanta
Sukas, J., AAS, Nov. 1866, Fort Dodge
Taylor, Blair D., AS, Oct.–Dec. 1875, Jan.–May, Oct.–Dec. 1876, Jan.–May 1877, Jan.–May 1878, Fort Rice; Feb.–July 1879, Fort A. Lincoln
Taylor, H. V., AAS, June–Sept. 1871, Darlington
Taylor, M. E., AS, Dec. 1871, Jan. 1872, Huntsville; Jan.–April 1876, McComb City; Jan. 1876, Colfax
Tilton, H. R., AS, Nov.–Dec. 1866, Jan.–Dec. 1867, Jan.–Oct. 1868, Nov.–Dec. 1869, Jan.–May and Oct.–Nov. 1870, Fort Lyon; Nez Perce Campaign Aug.–Oct. 1877
Tompkins, William A., AAS, Mar.–Nov. 1871, Yorkville; Dec. 1871, Unionville
Tramaine(?), William, AS, Jan.–Mar. 1871, Fort Dodge
Turner, F. H., AS, Nov.–Dec. 1866, Jan.–Dec. 1867, Jan.–May 1868, Fort Wallace
Turner, S. S., AAS, Jan.–Dec. 1881, Jan.–Mar. 1882, Fort Buford; May, Dec. 1882, detached service with Company F, Seventh Cavalry on Upper Yellowstone River; June–Nov. 1882, Fort Buford; Jan.–May 1883, detached service to Poplar River; June–Aug. 1883; Sept.–Dec. 1883, Jan.–Dec. 1884, Fort Buford
Vickery, Richard, AS, Dec. 1872, Jan. 1873, Jackson Barracks
Warnock, J. T., AAS, Dec. 1874, Opelika
Weeds, James F., Surgeon, June–Dec. 1872, Jan.–Feb. 1873, Nashville; Feb.–May 1875, Fort A. Lincoln
West, Theodore L., AAS, April 1871, Elizabethtown; May–June 1871, Mt. Vernon
Wierick, S. T., AAS, Dec. 1879, detached service; Jan.–Feb. 1880, Mar.–Dec. 1880, Jan.–June 1881, Fort Yates; detached service with Seventh Cavalry recruits, Aug.–Dec. 1881, Jan.–May, July–Oct. 1882, Fort A. Lincoln; detached service with Seventh Cavalry, June 1882
Wiggins, A. Y., AAS, Nov.–Dec. 1867, Jan.–May 1868, Fort Wallace
Williams, E. D., AAS, Aug.–Sept. 1867, Fort Wallace

Williams, John W., AS, Sept.–Dec. 1873, Jan.–Mar., May, Nov.–Dec. 1874, Fort Rice; April 1874 detached service; Black Hills Expedition 1874; Oct. 1874 temporary duty at Fort Yankton; Jan.–Sept. 1875, Fort Rice

Wilson, A. D., AS, Nov.–Dec. 1866, Jan.–June 1867, Fort Dodge

Wilson, William, AS, Nov.–Dec. 1880, Jan.–Dec. 1881, Jan.–Dec. 1882, Jan.–Dec. 1883, Jan.–Oct. 1884, Fort Meade

Witherspoon, John B., AAS, June–July 1871, Fort Sumter

Wolverton, W. A., AS, July–Dec. 1877, Jan.–Dec. 1878, Jan.–April, Nov.–Dec. 1879, Jan.–Dec. 1880, Jan.–Dec. 1881, Jan.–Oct. 1882, Fort A. Lincoln

Woodhull, A. A., AS, Mar.–May 1868, Fort Leavenworth; Oct.–Dec. 1870, Fort Lyon

Posts Affiliated with the Seventh Cavalry and Surgeons Stationed There

CENTRAL PLAINS

Fort Riley, Kansas

Forwood, W. H., AS, Sept., Dec. 1866, Jan.–Mar. 1867

Cinker(?), Augustus, AAS, Dec. 1866

Crandall, James B., AAS Jan.–Feb. 1867

Hartsuff, A., Surgeon, Dec. 1884

Fort Leavenworth, Kansas

Magruder, Daniel or David, Surgeon, Nov.–Dec. 1867, Jan.–Aug., 1868, Mar.–May, Oct.–Nov. 1869, Jan.–Aug. 1870

Perin(?), Glover, Surgeon, 1870 Sept.–Dec. 1870, Jan.–Feb. 1871

Lippincott, Henry, AS, Nov.–Dec. 1867, Oct.–Dec. 1869, Jan.–April, Nov.–Dec. 1870, Jan.–Feb. 1871

Renick, William, AAS, Dec. 1867, Jan.–Mar. 1868

Woodhull, A. A., AS, Mar.–May 1868

Fitzgerald, A., AS, Mar. 1869

Fryer, Benjamin, Surgeon, Nov.–Dec. 1881, Jan.–Dec. 1882, Jan.–Dec. 1883, Jan.–July 1884

Biart, Victor, Surgeon, Nov. 1881–May 1883

Middleton, J. V. D., Surgeon, Sept.–Dec. 1883, Jan.–Dec. 1884

Barlow, William, AAS, Feb.–Dec. 1882, Jan.–Dec. 1883, Jan.–Dec. 1884

McCall, W. P., AAS, July–Aug. 1884
Middleton, Passemore, Surgeon, Sept.–Dec. 1884

Fort Dodge, Kansas
Wilson, A. D., AS, Nov.–Dec. 1866, Jan.–June 1867
Sukas, J., AAS, Nov. 1866
Crandall, J. B., AAS, Nov. 1866
DeGraw, C. S., AS, Jan.–Dec. 1867, Jan.–Feb., June 1868, May 1869
Fitch, A. F., AAS, Sept.–Dec. 1867, Jan.–April 1868, April 1869
Forwood, W. H., AS, Dec. 1867, Jan.–Mar. 1868
Tramaine(?), William, AS, Jan.–Mar. 1871

Fort Hays, Kansas
Fitch, A. J., AAS, William Buchanan, AS, Oct.–Dec. 1869, Jan.–Mar. 1870
Meacham, Abel, AS, Oct.–Dec. 1870
Delany Alfred, AS, Jan.–April 1871

Fort Harker, Kansas
Sternberg, George, AS, Nov.–Dec. 1866, Jan., Mar. 1867
Chase, Thomas, AAS Dec. 1866–Mar. 1867, Mar. 1868–Dec. 1869
Fryer, Benjamin E., AS, Sept. 1867–Feb. 1871
Westerling, Richard, AAS, Dec. 1867
Collins, J. H., AAS, Dec. 1869–Feb. 1870

Fort Ellsworth, Kansas
Chase, V. B., AAS, Oct. 1866

Fort Fletcher, Kansas
Oct. 1866, no surgeon assigned

Fort Wallace, Kansas
Turner, F. H, AS, Nov.–Dec. 1866, Jan.–Dec. 1867, Jan.–May 1868
Williams, E. D., AAS, Aug.–Sept. 1867
Wiggins, A. Y., AAS, Nov.–Dec. 1867, Jan.–May 1868
Sheaver, M. M., AAS, Nov.–Dec. 1869, Jan.–Dec. 1870, Jan.–April 1871
Howard, W. King, AS, Oct.–Dec. 1870, Jan.–April 1871

Fort Larned, Kansas
Forwood, W. H., AS, July–Sept. 1868

Fort Lyon, Colorado
Tilton, H. R., AS, Nov.–Dec. 1866, Jan.–Dec. 1867, Jan.–Oct. 1868, Nov.–Dec. 1869, Jan.–May and Oct.–Nov. 1870
Shiffmen, B., AAS, May–June 1867
Fitzgerald, J. W., AAS, Sept.–Dec. 1867, Jan.–April 1868
Renick, William H., AAS, Nov.–Dec. 1869, Jan.–May 1870
Woodhull, A. A., AS, Oct.–Dec. 1870

Fort Morgan, Colorado
Brown, J. Morris, AS, Nov.–Dec. 1866, Jan.–May 1867

Fort Reynolds, Colorado
No return for June 1867
Brown, J. Morris, AS, July–Nov. 1867
Hilliard, E. D., AAS, Nov.–Dec. 1867
Miller, George M., AAS, Jan.–July 1868

RECONSTRUCTION SOUTH

Elizabethtown, Kentucky
Middleton, Passemore, AS, April–May and July 1871
West, Theodore L., AAS, April 1871
Pope, Benjamin F., AS, Aug. 1871–Feb. 1873

Chester, South Carolina
No surgeon on post returns, Mar. 1871
Skinner, F. C., AAS, April 1871
Lytton, J. F., AAS, May, Nov.–Dec. 1871, Jan.–Feb. 1872

Taylor Barracks, Louisville, Kentucky
Milham, John J., AS, Feb.–Dec. 1871, Jan.–Dec. 1872, Jan.–Mar. 1873

Unionville, South Carolina
No return for Mar.–April 1871
Harvey, J., AAS, May–Nov. 1871
Tompkins, William A., AAS, Dec. 1871

Ruger, H. H., AAS, Jan. 1872, Mar.–Dec. 1872, Jan.–Feb. 1873
No return for Feb. 1872

Rutherfordton, North Carolina
Rector, Pierson, AAS, June–Dec. 1871, Jan.–Feb. 1872

Spartanburg, SC
Russell, W. T., AAS, Mar.–April 1871
Ruger, H. H., AAS, May–Dec. 1871, Jan. 1872
Cronkhite, H. M., AS, Feb.–Dec. 1872, Jan.–Feb. 1873

Mt. Vernon, Kentucky
No return found for Mar. 1871
Redd, R. G., AAS, April, July–Aug. 1871
West, Theodore, AAS, May–June 1871

Columbia, South Carolina
Bartholf, J. K., AAS, June, Sept.–Oct. 1871
Robert, T. N., AAS, Sept.–Oct. 1871

Meridian, MS
Collins, H. C., AAS, July–Oct. 1871

Bagdad, Kentucky
O'dell, R. W., AAS, Mar.–Aug. 1871

Yorkville, South Carolina
Tompkins, William, AAS, Mar.–Nov. 1871
Krine, T. C., AAS, Nov. 1871
Gibson, Joseph, AS, Dec. 1872, Jan.–May 1872
Harvey, John, AAS, Dec. 1872, Jan.–Feb. 1872
Redd, R. G., AAS, June–Dec. 1872, Jan.–Feb. 1873

Fort Sumter, South Carolina
Witherspoon, John B., AAS, June–July 1871

Nashville, Tennessee
Weeds, James F., Surgeon, June–Dec. 1872, Jan.–Feb. 1873

Shelbyville, Kentucky
O'dell, R. W., AAS, Sept.–Dec. 1871, Jan.–Nov. 1872
Wagner, R. B., AAS, Dec. 1872

Winsboro, South Carolina
Krine, T. C., AAS, June–Sept. 1871

Darlington, South Carolina
Taylor, H. V., AAS, June–Sept. 1871

Opelika, Alabama
Barnette, J. B., AAS, Mar.–June 1872
Beach, S. S., AAS, July–Dec. 1872
Mann, A. H., AAS, Jan.–Feb. 1873
Warnock, J. T., AAS, Dec. 1874
Owsley, W. T., AAS, Jan.–April 1875

Lincolnton, North Carolina
Harvey, John, AAS, April–Sept. 1872

Huntsville, Alabama
Taylor, M. E., AS, Dec. 1871, Jan. 1872

Jackson Barracks, Louisiana
Hubbart, V. Buren, AS, Dec. 1872, Jan.–Feb. 1873
Vickery, Richard, AS, Dec. 1872, Jan. 1873
Meyer, George D., AAS, Dec. 1872, Jan. 1873
Manderville, W. B., AAS, Feb. 1873

Shreveport, Louisiana
Kinoblauch, L. F., AAS, Oct.–Dec. 1874, Jan.–Dec. 1875, Jan.–April 1876

Memphis, Tennessee
No return for Mar. 1873

Atlanta, Georgia
Smith, Andrew K., Surgeon, Aug. 1871
No return for Sept. 1871

Charlotte, North Carolina
Harvey, John, AAS, Oct.–Dec. 1872, Jan.–Feb. 1873
Rector, P., AAS, Feb. 1873

Greensboro, Alabama
Beach, S. S., AAS, Oct.–Nov. 1874

McComb City, Mississippi
Taylor, M. E., AAS, Jan.–April 1876

Livingston, Alabama
Beach, S. S., AAS, Oct.–Dec. 1874, Jan.–April 1875

Colfax, Louisiana
O'dell, William, AAS, Oct.–Dec. 1874, Jan.–Dec. 1875
Taylor, M. E., AS, Jan. 1876

New Orleans, Louisiana
No return for Mar. 1873
Manderville, William, AAS, Oct.–Dec. 1874, Jan.–Mar. 1875

Oxford, Mississippi
Bryan, B. J., AAS, Dec. 1872, Jan.–Feb. 1873

Laurenville, South Carolina
Frynham, John F., AAS, Aug.–Dec. 1872

Newberry, South Carolina
Lytton, J. F., AAS, Dec. 1872, Jan.–Feb. 1873

Montgomery, Alabama
Nov. 1872: see Opelika, Alabama, moved to support sheriff between Nov. 28 and Dec. 22 then returned to Opelika.

Lebanon, Kentucky
Price, C. E., AAS, Nov.–Dec. 1872, Jan.–Feb. 1873

NORTHERN PLAINS

Fort Snelling/Saint Paul, Minnesota

Heger, Anthony, Surgeon, April–Dec. 1873, Jan.–Sept. 1874

Fort Abraham Lincoln, North Dakota

Boughton, J. Frazer, AAS, Sept. 1873
Harvey, John, AAS, Sept.–Oct. 1873
La Bare, John, AAS, Oct.–Dec. 1873, Jan.–Oct. 1874
Davis, F. H., AAS, assigned to Cavalry Barracks, Dec. 1873, Jan.–Mar. 1874
Marselis, N. H., AAS, Nov.–Dec. 1874, Jan.–Feb. 1875
Weeds, James, Surgeon, Feb.–May 1875
Lord, George E., AAS, Black Hills Expedition May–July 1875
Du Bose, E. W., AAS, Black Hills Expedition June 1875; Fort Lincoln, July–Aug. 1875, April and June 1878
Byrne, C. C., AS, July–Sept. 1875
Redd, R. G., AAS, Sept.–Dec. 1875, Jan.–Sept., Nov.–Dec. 1876, Jan.–July 1877
Middleton, J. V. D., AS, Oct.–Dec. 1875, Jan.–Sept. 1876; detached service to Standing Rock Oct. 1876; Fort Lincoln, Nov.–Dec. 1876, Jan.–Mar. 1877
Kinsman, J. H., AS, Aug.–Oct. 1876
Gardner, Edwin F., AAS, July 1877
Wolverton, W. A., AS, July–Dec. 1877, Jan.–Dec. 1878, Jan.–April, Nov.–Dec. 1879, Jan.–Dec. 1880, Jan.–Dec. 1881, Jan.–Oct. 1882
Harvard, Valery, AS, in field with Seventh Cavalry, May–Oct. 1877; Fort Lincoln, Nov.–Dec. 1877
Paulding, Holmes O., AS, in field with Seventh Cavalry, July–Nov. 1877; Fort Lincoln, Dec. 1877, May–June 1878; in field with Seventh Cavalry, July–Sept. 1878; Fort Lincoln, Nov. 1878
Davis, William B., AAS, in field with Seventh Cavalry, Nov. 1877
Bell, Ralph, AAS, Nov. 1878
Taylor, Blair D., AS, Feb.–July 1879
Lloyd, Frederick, AAS, Sept.–Dec. 1879, Mar. 1880, Feb. 1882
Pleasant, Thomas H., AAS, May–Nov. 1880
Benham, R. B., AS, Jan.–April 1881
Werick, S. T., AAS, May–June 1881; detached service with Seventh Cavalry recruits, Aug.–Sept. 1881; Fort Lincoln, Oct.–Dec. 1881, Jan.–May, July–Oct. 1882; detached service with Seventh Cavalry, June 1882

Fort Rice, North Dakota

William, John W., AS, Sept.–Dec. 1873, Jan.–Mar., May, Nov.–Dec. 1874; detached service, April 1874; with Black Hills Expedition, June–Sept. 1874; temporary duty at Fort Yankton, Oct. 1874; Fort Rice, Jan.–Sept. 1875

Allen, S. J., AAS, Sept.–Dec. 1873, Jan.–April 1874

Davis, F. H., AAS, June–Dec. 1874, Jan.–April 1875

Taylor, Blair D., AS, Oct.–Dec. 1875, Jan.–May, Oct.–Dec. 1876, Jan.–May 1877, Jan.–May 1878

Davis, Thomas B., AAS, Oct.–Dec. 1876

Fort Totten, North Dakota

Ferguson, James L., AAS, Oct.–Dec. 1873, Jan.–Mar., Nov.–Dec. 1874, Jan.–April, Aug.–Dec. 1875, Jan.–Mar. 1876

De Wolf, James, AAS, Nov.–Dec. 1875, Jan.–Feb. 1876

Ruger, H. H., AAS, Nov.–Dec. 1876, Jan.–July, Nov.–Dec. 1877, Jan.–Mar., June–Oct., Dec. 1878, detached service in the field, July–Sept. and Nov. 1878; Fort Totten, Jan.–Dec. 1879, Jan.–Dec. 1880, Jan.–Dec. 1881, Jan.–June, Aug.–Dec. 1882, Jan.–Mar. 1883

Davis, William B., AS, Jan.–Mar., June–Dec. 1878, Jan.–June, Aug.–Dec. 1879, at Fort Buford; July 1879, Jan.–May, July–Dec. 1880, detached service; June 1880, Jan.–Oct. 1881, June–Dec. 1882, Jan.–Dec. 1883, Jan.–Dec. 1884

Shaw, James, AAS, Sept.–Oct. 1874

Fort Randall, South Dakota

Manderville, William, AAS, May 1875

Kimball, J. A., AS, June 1875; on detached service with Seventh Cavalry, July 1875

Byrnes, J. C., AAS, July–Sept. 1875

Fort Buford, North Dakota

Crayton, Louis W., AS, Oct.–Dec. 1880, Jan.–Dec. 1881, Jan.–Oct. 1882

Turner, S. S., AAS, Jan.–Dec. 1881, Jan.–Mar., May, Dec. 1882; detached service with Company F Seventh Cavalry on Upper Yellowstone River, June–Nov. 1882; Fort Buford, Jan.–May 1883; detached service to Poplar River, June–Aug. 1883; Fort Buford, Sept.–Dec. 1883, Jan.–Dec. 1884

Johnson, R. W., AS, Nov.–Dec. 1882, Jan.–Dec. 1883, Jan.–Dec. 1884

Camp Ruhlen/Fort Meade, South Dakota

Beechemin, Louis, AS, Jan.–April 1878, Aug.–Dec. 1878, Jan.–Dec. 1879, July–Oct. 1880, Jan.–April 1881

Bell, Ralph, AAS, Mar.–Oct. 1879

Irwin, Bernard D. J., AS, May 1880

Loring, Frederick, AAS, Sept. 1880

Simons, J. A., AAS, Sept.–Dec. 1880, Jan.–Aug. 1881

Wilson, William, AS, Nov.–Dec. 1880, Jan.–Dec. 1881, Jan.–Dec. 1882, Jan.–Dec. 1883, Jan.–Oct. 1884

Freeman, J. W., AAS, Oct.–Dec. 1881, Jan.–Dec. 1882; detached service with Seventh Cavalry, June–July 1882; Jan.–May 1883

Sanderson, J. L., AAS, Nov.–Dec. 1882, Jan.–Dec. 1883, Jan.–Dec. 1884

Sabin, W. E., AAS, Feb.–Dec. 1884; at wood camp, July 1884

McQuerry, George, AS, Oct.–Dec. 1884

Yankton, South Dakota

No return for April 1873

Fort Abercrombie, North Dakota

Hatch, C. W., AAS, Nov.–Dec. 1876

Davis, Thomas B., AAS, Jan.–Mar. 1877

Standing Rock/Fort Yates, North Dakota

Maus, Louis M., AS, Nov.–Dec. 1877, Jan.–Dec. 1878, Jan.–Oct., Nov. 1879, Jan.–Dec. 1880, Jan.–April 1881

Ferguson, James L., AAS, Nov.–Dec. 1877, Jan.–Mar., May–Aug., Oct.–Dec. 1878, detached service; April and Sept. 1878, Jan.–June 1879

Wierick, S. T., AAS, Dec. 1879, detached service; Jan.–Feb. 1880, Mar.–Dec. 1880, Jan.–April 1881

Bushnell, George, AS, Mar.–Dec. 1881, Jan.–Sept. 1882

Deeble, H. M., AAS, Aug.–Dec. 1881, Jan.–Mar., July–Dec. 1882, Jan.–Dec. 1883, Jan.–April, June–Dec. 1884

Alden, Charles, AS, Jan.–Dec. 1883, Jan.–Sept. 1884

Goddard, C. E., AS, Nov.–Dec. 1884

EXPEDITION SURGEONS

Hancock Expedition, Summer 1867, Kansas

Lippincott, Henry, AS

Coates, Isaacs, AAS

Washita and Southern Plains, Fall/Winter 1868
Lippincott, Henry, AS
Renick, William, AAS

Northern Pacific Railroad Surveying Expedition/Yellowstone Expedition, 1873
Kimball, James P., Surgeon
Ruger, H. H., AAS
Harvey, Johny, AAS
La Bare, John, AAS
Allen, S. J., AAS
Hoffman, W. J., AAS
Burkwell, M. C., AAS

Black Hills Expedition, 1874
Williams, John W., AS
Allen, S. J., AAS
Bergen, Andrew C., AAS

Sioux War, Little Bighorn, 1876
Lord, George E., AS
De Wolf, James, AAS
Porter, Henry R., AAS

Nez Perce Campaign, 1877
Tilton, Henry, Surgeon
Gardner, Edwin F., AS
Fitzgerald, A., AS

Glossary of Medical Terms

P. Willey and Patrick J. Collison

Most definitions presented here are abstracted from *Dorland's Pocket Medical Dictionary* (McCullough 1982) and James Byars Carter (1988). Many definitions, however, employ the meanings of the terms in the twentieth and twenty-first century. To extend the meaning of terms to their use in the nineteenth century, we included earlier definitions from Frank R. Freemon (1998) and Rudy's List of Archaic Medical Terms (http://www.antiquusmorbus.com/english/english.htm).

abrasion—Injury caused by rubbing or scraping soft tissues with more durable materials.
abscess—Restricted collection of pus in a tissue, organ, or other limited space. Usually associated with swelling and pain.
acne—Skin eruption of pimples or tubercles on the face.
acute—Form of a disease that has a sudden onset and severe expression and may be relatively brief in duration. Contrast with chronic.
alcoholism—Persistent or lengthy episodes of excessive alcohol consumption.
allopathic—Related to one of the major early-nineteenth-century orientations to medicine, which applied toxic drugs and practiced bleeding as part of its "heroic" treatments.
amputation—Removal of an appendage or portion of a limb.
analgesic—Drug that relieves pain, "painkiller."
anemia—Condition of having inadequate numbers of red blood cells, limiting oxygen carry-capacity of the red blood cells.

anesthetic—Drug that produces anesthesia, a temporary loss of normal sensation.

aneurism—Swelling, ballooning, or saculation of a blood vessel.

ankylosis—Fusion of adjacent bones or abnormal stiffness of a joint. Spelled "anchylosis" in most nineteenth-century records.

anthrax—Infectious, often fatal disease caused by *Bacillus anthracis*. Indications include flu-like symptoms leading to severe respiratory distress, intestinal symptoms including diarrhea and vomiting blood, or skin lesions.

anthropology—Holistic study of humans, employing biological, linguistic, social, and historical perspectives.

anthropometry—Measurement of human body dimensions.

antibacterial—Antiseptic substance or material that kills, combats, or inhibits bacteria.

antiperiodic—Disruption of the regular reappearance of disease symptoms. Refers to the treatment of symptoms attributed to malaria.

antiphlogistics—Medications reducing inflammation or fever.

antipyretic—Drug that diminishes or suppresses fever.

antiseptic—Substance or material that diminishes growth of microorganisms, combating infection and decay.

antispasmodic—Substance or material that diminishes or alleviates muscle spasms, particularly smooth muscle activity in the intestine.

antitoxin—Substance or material that counteracts the effects of toxins.

anxiety—Subjectively unpleasant feelings of uneasiness, dread, and psychic turmoil.

aphonia—Inability to make vocal sounds or speak, sometimes associated with laryngitis.

ascites—Gathering of fluid in abdominal cavity. Also known as dropsy of peritoneum.

asphyxia—Unconsciousness from lack of oxygen.

asthma—Uncontrolled spasms of the bronchi, resulting in wheezing and labored breathing.

auscultation—Act of listening to sounds produced by the body, usually as part of a physical examination (for example, auscultation of the breath sounds in the lungs with a stethoscope or auscultation of bowel sounds).

auscultation, direct—Placing ear against patient's chest to listen to breathing sounds.

auscultation, mediate—Listening to breath sounds indirectly, commonly involving a stethoscope.

autopsy—Postmortem examination of corpse to identify medical conditions, such as disease and cause of death.

benign—Nonlethal, having minimal effect, noninvasive.

bilious fever—A remitting fever especially during the summer and fall months thought to be related to a disorder of the biliary system, accompanied by vomiting or diarrhea.

bite—Result of teeth piercing and causing damage to tissues.

bleeding—Hemorrhage, letting of blood for medicinal purposes.

blunt force injury—Injury from broadly applied flat surfaces. Contrast with sharp force and gunshot injuries.

boil—Painful skin lesion with a central core filled with pus, which often begins with the infection of a hair follicle or gland. Now associated with *Staphylococcus*. Cf. furuncle.

botanical—One of the major nineteenth-century orientations to medicine, which emphasized treatment with plants and their derivatives.

Bright's disease—Diseases of the kidney.

bronchitis—Inflammation of the lower respiratory tract, especially the trachea and bronchi. Typified by a phlegm-filled cough.

bubo—Enlarged and painful lymph node, often in the groin, producing pus.

burn—Injury caused by exposure to heat.

cachectic—Suffering from intense, general ill health characterized by the loss of body mass. The end result of many chronic diseases, such as tuberculosis, cancer, and malnutrition.

calculus—Abnormal formation of calcium salts in the body. In the nineteenth-century medical records the term usually refers to urinary, gallbladder, lacrimal, and oral "stones," not the buildup of calcified deposits on teeth, as the term is often used today.

cancer—Malignant growth, tumor.

carbuncle—Infection of skin and adjacent underlying tissues, resulting in death of the tissues and concentration of boils. Similar to "boil" but deeper and larger, often with several exits. Sometimes a cluster of boils.

caries—Rottenness, decay, or deterioration, usually of a tooth or bone.

casualty—Person killed or injured; a soldier missing from service.

cataract—Opacity of lens or capsule of the eye.

catarrh—Phlegm-filled discharge, usually from nose and throat, accompanied by cold-like symptoms. May originate from any mucus membrane (for example, bladder or stomach).

catarrh, pulmonary—Bronchitis in nineteenth-century medical records.

category of death—Broad groups of causes of fatal illnesses and injuries grouped together. Contrast with cause of death.

cathartic—Substance or material that produces evacuation of bowels, purgative.

catheter—Flexible tube inserted into the body to remove fluids.

cause of death—Specific illness or injury producing death. Contrast with category of death.

cephalgia—Headache.

cereum impaction—Ear wax lodged in ear canal.

chancre—Painless hard sore or ulcer caused by syphilis (first definitive symptom).

chicken pox—Skin eruptions and fevers caused by herpes zoster. Contagious.

chills—Cyclical sensation of feeling too cold, even in normal ambient temperatures, usually with accompanying shivering. During the nineteenth century, this symptom was often associated with malarial fevers.

cholera—Acute waterborne, bacterial, epidemic disease causing vomiting, profuse diarrhea, and cramps.

cholera, epidemic—Acute, profuse vomiting, cramps, and diarrhea, often leading to dehydration and electrolyte imbalance. May be life threatening. Now associated with *Vibrio cholera* bacterium, transmitted by eating food or drinking water tainted by an infected person's feces.

cholera infantum—Intestinal disruption among infants.

cholera morbus—Acute gastroenteritis, characterized by cramps, vomiting, and diarrhea. Usually occurs in spring and fall. Terms used in the nineteenth and early twentieth centuries include nonepidemic cholera and other gastrointestinal diseases with symptoms similar to cholera.

cholesteatoma—Cyst-like growth that destroys bones of the middle ear and mastoid.

chronic—Form of a disease that persists for a relatively long period or recurs periodically. Contrast with acute.

colic—Sharp, severe abdominal pain.

coma—Total, profound, deep unconsciousness and inability to be roused from that state.

communicable disease—Illness spread from person to person, infectious disease.

concussion—Sudden impact to the brain, causing damage to tissues surrounding it. Often accompanied by unconsciousness.
congenital—Describing a condition that is present from birth or resulting from a developmental alteration; "birth defects."
congestive heart failure—Excessive blood pooling in heart that occurs when it cannot provide sufficient pumping action to maintain blood flow to meet the needs of the body. Symptoms include shortness of breath, leg swelling, and fatigue.
conjunctivitis—Inflammation of the eye or tissues immediately surrounding the eye, such as the eyelid. Frequently caused by microorganisms and may be contagious (for example, "pink-eye"). Allergic reaction may also cause conjunctivitis.
constipation—Infrequent and/or difficult bowel movements.
constitutional diseases—Class of disease involving the entire body, not limited to one portion.
consumption—Tuberculosis of the lungs. As employed in the nineteenth-century medical records, the term was generally reserved for the advanced stages of tuberculosis, with loss of weight and exhaustion. Now associated with the bacterium *Mycobacteria tuberculosis*. Cf. phthisis.
contagionism—One of the major nineteenth-century approaches to medicine that attributed diseases to infections caused by contact or vapors. Contrast with miasmatism.
contusion—Bruise, crushed soft tissues often resulting from blunt force trauma and other forces. Appears as "contusio" in some nineteenth-century records.
convulsions—Involuntary, rhythmic, violent muscle contractions, often accompanied by unconsciousness.
cough—Loud expiration of air from the lungs.
cramps—Sudden muscular contractions and associated pain.
cupping—Application of a cup to skin, creating suction.
curette—Spoon-shaped surgical instrument used to remove diseased tissucs.
cyst—Abnormal, discrete fluid-filled mass of membrane surrounded by other tissues, generally a benign mass.
deafness—Inability to hear ordinary sounds.
debility—Weakness, feebleness, inability to perform ordinary tasks.
degenerative—Associated with wear, tear, and time, deterioration.
delirium—Brief mental derangement or disturbance.
delirium tremens—Acute mental derangement with accompanying shakes and sweats and sometimes seizures. Typically associated

with cessation of frequent and voluminous alcohol intake but may occur during a period of excessive alcohol consumption.

dementia—Disorientation often due to physical causes.

demography—Statistical study of populations concentrating on births, deaths, age, sex, marriage, divorce, and other parameters.

diabetes—Illness associated with symptoms of extensive thirst and copious urine production.

diarrhea—Watery, frequent stools due to gastrointestinal problems, indicating inadequate time for the intestine to absorb water and diminished value of ingested food. May be acute or chronic.

diathesis—Hereditary susceptibility, vulnerability, or predisposition to a disease.

diathetic diseases—Ailments involving hereditary susceptibility or vulnerability, including rheumatism, tumor, cancer and epithelioma, dropsy, and anemia. One of two subdivisions of the constitutional disease class.

dietic diseases—Illnesses involving either underconsumption of substances (such as starvation and scurvy) or overconsumption (for example, alcoholism). One of the three subdivisions of the zymotic disease class.

digestive disorders—Diseases including inflammations (for example, of stomach, bowels, and peritoneum), bleeding (hemorrhage of stomach and bowels), and degenerative alterations (such as piles).

diphtheria—Acute inflammation of the throat that produces a false membrane attached to the normal underlying tissue. Now known to be caused by the bacterium *Corynebacterium diptheriae.*

dislocation—Severe displacement of a joint, resulting in torn tendons, ligaments, and/or disruption of the joint capsule. More severe than a sprain. Cf. luxation.

dropsy—Abnormal fluid buildup in tissues or a body cavity; edema.

dysentery—Inflammation of the intestines, typified by cramps and runny, bloody, pus-filled feces, resulting from ulcerations of the intestine. The condition has a variety of causes, but many nineteenth-century cases probably were caused by *Entamoeba histolytica* (an amoeba) or *Shigella* sp. (a genus of bacteria). Exacerbated by unsanitary conditions, amoebic dysentery enters the digestive system via food or water.

dyspepsia—Acid indigestion often associated with heartburn or nausea.

dyspnea—Abnormal shortness of breath, requiring labored breathing.

dysuria—Difficult or painful urination.

earache—Ear pain from infection.

eclectic—One of the major nineteenth-century orientations to medicine, requiring formal training and involving botanical treatments. Contrast with homeopathic and botanical.
ecthyma—Ulcerative skin infection, most often located on the lower legs or forearms.
edema—Fluid buildup in tissue or an organ.
elevator—Surgical instrument used to raise tissues to remove underlying bone or teeth.
emetic—Substance or material that produces vomiting.
emphysema—Breakdown of the lungs' alveoli, loss of their elasticity, and accumulation of air in the lungs. Associated with cough, shortness of breath, and inadequate oxygenation of the blood.
empyema—Abnormal accumulation of pus in a cavity, particularly the pleura.
endemic—Occurring persistently or consistently in a region or group. Contrast with epidemic.
endocarditis—Inflammation of the inner surface of heart or its valves.
endoscopy—Examination of organs using an endoscope, an instrument that provides a view of the interior of an organ.
enema—Fluid squirted into the anus.
enteric—Related to the small intestine.
enteritis—Inflammation of the intestine, "intestinal flu."
enthetic diseases order—Illnesses involving "morbid matters" introduced into the body. Sexually transmitted diseases dominate the order. One of three subdivisions of zymotic disease class.
epidemic—Disease that occurs erratically in high frequency then is absent for significant periods before another outbreak occurs (for example, "epidemic catarrh"). Contrast with endemic.
epidemiology—Distribution and occurrence of disease in a group or population. Often emphasizes demographic variables, such as age, nativity, height, and sex.
epilepsy—Neurological impairment, in its severe form typified by periodic seizures and loss of consciousness.
epistaxis—Nosebleed.
epistemology—Study and theory of knowledge, emphasizing the limits of knowledge.
epithelioma—Tumor involving the epithelium, specifically skin and related tissues.
erysipelas—Infectious disease of skin, other superficial tissues, or mucous membranes. Localized superficial inflammation of skin due to acute infection. Symptoms include distinct redness and swelling. Now usually attributed to the bacteria *Staphylococcus*

and *Streptococcus*, which cause destruction of tissues and pus production.

etiology—Systematic study of cause(s) or origin of disease.

excision—Removal by cutting.

expectorants—Medicines that cause spitting or coughing up of mucus and other materials.

exsanguination—Extensive blood loss resulting in death.

fatigue—Exhaustion, tiredness.

febrile—Marked by fever, having elevated body temperature.

fever—Elevated body temperature. Especially notable in remittent and intermittent fevers.

fistula—Abnormal opening or hollow passage connecting internal with external structures.

fracture—Break, split, or separation, usually of a bone.

fracture, comminuted—Break of a bone into many small pieces.

fracture, compound (open)—Break of a bone that perforates the skin, with contact between the broken bone and the outside environment.

fracture, simple (closed)—Break of a bone that remains internal, with no contact between the broken bone and outside environment.

frostbite—Injury to tissues caused by freezing. The body portions farthest from the heart, including the fingers and toes, and those most frequently exposed, including the nose and ears, are most often frostbitten.

furuncle—Painful localized skin lesion, often from infection of a hair follicle. Cf. boil.

gangrene—Death of tissue, usually severe and involving associated bacterial infestation and odorous decomposition.

gastrectomy—Surgical removal of the stomach.

gastrointestinal—Related to the lower digestive tract, including the stomach and intestine (GI tract).

germ theory of disease—Concept that specific microorganisms cause particular diseases.

gleet—Thin discharge, especially associated with chronic inflammation of urethra, often caused by gonorrhea and associated with an accompanying urethral discharge.

gonorrhea—Sexually transmitted bacterial disease. Primary symptoms include inflammation of urethra, painful urination, and pus-filled discharge. Untreated, as it was in the nineteenth century, the disease may eventually cause a stricture of the urethra and affect joints and skin.

gout—Form of arthritis that periodically attacks a joint then disappears, often involving the large toe.

gravel—Kidney stones.

gunshot wound—Injury resulting from bullets, pellets, or other firearm-related discharges.

headache—Head pain, also known as cephalgia.

heart disease—Any of a number of cardiac-related problems, including structural or functional abnormality of valves, hypertrophy, aortic obstruction, "irritable" heart, and palpitation.

hematologic—Related to blood and its production.

hemoptysis—Coughing of blood, usually initiated by bronchial or pulmonary bleeding.

hemorrhage—Bleeding, blood discharge.

hernia—Protrusion of tissues beyond the anatomical wall that normally contains them.

heroic treatment—Manner of administering medical therapy that involved increasing dosages and intensity of treatment to the point that demonstrable physiological effects were evident in the patient. During the first half of the nineteenth century, it usually included depleting heroic treatment with bleeding, cathartics, and emetics. Later in the century stimulative heroic treatment was preferred, using alcohol, iron compounds, and "high diet" to invigorate patients.

herpes—Eruptive skin disease.

homeopathic—One of the major nineteenth-century medical orientations, embracing the view that diseases are caused by disruption of the spirit rather than by physical causes. Treatments typically involved the law of similar, "like cures like," and the administration of substances diluted to infinitesimal amounts. This school stressed the ability of nature alone (rather than aggressive medical intervention) to cure disease. Contrast with eclectic and botanical.

homicide—Killing another person.

hospital gangrene—Gangrene associated with open wounds or ulcers occurring in hospitals and other crowded conditions.

humors—Medical system attributing illness to imbalance of bodily fluids: the four humors, which classically consist of blood, yellow and black bile, and phlegm.

hydrocele—"Pooling" of fluids. Often used to describe fluid buildup along the spermatic cord in the scrotum.

hydrophobia—Rabies.

hydrothorax—Abnormal concentration of fluids between pleural linings.

hyoid—Bone in the anterior neck, serving as muscle attachment for tongue and throat.

hypertrophy—Abnormal enlargement, "over-growth" of an organ.

hyperventilation—Fast and deep breathing, "over breathing."

hypodermic—Under, below the skin.

idiopathic—Of uncertain origin or etiology.

incised wound—Injury produced by a bladed object, resulting in cut, chopped, or sliced tissue.

incontinence—Involuntary passing of bodily excretions, loss of sphincter control. In the nineteenth-century medical records urinary incontinence is most frequently mentioned. It may be caused by urinary diseases or damage to the associated tissues.

inebriation—Condition of being drunk, intoxicated. Usually indicates a temporary, nonchronic condition. Contrast with alcoholism.

infectious disease—Illness caused by organisms.

inflammation—Redness, pain, elevated temperature, and swelling. Depending on the anatomical location of the inflammation, it can be of little consequence or extremely critical. In the nineteenth-century medical records inflammations affected the pleura, lungs, testicle, and other key organs.

influenza—Viral infection mostly affecting the respiratory tract and characterized by fever and chills.

insanity—Significant mental illness with persistent derangement.

insomnia—Inability to fall asleep or stay asleep for an adequate time.

integumentary system—Anatomical tissues that include superficial anatomical structures, particularly skin, nails, and other associated external structures.

intermittent fever—Nineteenth-century term usually associated with the malarial symptoms, indicating the cyclical commencing and halting of symptoms. Malaria is caused by protozoa that are passed to humans by bites of infected mosquitoes.

intermittent fever, congestive—Severe, serious form of malaria that may lead to collapse of lungs and death.

intermittent fever, quartan—Form of malaria with shaking chills in four-day cycles.

intermittent fever, quotidian—Form of malaria with shaking chills occurring daily.

intermittent fever, tertian—Form of malaria with shaking chills every other day.

intravenous—Inside a vein.

intrinsic—Inherent in or a property of. Examples of an person's intrinsic variables include age, sex, height, and birthplace.

iritis—Inflammation of the iris of the eye. May be caused by blunt trauma to eye or by infection, such as tuberculosis, syphilis, or herpes.

itch—Irritation of skin with associated itching sensation.

jaundice—Accumulation of bile in the circulatory system, characterized by yellow skin and eyes. Caused by liver diseases.

laceration—Traumatic tearing, mangling, or ripping of soft tissues. Contrast with puncture wound and incised wound.

lancinating—Piercing. Usually associated with a piercing pain.

laryngectomy—Surgical removal of the larynx.

laryngitis—Inflammation of the larynx, the upper throat including the "voice box" and adjacent structures. Characterized by hoarseness.

laryngoscope—Medical instrument for examining the larynx.

larynx—"Voice box."

ligation—Tying or restricting a vessel.

local diseases—Class of diseases related to specific anatomical systems, including orders that involve the nervous system, circulatory system, and respiratory organs.

luxation—Dislocation.

malaria—Illness whose symptoms consist of cycles of high fever and shaking chills.

mania—Mental derangement involving an extremely excited, agitated mental state.

manic-depression—Psychological state involving wide mood swings from depression to elation. Now generally considered bipolar disorder.

measles—Viral infection typified by respiratory problems, formation of raised red, pus-containing "pimples" and elevated temperature.

melancholia—Persistent mental depression, despondency, and despair, sometimes including delusions. Considered a subdivision of mania in the nineteenth century. Treatment consisted of variety of approaches, including opium to calm agitation and for insomnia as well as hospitalization in an asylum for more severe cases (Jackson 1986:394).

meningitis—Inflammation of tissues surrounding the brain and spinal cord.

miasmas—Malarias and malaria-like conditions.

miasmatism—View that diseases were caused by airborne poisons. One of the major nineteenth-century approaches to medicine. Contrast with contagionism.

microbe—Microscopic, single-celled organism.

microorganism—Microscopic single-celled or multicelled organism.

migraine—Severe, incapacitating, often periodic headache.

miliary—Characterized by lesions resembling millet seeds typically associated with disseminated tuberculosis.

morbidity—Illness, related to disease. Contrast with mortality.

mortality—Death. Contrast with morbidity.

mumps—Viral disease characterized by swelling of the parotid glands (in cheeks), associated with painful swallowing and moderate fever.

myopia—Nearsightedness (objects can be seen clearly only when close to the viewer).

nausea—Unpleasant sensation often associated with vomiting.

necrosis—Abnormal dying and sloughing away of tissue.

neuralgia—Pain coursing along a nerve. Many different causes, including anemia, malaria, and syphilis.

neurasthenia—Nervousness. Disease of nervous system resulting in chronic fatigue, disorientation, and dull pain. "Exhaustion of the nervous system."

neuropathy—Disease of a nerve or the nervous system.

neurosis—Psychological state involving stressful mental disturbance.

neurosyphilis—Advanced syphilis attacking nerves, brain, and surrounding tissues.

night blindness—Limited vision in darkness with normal vision in daylight. Now associated with inadequate Vitamin A.

nosology—Organization and categorization of diseases.

nostalgia—Longing for home. In the nineteenth century it was considered a severe form of melancholia.

nostrum—Patent medicine, ineffective.

ophthalmia—Severe inflammation of eye. May produce pus and may result from gonorrhea.

ophthalmic—Associated with or related to the eye.

ophthalmology—Medical specialty related to illnesses of the eye.

ophthalmoscope—Medical instrument for examining the eye's interior.

orchitis—Inflammation of a testicle. Indicative of a bacterial infection or a secondary effect of mumps, syphilis, or gonorrhea.

orthopedic—Type of surgery to correct skeletal and muscular dysfunctions.
osteology—Study of the skeleton and what bones indicate about the deceased person and past populations.
otitis—Inflammation of the inner, middle, or external ear, involving pain and fluid discharge.
otolaryngology—Medical specialty related to illnesses involving the ear, nose, and throat.
otorrhea—Fluid discharge from the ear.
ozena—Chronic inflammation of nasal membranes with wasting away and resultant crusting and foul odor.
paleopathology—Study of past diseases, generally based on skeletal or mummified remains.
palliative—Treatment to relieve disease symptoms rather than striking at the cause or curing the disease itself.
palpitation—Abnormal heartbeats, usually involving increased heart rate or skipped beats.
palsy—Inability to move, impairment of movement.
pandemic—Periodic, geographically widespread epidemic illness.
paralysis—Inability to move, impairment of movement, loss of motor control. In the nineteenth century the term may include deranged mental states.
parasitic diseases—Class of diseases caused by organisms. For much of the nineteenth century parasitic diseases involved ailments whose causative organisms could be observed without recourse to microscopic examination or histological samples.
pathogen—Agent that causes or produces disease.
pathogenesis—Start or process of a disease.
pectoriloquy—Vocalization heard on auscultation over areas of the lung. The procedure tests for abnormal resonance caused by edema or consolidation. The resulting condition is also known as whispered pectoriloquy or bronchophony.
percussion—Striking an organ with fingertips, resulting in sounds that permit interpreting normal and pathological conditions.
pericarditis—Inflammation of the pericardium, the tissue lining surrounding the heart.
pericardium—Tissue sac that surrounds the heart.
periosteum—Tissue covering a bone surface.
periostitis—Inflammation of the membrane attached to bone surfaces.
peritonsillar—Near the tonsils.
pharmaceutical—Related to drugs or pharmacy.

pharmacopoeia—Treatise on the preparation and use of drugs.

pharyngitis—Inflammation of the tissues in the upper respiratory tract, especially those at the back of the nasal passage and upper throat.

pharynx—Throat.

phthisis—Pulmonary tuberculosis, consumption, wasting away, emaciation. Often associated with advanced and rapid progression of the disease.

piles—Hemorrhoids. Enlargement of vein or veins near anus.

plague—Severe, acute contagious disease.

pleura—Tissues that surround the lungs.

pleurisy—Inflammation of the pleura, which surround the lungs. Symptoms include chills, cough, fever, and pain. Same meaning as pleuritis.

pleuritis—Inflammation of the pleura, which surround the lungs. Symptoms include chills, cough, fever, and pain. Same meaning as pleurisy.

pleurodynia—Sudden, seizure-like pain in the areas between the ribs. "False pleurisy."

pneumonia—Acute inflammation of the lungs, resulting in fluid buildup. Symptoms include thorax pain, cough, and difficulty breathing.

poisoning—Illness from exposure to a toxic substance. Most often in the post-Civil War Seventh Cavalry medical records poisoning involves the genus *Rhus* (poison ivy/oak). The diagnosis is also associated with rattlesnake and insect bites, cactus spines, and ingestion of opium or laudanum.

Post–Traumatic Stress Disorder (PTSD)—Alterations in normal behavior and physiology following traumatic events or stress.

primary—Occurring first or foremost, undeveloped.

prophylaxis—Prevention or preventative treatment of disease.

prostatitis—Inflammation of the prostate gland.

prostration—Extreme lack of energy or power.

psychogenic—Of psychological origin, resulting from psychological causes.

puerile—Childlike, including short, frequent respirations.

pulmonary disease—Illness involving the respiratory system, particularly the lungs.

puncture wound—Injury produced primarily by a piercing action of a tool or instrument. Contrast with laceration and incised wound.

purging—Cathartic evacuation produced by medicine.

purpura—Skin spotted with purple areas, caused by several disorders.

purulent—Associated with pus or pus production.

pyemia—Blood infection associated with pus-filled abscesses, previously thought to be caused by absorption of pus into blood. Subdivision of septicemia.

quinine—Medicine for prevention and treatment of malaria.

quinsy—Abscess near back of mouth and top of throat near tonsils, a collection of pus between the tonsil and pharyngeal constrictor muscle. Cf. tonsillitis.

rales—High-pitched breath sounds caused by fluid in small air passages. Described as a moist crackling sound.

raspatory—Surgical instrument for scraping or abrading.

remittent fever—Cycling of greater and lesser shaking chills similar to and most likely caused by malarial agent. The patient improves rapidly. Symptoms regularly diminish but do not disappear with periodic remissions.

respiratory—Related to the act of breathing, involving lungs and related anatomical structures, such as the larynx, bronchi, and pleura.

retention—Retaining substances, usually urine in nineteenth-century records.

retinitis pigmentosa—Disease involving retina and leading to blindness.

revulsives—Counterirritant medicines. Also bloodletting distant from the part affected by disease.

rheumatic fever—Infectious disease involving pain and fever that inflames joints and heart valves. An inflammatory disease following streptococcus infection.

rheumatism—Joint, muscle, and tendon aches and pains.

rhinorrhea—Discharge from the nasal passage.

ronchi—Coarse rattling sound caused by secretions in the bronchi and larger air passages.

rongeur—Surgical instrument for cutting bone in bite-like pieces.

scald—Burn from contact with steam or hot liquids.

scalpel—Surgical knife.

scarlet fever—Infectious disease whose symptoms include bright red rash spread over body. Transmitted by inhalation.

scrofula—Inflammation occurring in the lymph nodes, especially those of the neck. May develop into abscesses and draining tracts. A symptom of tuberculosis.

scurvy—Fatigue and excessive bruising, symptoms now associated with inadequate Vitamin C.

sebaceous—Related to oil or oil glands.
sepsis—Catastrophic health condition caused by bacterial toxins or their products.
sequela—Subsequent condition, resulting symptom or condition caused by a previous injury or disease.
sexually transmitted infections (STIs)—Infectious diseases typically transmitted by sexual contact. Syphilis and gonorrhea were the two recognized STIs in the nineteenth century.
sharp force trauma—Cut, chop, or slice resulting from contact with a bladed tool.
sinusitis—Inflammation of sinus.
smallpox—Highly contagious disease whose early symptoms include chills and fever, followed by skin pustules distributed in a centrifugal manner. Vaccine was known in the nineteenth century and used to prevent development of the disease.
somatic—Related to the body, caused by biological factors.
sprain—Wrenching, pulling, or twisting of a joint with partial breaking or tearing of ligaments or other joint attachments. Less severe than a dislocation.
starvation—Prolonged inadequate nutritional intake.
stethoscope—Medical instrument for examining the chest, particularly heartbeats.
sthenic—Overly strong, energetic, or excited state.
strain—Injury from overuse or exertion.
stricture—Narrowing or closing of an anatomical passage.
stye—Pus-producing inflammation of an oil-producing eyelid gland.
subluxation—Partial dislocation, sprain.
suicide—Purposefully killing oneself.
sunstroke—Exposure to heat resulting in elevated temperature and convulsions. Sunstroke was sometimes associated with mental derangement in the nineteenth century.
suppurative—Associated with pus.
synovitis—Inflammation of membrane capsule that surrounds major movable joints.
syphilis—Sexually transmitted or congenital disease caused by a bacterium.
syphilis, constitutional—Disease whose symptoms usually involve fever and malaise. Associated with secondary syphilis (and perhaps the tertiary stage of syphilis infection).
syphilis, primary—Early stage of syphilis infection, typified by an initial painless chancre. Duration two weeks to three months.

syphilis, secondary—Middle stage of syphilis infection, appearing two to six months after primary syphilis. Displays systematic involvement, typified by skin rashes, particularly on palms and soles, elevated body temperature, and muscular and joint aches. Duration two weeks to six months.

syphilis, tertiary—Advanced stage of syphilis, which may invade bones, heart, and other organs.

tachycardia—Pathologically rapid heartbeat.

tactile fremitus—Vibration felt on the patient's chest during low frequency vocalization.

tapeworm—Intestinal flatworm parasites.

therapeutics—Healing, treatment of a disease (particularly with medications).

thyroid cartilage—Shield-shaped cartilage in the neck that encloses the larynx, located deep and above the thyroid gland.

titration—Laboratory process involved in identifying the concentration of a chemical.

tonsillectomy—Removal of tonsils.

tonsillitis—Inflammation of tonsils.

toothache—Pain associated with teeth or adjacent structures.

tracheal rings—C-shaped cartilaginous rings forming the trachea.

tracheostomy—Surgical opening of trachea through the front of the neck.

trauma—Physical injury by force, temperature, or caustic agents.

trephanation—Surgical opening of the skull that reveals the brain and surrounding tissues.

tubercular diseases—Illnesses manifested by persistent infections now associated with *Mycobacterium tuberculosis*. Symptoms include a slow wasting or "consumption." Another form of tubercular disease, scrofula, was manifested as inflammation of the neck lymph glands. One of two subdivisions of the constitutional disease class.

tuberculosis—Persistent infection involving slow wasting (consumption) or inflammation of neck lymph glands (scrofula). Caused by *Mycobacterium*.

tumor—Abnormal new growth of a group of cells.

tympanic membrane—Eardrum.

typhoid fever—Disease whose symptoms include intestinal inflammation and ulceration, abdominal pain, headache, and delirium. Often fatal. Caused by the bacterium *Salmonella typhi*, usually passed by contamination of food or water by feces. The name derives from the similarity of its symptoms to those of typhus.

typhoid malarial (typhomalarial) fever—Illness in which patient has symptoms of malaria and typhoid fever.

typhus, typhus fever—Headache, fever, and rash. Causative agent is a rickettsia (one of several small bacteria), passed from fleas via person-to-person or rat-to-person contact.

ulcer—Open, oozing sore.

universalism—In nineteenth-century medicine the belief that human physiology, diseases, and treatments were basically the same for all individuals, regardless of geographic, social, or ethnic background. Contrasted with specificism, which postulated regional differences in human responses to illness and treatment. European physicians tended to promote universalism, while American practitioners, especially in the South and West, clung to specificism.

urethritis—Inflammation of the urethra.

vaccination—Procedure involving administering weakened pathogenic agents to a patient to confer immunity from the disease. In the mid-nineteenth century the only vaccination available was against smallpox.

valvular heart disease—Pathological alterations of the valves of the heart.

varicocele—Swelling of the scrotum caused by enlargement of the spermatic cord, taking on the characteristics of a "bag of worms."

varicose veins—Abnormally swollen and sometimes ruptured veins, most often located in the leg.

varioloid—Mild form of smallpox among persons who have previously had the disease or been vaccinated against it.

venereal diseases—Infectious diseases transmitted through sexual contact, including gonorrhea and syphilis.

vomiting—Ejection of stomach contents through the oral passage.

wheezing—High-pitched expiratory sounds produced by partial obstruction of small airways, such as in asthma.

whitlow—Painful infection of the thumb or fingertips that may involve tendons and the spongy portions of the distal phalanges. The disease prevails in unhygienic conditions. Synonyms: felon, onychia, paronychia.

whooping cough—Infection by *Bordetella pertussis*, whose symptoms include respiratory irritation and discharge and coughs that terminate in "whoops."

yellow fever—Acute infectious disease caused by mosquito-carried virus. Symptoms include vomiting and especially high fever and jaundice, hence the name.

zymotic diseases—Nineteenth-century class of diseases thought to involve fermentation-caused illnesses, including miasmas (malarias).

References Cited

Adams, Kevin

2009 *Class and Race in the Frontier Army: Military Life in the West, 1870–1890*. Norman: University of Oklahoma Press.

Adjutant General's Office

1909 *Circular Showing the Distribution of Troops of the Line of the United States Army, January 1, 1866 to June 30, 1909*. Washington, D.C.: Government Publishing Office.

Agnew, Jeremy

2008 *Life of a Soldier on the Western Frontier*. Missoula, Mont.: Mountain Press.

American Psychiatric Association (APA)

2013 *Diagnostic and Statistical Manual of Mental Disorders*. 5th ed. Washington, D.C.: American Psychiatric Publishing.

Anonymous

1921 *A Half Century of Public Health*. Ed. M. P. Ravenel. New York: American Public Health Association.

1976 "The State and Public Welfare in Nineteenth-Century America: Five Investigations, 1833–1877." In *Social Problems and Social Policy*, ed. G. N. Grob. The American Experience Series. New York: Arno Press.

Arms, L. R.

1991 *A Short History of the NCO*. Fort Bliss, Tex.: U.S. Army Museum of the Noncommissioned Officer.

Asch, Morris J.
1883 "Army Medical Service." *New York Medical Journal* 37:203–204.

Ashburn, P. M.
1929 *A History of the Medical Department of the United States Army.* New York: Houghton Mifflin Company.

Aufderheide, Arthur C., and Conrado Rodríguez-Martín (editors)
1998 *The Cambridge Encyclopedia of Human Paleopathology.* New York: Cambridge University Press.

Autino, Beatrice, Alice Noris, Rosario Russo, and Francesco Castelli
2012 "Epidemiology of Malaria in Endemic Areas." *Mediterranean Journal of Hematology and Infectious Diseases* 4. no. 1:1–11.

Baker, Brenda J., and Maria A. Liston
1995 "Infection in Eighteenth-Century Military Remains at Fort William Henry." *American Journal of Physical Anthropology,* Supplement 20:61.

Ballenger, J. J. (editor)
1977 *Diseases of the Nose, Throat, and Ear.* Philadelphia, Pa: Lea and Febiger.

Barnes, Joseph K.
1870 *The Medical and Surgical History of the War of the Rebellion, 1861–1865, Part I, Volumes 1 and 2, Medical History.* Washington, D.C.: Government Printing Office.
1888 *The Medical and Surgical History of the War of the Rebellion, 1861–1865, Part III, Volume I, Medical History.* Washington, D.C.: Government Printing Office.

Barrett, R., C. W. Kuzawa, T. McDade, and G. J. Armelagos
1998 "Emerging and Reemerging Infectious Diseases: The Third Epidemiological Transition." *Annual Review of Anthropology* 27:247–71.

Barry, John M.
2004 *The Great Influenza: The Epic Story of the Deadliest Plague in History.* New York: Penguin Books.

Bartholow, Robert
1863 *A Manual of Instructions for Enlisting and Discharging Soldiers.* Philadelphia, Pa.: J. B. Lippincott.

Barton, R.
2009 "Help for PTSD, Combat Reactions." http://www.dcmilitary.com/stories/020509/standard_28148.shtml.

Battle of Marathon, 490 BC
2006 http://www.eyewitnesstohistory.com.

Benenson, Abram S.
1984 "Immunization and Military Medicine." *Reviews of Infectious Diseases* 6(1):1–12.

Bernstein, N.
1972 *The First One Hundred Years: Essays on the History of the American Public Health Association*. Washington, D.C.: American Public Health Association.

Bielicki, Tadeusz, and Zygmunt Welon
1982 "Growth Data as Indicators of Social Inequalities: The Case of Poland." *Yearbook of Physical Anthropology* 25:153–67.

Billings, John S.
1974 *A Report on the Hygiene of the United States Army: With Descriptions of Military Posts*. Circular No. 8, Surgeon General's Office. Reprint of 1875 edition, New York: Sol Lewis.

Bismarck Weekly Tribune
1876–77 "Monthly Weather Synopses: October 1876 through March 1877." Microfilm Rolls 5906–5908.

Blair, Joseph R., Richard Schatzki, and Kenneth D. Orr
1957 "Sequelae to Cold Injury in One Hundred Patients: Follow-up Study Four Years after Occurrence of Cold Injury." *Journal of the American Medical Association* 163(14):1203–1208.

Bleakley, Hoyt
2010 "Malaria Eradication in the Americas: A Retrospective Analysis of Childhood Exposure." *American Economic Journal: Applied Economics* 2:1–45.

Bodenhamer, David J.
1981 "Law and Disorder in the Old South: The Situation in Georgia, 1830–1860." In *From the Old South to the New: Essays on the Transitional South*, ed. W. F. Fraser, Jr., and W. B. Moore, Jr., 108–19. Westport, Conn.: Greenwood Press.

Bollet, Alfred Jay
1991 "Rheumatic Diseases among Civil War Troops." *Arthritis and Rheumatism* 34(9):1197–1203.
2002 *Civil War Medicine: Challenges and Triumphs*. Tucson, Ariz.: Galen Press.

Boyle, Wade
1991 *Official Herbs: Botanical Substances in the United States Pharmacopoeias, 1820–1990*. East Palatine, Ohio: Buckeye Naturopathic Press.

Bradley, James H.
1961 *The March of the Montana Column: A Prelude to the Custer Disaster*. Norman: University of Oklahoma Press.
Bretlinger, Paula E.
2006 "Health, Human Rights, and Malaria Control: Historical Background and Current Challenges." *Health and Human Rights* 9(2):10–38.
Brinton, John H.
1896 "Address: Closing Exercises of the Session 1895–96, Army Medical School." *Journal of the American Medical Association* 26 (1896):599–605.
Brown, Richard Maxwell
1969 "Historical Patterns of Violence in America." In *The History of Violence in America*, ed. H. D. Graham and T. R. Gurr, 45–87. New York: Praeger.
1970 *American Violence*. Englewood, N.J.: Prentice-Hall.
Burgess, John E., and F. Macfarlane
2009 "Retrospective Analysis of the Ethnic Origins of Male British Army Soldiers with Peripheral Cold Weather Injury." *Journal of the Royal Army Medical Corps* 155(1):11–15.
Butler, Anne M.
1985 *Daughters of Joy, Sisters of Misery: Prostitutes in the American West, 1865–90*. Urbana: University of Illinois Press.
Caldwell, Mark
1988 *The Last Crusade: The War on Consumption 1862–1954*. New York: Atheneum.
Candler, William H., and Hazel Ivey
1997 "Cold Weather Injuries among U.S. Soldiers in Alaska: A Five-Year Review." *Military Medicine* 162(12):788–91.
Carroll, John M. (editor)
1979 *The Medal of Honor: Its History and Its Recipients for the Indian Wars*. Mattituck, N.Y.: J. M. Carroll.
Carroll, John M., and Lawrence A. Frost (editors)
1976 *Private Theodore Ewert's Diary of the Black Hills Expedition of 1874*. Piscataway, N.J.: CRI Books.
Carter, James Byars
1988 "Disease and Death in the Nineteenth Century: A Genealogical Perspective." *National Genealogical Society Quarterly* 76:289–301.

Chandler, Melbourne C.
1960 *Of Garry Owen in Glory: The History of the Seventh United States Cavalry Regiment*. Annandale, Va.: Turnpike Press.

Chang, Dow
2008 "Comparison of Crash Fatalities by Sex and Age Group." NHTSA's National Center for Statistics and Analysis, Traffic Safety Facts, DOT HS 810853. www-nrd.nhtsa.dot.gov/Pubs/810853.pdf.

Chuinard, E. G.
1979 *Only One Man Died: The Medical Aspects of the Lewis and Clark Expedition*. Glendale, Calif.: A. H. Clark.

Chun, Clayton K. S.
2004 *US Army in the Plains Indian Wars, 1865–91*. Long Island City, N.Y.: Osprey.

Coffman, Edward M.
1986 *The Old Army: A Portrait of the American Army in Peacetime, 1784–1898*. New York: Oxford University Press.

Cohan, Katie
2011 "'The Bitter, Freezing Hours of Night': An Investigation of Cold Injury Susceptibility in the Post-Civil War Seventh Cavalry." MA thesis, Department of Anthropology, California State University, Chico.

Collison, Patrick J.
2011 "Otolaryngologic Diseases of the 7th Cavalry, 1867–1883." Hardin, Mont.: Brian C. Pohanka 25th Annual Symposium, Custer Battlefield Historical and Museum Association.

Communicable Disease Center
2012 Electronic source, www.cdc.gov/std/stats12/gonorrhea.htm.

Cook, Charles M.
1987 "The Little Big Horn Survivors." MS in possession of the authors.

Courtwright, D. T.
1996a "Violence in America." *American Heritage* 47:36–40.
1996b *Violent Land: Single Men and Social Disorder from the Frontier to the Inner City*. Cambridge, Mass.: Harvard University Press.

Cozzens, Peter
2004 *Eyewitnesses to the Indian Wars, 1865–1890: The Long War for the Northern Plains*. Mechanicsburg, Pa.: Stackpole Books.

Crosby, Alfred W.
1993 "Influenza." In *The Cambridge History of Human Disease*, ed. Kenneth F. Kiple, 807–11. New York: Cambridge University Press.

Cullen, Karen A., and Paul M. Arguin
2013 "Malaria Surveillance—United States, 2011." *Centers for Disease Control and Prevention, Morbidity and Mortality Weekly Report*. 62, no. 5:1–17.

Custer, Elizabeth B.
1885 *Boots and Saddles: Life in Dakota with General Custer*. New York: Harper and Row.
1893 *Tenting on the Plains*. New York: Charles L. Webster.
2006 *Boots and Saddles: Life in Dakota with General Custer*. New York: Barnes and Noble.

Custer, George Armstrong
1874 *My Life on the Plains or, Personal Experiences with Indians*. New York: Sheldon and Company.

Daanen, Hein A.
2003 "Finger Cold-Induced Vasodilation: A Review." *European Journal of Applied Physiology* 89:411–26.

Daily, Edward
1995 *From Custer to MacArthur: The 7th Cavalry (1866–1945)*. Paducah, Ky.: Turner Publishing.

Dean, Eric T.
1997 *Shook over Hell: Post-Traumatic Stress, Vietnam, and the Civil War*. Cambridge, Mass.: Harvard University Press.

DeGroot, David W., John W. Castellani, Jeffrey O. Williams, and Paul J. Amoroso
2003 "Epidemiology of U.S. Army Cold Weather Injuries, 1980–1999." *Aviation, Space and Environmental Medicine* 74(5): 564–70.

Devine, Shauna
2014 *Learning from the Wounded: The Civil War and the Rise of American Medical Science*. Chapel Hill: University of North Carolina Press.

Dubos, Rene, and Jean Dubos
1996 *The White Plague: Tuberculosis, Man, and Society*. New Brunswick, N.J.: Rutgers University Press.

Duffin, Jacalyn
1993 "Pneumonia." In *The Cambridge History of Human Disease*, ed. Kenneth F. Kiple, 938–42. New York: Cambridge University Press.

Duffy, J.
1978 "Social Impact of Disease in the Late 19th Century." In *Sickness and Health in America: Readings in the History of Medicine and Public Health*, ed. J. W. Leavitt and R. L. Numbers, 395–402. Madison: University of Wisconsin Press.
1990 *The Sanitarians: A History of American Public Health*. Urbana: University of Illinois Press.

Dunglison, Robley
1866 *A Dictionary of Medical Science*. Philadelphia, Pa: Henry C. Lea.

Eckroth, David
2013 *Colonel Stanley and Lt. Col. Custer's Expedition on the Yellowstone, 1873*. Billings, Mont.: Frontier Heritage Alliance for the American Battlefield Protection Program.

English, Peter C.
1989 "Emergence of Rheumatic Fever in the Nineteenth Century." *Milbank Quarterly* 67:33–49.

Etulain, Richard W.
2006 *Beyond the Missouri: The Story of the American West*. Albuquerque: University of New Mexico Press.

Ewing, Charles B.
1894 "The Selection and Physical Examination of the Recruit." In *Transactions of the Third Annual Meeting of the Military Surgeons of the National Guard of the United States*, 166–92. St. Louis: Buxton and Skinner Stationery Company.

Faust, Ernest Carroll
1951 "The History of Malaria in the United States." *American Scientist* 39(1):121–30.

Finkel, David
2013 "The Military Life: The Return." *New Yorker*, September 9, 2013, 36–40.

Fisher, John C., and Carol Fisher
2011 *Food in the American Military: A History*. Jefferson, N.C.: McFarland and Company.

Flannery, Michael A.
2004 *Civil War Pharmacy*. Binghamton, N.Y.: Hawthorne Press.

Freemon, Frank R.
1998 *Gangrene and Glory: Medical Care during the American Civil War*. Teaneck, N.J.: Fairleigh Dickinson University Press.

Frost, Lawrence
1964 *The Custer Album*. Seattle, Wash.: Superior Publishing.

Gage, T. B.
2005 "Are Modern Environments Really Bad for Us?: Revisiting the Demographic and Epidemiologic Transitions." *Yearbook of Physical Anthropology* 48:96–117.

Garlington, E. A.
1896 "The Seventh Regiment of Cavalry." In *The Army of the United States*, ed. T. F. Rodenbough and W. L. Haskin, 251–67. New York: Maynard, Merrill and Company.

Giesbrecht, Gordon G., and James A. Wilkerson
2006 *Hypothermia, Frostbite and Other Cold Injuries: Prevention, Survival, Rescue and Treatment*. 2nd ed. Seattle, Wash.: Mountaineers Books.

Gillett, Mary C.
1989 "United States Military Surgeons and the Big Horn-Yellowstone Expedition of 1876." *Montana: The Magazine of Western History* 39(1):16–27.
1995 *The Army Medical Department 1865–1917*. Washington, D.C.: U.S. Government Printing Office.

Goff, Alaina K.
n.d. *Report of Skeletal Remains Excavated at Fort Craig Post Cemetery, Fort Craig Project, New Mexico, Upper Colorado Region*. Albuquerque, N.Mex.: Bureau of Reclamation.

Goode, Erica
2009 "After Combat, Victims of an Inner War." *New York Times* August 1, 2009, A1.

Gove, Philip Babcock (editor)
2002 *Webster's Third New International Dictionary of the English Language: Unabridged*. Springfield, Mass.: Merriam Webster.

Gray, John
1976 *Centennial Campaign: The Sioux War of 1876*. Fort Collins, Colo.: Old Army Press.

Green, Samuel, and Neil J. Salkind
2010 *Using SPSS for Windows and Macintosh: Analyzing and Understanding Data*. Boston: Prentice Hall.

Greene, Jerome
1981 "The Composite Army Bunk." *Military Collector and Historian* 33(3):103–107.
2008 *Washita: The U.S. Army and the Southern Cheyennes, 1867–1869*. Norman: University of Oklahoma.
2014 *American Carnage: Wounded Knee, 1890*. Norman: University of Oklahoma Press.

Greene, Jerome A. (editor)
1993 *Battles and Skirmishes of the Great Sioux War, 1876–1877: The Military View*. Norman: University of Oklahoma Press.

Grossman, D.
1996 *On Killing*. Boston: Little, Brown and Company.
2000 "The Morality of Bombing: Psychological Responses to "Distant Punishment." Warrior Science Group: www.killology.com/art_bombing.htm.

Gurda, J.
2006 *The Making of Milwaukee*. 3rd ed. Brookfield, Wisc.: Milwaukee County Historical Society.

Haines, Michael R.
2000 "The White Population of the United States, 1790–1920." In *A Population History of North America*, ed. Michael R. Haines and Richard H. Steckel, 305–69. Cambridge: Cambridge University Press.

Hanson, Jeff, and David H. Greenwald
2004 *Fort Craig Post Cemetery Report, Socorro County, New Mexico*. Albuquerque, N.Mex.: Bureau of Reclamation.

Harstad, Peter T.
1960 "Sickness and Disease on the Wisconsin Frontier: Malaria, 1820–1850." *Wisconsin Magazine of History* 43(2):83–96.

Hedren, Paul L.
2011 *Great Sioux War Orders of Battle, How the United States Army Waged War on the Northern Plains, 1876–1877*. Norman: University of Oklahoma Press.

Hess, Earl J.
1997 *The Union Soldier in Battle: Enduring the Ordeal of Combat*. Lawrence: University of Kansas Press.

Higgins, Rosanne L.
2003 "Children of the Poor: Infant Mortality in the Erie County Almshouse during the Mid-Nineteenth Century." In *Human Biologists in the Archives: Demography, Health, Nutrition and Genetics in Historical Populations*, ed. Ann Herring and Alan C. Swedlund, 78–95. New York: University of Cambridge Press.

Hoeprich, Paul D. (editor)
1977 *Infectious Diseases: A Modern Treatise of Infectious Processes*. Hagerstown, Md.: Harper and Row.

Hoig, Stan
1979 *The Battle of the Washita*. Lincoln: University of Nebraska Press, Lincoln.

Holmes, Oliver Wendell
1860 "Currents and Countercurrents in Medical Science: An Address Delivered before the Massachusetts Medical Society at the Annual Meeting, May 30, 1860." In *Medical Essays*, 121–44. Whitefish, Mont.: Kessinger Publishing.

Hyams, K. C., F. S. Wignall, and R. Roswell
1996 "War Syndromes and Their Evaluation: From the U.S. Civil War to the Persian Gulf War." *Annals of Internal Medicine* 125(5):398–405.

International Statistical Classification of Diseases and Related Health Problems
See World Health Organization.

Jackson, Stanley W.
1986 *Melancholia and Depression: From Hippocratic Times to Modern Times*. New Haven, Mass.: Yale University Press.

Jensen, Richard E., R. Eli Paul, and John E. Carter
1991 *Eyewitness at Wounded Knee*. Lincoln: University of Nebraska Press.

Johnson, Eric S.
2012 *No Greater Calling: A Chronological Record of Sacrifice and Heroism during the Western Indian Wars, 1865–1898*. Atglen, Pa.: Schiffer Publishing.

Jones, Edgar
2006 "Historical Approaches to Post Combat Disorders." *Philosophical Transactions of the Royal Society* B, 361:533–42.

Jones, Edgar, Robert Hodgins-Vaermaas, Helen McCrartney, Brian Everitt, Charlotte Beech, Denise Poynter, Ian Palmer, Kenneth Hymas, and Simon Wessely
2002 "Post-Combat Syndromes from the Boer War to the Gulf War: A Cluster Analysis of Their Nature and Attribution." *British Medical Journal* 324:1–7.

Jones, Edgar, and Simon Wessely
2001 "Psychiatric Battle Casualties: An Intra- and Interwar Comparison." *British Journal of Psychiatry* 178:242–47.

Kaplan, Bernice A.
1988 "Migration and Disease." In *Biological Aspects of Human Migration*, ed. C. G. N. Mascie-Taylor and G. W. Lasker, 216–45. Cambridge: Cambridge University Press.

Kautz, August V.
2001 *The 1865 Customs of Service for Non-Commissioned Officers and Soldiers*. Mechanicsburg, Pa.: Stackpole Books.

Originally published in 1865 as *Customs of Service for Non-Commissioned Officers and Soldiers as Derived from Law and Regulations Practiced in the Army of the United States*. Philadelphia, Pa.: J. B. Lippincott.

Kinsley, Maxine Schuurmans
2007 *Roots in Dakota Soil: Prairie Cemeteries of Bon Homme County, South Dakota*. Sioux Falls, S.D.: Pine Hill Printery.

Knapik, Joseph J., Michelle Canham-Chervak, Keith Hauret, Mary Jo Laurin, Edward Hoedebecke, Stephen Craig, and Scott J. Montain
2002 "Seasonal Variation in Injury Rates during US Army Basic Combat Training." *Annals of Occupational Hygiene* 46(1):15–23.

Knudson, Ronald J.
1993 "Emphysema." In *The Cambridge History of Human Disease*, ed. Kenneth F. Kiple, 706–708. New York: Cambridge University Press.

Komlos, John
1984 "The Height and Weight of West Point Cadets: Dietary Change in Antebellum America." *Journal of Economic History* 47:897–927.
1989 *Nutrition and Economic Development in the Eighteenth-Century Habsburg Monarchy: An Anthropometric History*. Princeton, N.J.: Princeton University Press.

Kraft, Louis
1995 *Custer and the Cheyennes*. El Segundo, Calif.: Upton and Sons.

Kramer, Howard D.
1948 "Effect of the Civil War on the Public Health Movement." *Mississippi Valley Historical Review* 35(3):449–62.

Larkin, Scott
2011 Personal communication, February 24, 2011. Fort Abraham Lincoln Foundation, Mandan, N.Dak.

Larrey, Dominique Jean
1814 *Memoirs of Military Surgery, and Campaigns of the French Armies, on the Rhine, in Corsica, Catalonia, Egypt, and Syria; at Boulogne, Ulm, and Austerlitz; in Saxony, Prussia, Poland, Spain, and Austria*. Baltimore, Md.: Joseph Cushing.

Last, John
1963 "The Iceberg: Completing the Clinical Picture in General Practice." *Lancet* 6 (July):28–31.

Leavitt, J. W.
1978 "Politics and Public Health: Smallpox in Milwaukee, 1894–1895." In *Sickness and Health in America: Readings in the History of Medicine and Public Health*, ed. J. W. Leavitt and R. L. Numbers, 403–13. Madison: University of Wisconsin Press.
1982 *The Healthiest City: Milwaukee and the Politics of Health Reform*. Princeton, N.J.: Princeton University Press.

Leckie, William H.
1963 *The Military Conquest of the Southern Plains*. Norman: University of Oklahoma Press.

Lee, Everett S.
1966 *A Theory of Migration*. Philadelphia: University of Pennsylvania Press.

Lipsky, M. S., and L. K. Sharp
2001 "From Idea to Market: The Drug Approval Process." *Journal of the American Board of Family Medicine* 14(5):362–67.

Liston, Maria A., and Brenda J. Baker
1995 "Trauma in Eighteenth-Century Military Remains at Fort William Henry." *American Journal of Physical Anthropology*, Supplement 20:135–36.
1996 "Reconstructing the Massacres at Fort William Henry, New York." *International Journal of Osteoarchaeology* 6:28–44.

Little, Michael A., and Paul T. Baker
1988 "Migration and Adaptation." In *Biological Aspects of Human Migration*, ed. C. G. N. Mascie-Taylor and G. W. Lasker, 167–215. Cambridge: Cambridge University Press.

MacLean, French L.
2011 *Custer's Best: the Story of Company M, 7th Cavalry at the Little Bighorn*. Alglen, Pa.: Schiffer Publishing.

Marlowe, D. H.
2000 "Psychological and Psychosocial Consequences of Combat and Deployment with Special Emphasis on the Gulf War." RAND: www.rand.org/pubs/monograph_reports/MR1018z11.html.

Mascie-Taylor, C. G. N., and G. W. Lasker (editors)
1988 *Biological Aspects of Human Migration*. Cambridge: Cambridge University Press.

Mattison, Ray H.
1954 "The Army Posts on the Northern Plains, 1865–1885." *Nebraska History* 35:17–44.

Mays, B., A. Parfitt, and M. J. Hershman
1994 "Treatment of Arrow Wounds by Nineteenth Century USA Army Surgeons." *Journal of the Royal Society of Medicine* 87:102–103.

McChristian, Douglas C.
1995 *The U.S. Army in the West, 1870–1880*. Norman: University of Oklahoma Press.
2007 *Uniforms, Arms, and Equipment: The U.S. Army on the Western Frontier, 1880–1892*. Norman: University of Oklahoma Press.

McCullough, Kathleen (editor)
1982 *Dorland's Pocket Medical Dictionary*. 23rd ed. Philadelphia, Pa.: W. Saunders Company.

McDermott, John D.
1997 "Were They Really Rogues? Desertion in the Nineteenth-Century U.S. Army." *Nebraska History* 78(4):165–74.

McDonald, M. A.
1958 "Treatment of Tonsillitis: A Therapeutic Trial of Phenoxymethyl Penicillin in a Food-Borne Epidemic of Tonsillitis." *British Medical Journal* 1:537–39.

McDowall, David, Colin Loftin, and Matthew Pate
2012 "Seasonal Cycles in Crime and Their Variability." *Journal of Quantitative Criminology* 28(3):389–410.

Miles, Nelson A.
1969 *Personal Recollections and Observations of General Nelson A. Miles*. New York: De Capo Press.

Milwaukee Health Department (MHD)
1876–77 *10th Annual Report of the Board of Health of the City of Milwaukee*. Milwaukee, Wisc.: Bray Brothers.
1877–78 *11th Annual Report of the Board of Health of the City of Milwaukee*. Milwaukee, Wisc.: Bray Brothers.
1892–93 *16th Annual Report of the Commissioner of Health of the City of Milwaukee*. Milwaukee, Wisc.: Edward Keogh Press.
1899–1900 *23rd Annual Report of the Commissioner of Health of the City of Milwaukee*. Milwaukee, Wisc.: Westlake, Delahunt and Smith Company.
1907 *31st Annual Report of the Commissioner of Health of the City of Milwaukee*. Milwaukee, Wisc.: Edward Keogh Press.

1912 *35th Annual Report of the Commissioner of Health of the City of Milwaukee.* Milwaukee, Wisc.: Bureau of Education and Publications of the Health Department.

Mitchell, Piers D.
2011 "Retrospective Diagnosis and the Use of Historical Texts for Investigating Disease in the Past." *International Journal of Paleopathology* 1:81–88.

Mokyr, J., and C. O. Grada
1994 "The Height of the British and the Irish c. 1800–1815: Evidence from Recruits to the East India Company's Army." In *Stature, Living Standards, and Economic Development: Essays in Anthropometric History*, ed. J. Kolmos, 39–59. Chicago: University of Chicago Press.

Murphy, James V., Paul E. Banwell, Anthony H. N. Roberts, and D. Angus McGrouther
2000 "Frostbite: Pathogenesis and Treatment." *Journal of Trauma: Injury, Infection and Critical Care* (January):171–78.

Murphy, Lawrence R.
1985 "The Enemy among Us: Venereal Disease among Union Soldier in the Far West." *Civil War History* 31(3):257–69.

National Institute of Health
2009 "PTSD: A Growing Epidemic." *NIH: The Magazine* 4(1):10–14.

National Institute of Mental Health
n.d. "Post–Traumatic Stress Disorder (PTSD)." www.nimh.nih.gov/health/topics/post-traumatic-stress-disorder-ptsd/index.shtml.

Nichols, Ronald H. (ed.)
2000 *Men with Custer: Biographies of the 7th Cavalry.* Hardin, Mont.: Custer Battlefield Historical and Museum Association.

Olch, Peter D.
1982 "Medicine in the Indian Fighting Army, 1866–1890." *Journal of the West* 21:32–41.

Omran, A. R.
1977 "Epidemiological Transition in the U.S." *Population Bulletin* 32:1–42.

Ortner, Donald J.
2003 *Identification of Pathological Conditions in Human Skeletal Remains.* 2nd ed. Amsterdam, Netherlands: Academic Press.

Otis, George Alexander

1871 *A Report of the Surgical Cases Treated in the Army of the United States from 1865 to 1871*. Washington, D.C.: Government Printing Office.

Owsley, Douglas W.

1994 *Bioarchaeology on a Battlefield: The Abortive Confederate Campaign in New Mexico*. Museum of New Mexico Office of Archaeological Studies, Archaeology Notes 142.

Owsley, Douglas W., and Karin S. Bruwelheide

2008 "Cranial Trauma in Historic Period Central and Northern Plains Indians." In *Skeletal Biology and Bioarchaeology of the Northwestern Plains*, ed. G. W. Gill and R. L. Weathermon, 212–25. Salt Lake City: University of Utah Press.

Parillo, Vincent N.

2003 *Strangers to These Shores: Migration to US*. 7th ed. Boston: Allyn and Bacon.

Persian Wars: The Battle of Marathon

2009 www.thenagain.info/Classes/Sources/Herodotus-Marathon.html.

Pfeiffer, Susan, and Ronald F. Williamson (editors)

1991 *Snake Hill: An Investigation of a Military Cemetery from the War of 1812*. Toronto, Canada: Dundurn.

Phillips, Shawn M.

2003 "Worked to the Bone: The Biomechanical Consequences of 'Labor Therapy' at a Nineteenth Century Asylum." In *Human Biologists in the Archives: Demography, Health, Nutrition and Genetics in Historical Populations*, ed. D. Ann Herring and Alan C. Swedlund, 96–129. New York: University of Cambridge Press.

Pohanka, Brian

1983 *A Summer on the Plains, 1870: From the Diary of Annie Gibson Roberts*. Mattituck, N.Y.: J. M. Carroll.

1989 "In Hospital at West Point: Medical Records of Cadets who Later Served with the Seventh Cavalry." *Little Big Horn Associates Newsletter* 23(4):5–7.

Portes, Alejandro, and Ruben G. Rumbault

2006 *A Portrait of Immigration in America*. 3rd ed. Berkeley: University of California Press.

Post, Peter W., Farrington Daniels, Jr., and Robert T. Binford, Jr.

1975 "Cold Injury and the Evolution of 'White' Skin." *Human Biology* 47(1):65–80.

Powell, Mary Lucas, and Della Collins Cook
2005 "Treponematosis." In *The Myth of Syphilis: The Natural History of Trepanematosis in North America*, ed. M. L. Powell and D. C. Cook, 9–62. Gainesville: University Press of Florida.

Powers, Rod
2005 "U.S. Military Desertion Military Rates." usmilitary.about.com/od/justicelawlegislation/a/desertionrates.htm.

Progulske, Donald R., and Frank J. Shideler
n.d. *Following Custer.* Bulletin 674 Agricultural Experiment Station. Brookings: South Dakota State University.

Rathbun, Ted A., and Steven D. Smith
1997 "Folly Island: An African-American Union Brigade Cemetery in South Carolina." In *In Remembrance: Archaeology and Death*, ed. David A. Poirier and Nicholas F. Bellantoni, 65–77. Westport, Conn.: Bergin and Garvey.

Ratliff, E. A.
1993 "Resaca de la Palma (41CF3): A Mass Grave from the Mexican-American War." *American Journal of Physical Anthropology* Supplement 16:162.

Ravenholt, R. T.
1993 "Encephalitis Lethargica." In *The Cambridge History of Human Disease*, ed. Kenneth F. Kiple, 708–12. New York: Cambridge University Press.

Reimers, David M.
2005 *Other Immigrants: The Global Origins of the American People.* New York: New York University Press.

Richards, P. B., and M. W. Kastell
1993 *Archaeological Excavations at the Almshouse Burial Ground, Milwaukee County Poorhouse, Wauwatosa, Wisconsin.* Reports of Investigation No. 333, Great Lakes Archaeological Research Center.

Rickey, Don
1963 *Forty Miles a Day on Beans and Hay: The Enlisted Soldier Fighting the Indian Wars.* Norman: University of Oklahoma Press.

Roberts, Gary L.
1976 "Violence and the Frontier Tradition." In *Kansas and the West*, ed. F. R. Blackburn, 96–111. Topeka: Kansas State Historical Society.

Robertson, Leon S.
1998 *Injury Epidemiology: Research and Control Strategies.* 2nd ed. New York: Oxford University Press.

Schneider, James V.
1988 *An Enigma Named Noonan*. Fort Wayne, Ind.: Privately published by the author.

Schroeder-Lein, Glenna R.
2008 *The Encyclopedia of Civil War Medicine*. Armonk, N.Y.: M. E. Sharpe.

Sciulli, Paul W., and Richard M. Gramly
1989 "Analysis of the Ft. Laurens, Ohio, Skeletal Sample." *American Journal of Physical Anthropology* 80:11–24.

Scott, Douglas D., Peter Bleed, and Stephen Damm
2013 *Custer, Cody and the Grand Duke: Camp Alexis and the Royal Buffalo Hunt in Nebraska*. Norman: University of Oklahoma Press.

Scott, Douglas, Melissa Connor, and Clyde Snow
1988 "Nameless Faces of Custer Battlefield." *Greasy Grass* 4:2–4.

Scott, Douglas, and Douglas Owsley
1991 "Oh, What Tales Bones Could Tell—and Often Do!" *Greasy Grass* 7:33–39.

Scott, Douglas D., and Clyde Collins Snow
1991 "Archaeology and Forensic Anthropology of the Human Remains from the Reno Retreat Crossing." *In Papers on Little Bighorn Battlefield Archeology: The Equipment Dump, Marker 7, and the Reno Crossing*, ed. Douglas D. Scott, 207–32. Reprints in Anthropology, vol. 42. Lincoln, Nebr.: J & L Reprint Company.

Scott, Douglas D., and P. Willey
1996 "Custer's Men Took Names to Their Graves: Experts Match Skeletons with Identities." *Greasy Grass* 12:20–28.

Scott, Douglas D., P. Willey, and Melissa A. Connor
1998 *They Died with Custer: Soldiers' Bones from the Battle of the Little Bighorn*. Norman: University of Oklahoma Press.

Sledzik, Paul S., and Peer H. Moore-Jansen
1991 "Dental Disease in 19th Century Military Skeletal Samples." In *Advances in Dental Anthropology*, ed. Mack A. Kelley and Clark Spencer Larsen, 215–24. New York: Wiley-Liss.

Sledzik, Paul S., and Lars G. Sandberg
2002 "The Effects of Nineteenth-Century Military Service on Health." In *The Backbone of History*, ed. Richard H. Steckel and Jerome C. Rose, 185–207. New York: Cambridge University Press.

Smith, Dale C.
1982 "The Rise and Fall of Typhomalarial Fever: I. Origins." *Journal of the History of Medicine and Allied Sciences* 37(2):182–220.

Smith, Stephen
1863 *Handbook of Surgical Operations*. New York: Balliere Brothers. Reprinted in 2009: LaVergne, Tenn.: Kessinger Publishing.

Snow, Clyde Collins, and John Fitzpatrick
1989 "Human Osteological Remains from the Battle of the Little Bighorn." In *Archaeological Perspectives on the Battle of the Little Bighorn*, ed. Douglas D. Scott, Richard A. Fox, Jr., Melissa A. Connor, and Dick Harmon, 243–82. Norman: University of Oklahoma Press.

Stallard, Patricia Y.
1978 *Glittering Misery: Dependents of the Indian Fighting Army*. Fort Collins, Colo.: Old Army Press.

Starr, Paul
1982 *The Social Transformation of American Medicine*. New York: Basic Books.

Statistical Package for the Social Sciences (SPSS)
2008 SPSS Statistics for Windows, Version 17.0. Chicago: SPSS.
2009 PASW Statistics for Windows, Version 18.0. Chicago: SPSS.
2011 SPSS Statistics for Windows, Version 20.0. Armonk, N.Y.: IBM Corporation.

Steegman, A. T., Jr.
1985 "18th Century British Military Stature: Growth Cessation, Selective Recruiting, Secular Trends, Nutrition at Birth, Cold, and Occupation." *Human Biology* 57:77–95.
1986 "Skeletal Stature Compared to Archival Stature in Mid-Eighteenth Century America: Ft. William Henry." *American Journal of Physical Anthropology* 71:431–35.

Steegman, A. T., Jr., and P. A. Haseley
1988 "Stature Variation in the British American Colonies: French and Indian War Records, 1755–1763." *American Journal of Physical Anthropology* 75:413–21.

Stevenson, Joan Nabseth
2012 *Deliverance from the Little Bighorn: Doctor Henry Porter and Custer's Seventh Cavalry*. Norman: University of Oklahoma Press.
Stewart, Edgar I.
1955 *Custer's Luck*. Norman: University of Oklahoma Press.
1972 "The Custer Battle and Widow Weeds." *Montana Magazine* 22(1):22–59.
Still, B.
1948 *Milwaukee: The History of a City*. Madison: Historical Society of Wisconsin.
Swedlund, Alan C., and D. Ann Herring
2003 "Human Biologists in the Archives: Demography, Health, Nutrition and Genetics in Historical Populations." In *Human Biologists in the Archives: Demography, Health, Nutrition and Genetics in Historical Populations*, ed. D. Ann Herring and Alan C. Swedlund, 1–10. New York: University of Cambridge Press.
Tate, Michael L.
1999 *The Frontier Army in the Settlement of the West*. Norman: University of Oklahoma Press.
Thatcher, Richard W., Ward T. McCraney, Douglas S. Kellogg, and William H. Whaley
1969 "Asymptomatic Gonorrhea." *Journal of the American Medical Association* 210(2):315–17.
Toynbee, Joseph
1860 *The Diseases of the Ear: Their Nature, Diagnosis, and Treatment*. London: Goodale Press.
Trampuz, Andrej, Matjaz Jereb, Igor Muzlovic, and Rajesh M. Prabhu
2003 "Clinical Review: Severe Malaria." *Critical Care* 7(4):315–23.
Trostle, James A.
1986 "Early Works in Anthropology and Epidemiology: From Social Medicine to the Germ Theory, 1840–1920." In *Anthropology and Epidemiology*, ed. C. Janes, R. Stall, and S. Gifford, 35–57. Dordrecht, Nederlands: Reidel Publishing Company.
U.S. Army Regulations
1881 *Regulations of the Army of the United States and General Orders in Force on the 17th of February, 1881*. Washington D.C.: Government Publishing Office.

U.S. Census Bureau
1872 *The Statistics of the Population of the United States, Embracing the Tables of Races, Nationality, Sex, Selected Ages and Occupations*. F. A. Walker, Superintendent of Census. Washington, D.C.: Government Publishing Office.
2012 "Transportation: Motor Vehicle Accidents." *Statistical Abstract of the United States*. www.census.gov/compendia/statab/cats/transportation/motor_vehicle_accidents_and_fatalities.html. Washington D.C.: Government Publishing Office.

Utley, Robert
1963 *Last Days of the Sioux Nation*. New Haven, Conn.: Yale University Press.
1967 *Frontiersmen in Blue: The United States Army and the Indian, 1848–1865*. New York: Macmillan and Company.
1973 *Frontier Regulars: The U.S. Army and the Indian, 1866–1890*. New York: Macmillan and Company.
1988 *Cavalier in Buckskin: George Armstrong Custer and the Western Military Frontier*. Norman: University of Oklahoma Press.

Utley, Robert M. (editor)
1977 *Life in Custer's Cavalry: Diaries and Letters of Albert and Jennie Barnitz, 1867–1868*. Lincoln: University of Nebraska Press.

Vestal, Stanley
1996 *The Missouri*. Lincoln, Nebr.: Bison Books.

Vilensky, Joel A., Paul Foley, and Sid Gilman
2007 "Children and Encephalitis Lethargica: A Historical Review." *Pediatric Neurology* 37(2):79–84.

Vogel, Steve
2013 "PTSD in the Spotlight at White House Medal of Honor Ceremony." *Washington Post*, August 26, 2013. http://www.washingtonpost.com/blogs/federal-eye/wp/2013/08/26/ptsd-in-the-spotlight-at-white-house-medal-of-honor-ceremony/.

Waldron, Tony
1994 *Counting the Dead: The Epidemiology of Skeletal Populations*. Chichester, U.K.: John Wiley and Sons.

Walker, L. G.
2008 *Dr. Henry R. Porter: The Surgeon Who Survived Little Big Horn*. Jefferson, N.C.: McFarland and Company.

Warner, John Harley
1997 *The Therapeutic Perspective: Medical Practice, Knowledge, and Identity in America, 1820–1885*. Princeton, N.J.: Princeton University Press.

Weathermon, Rick L.
2008 "Those Left Behind: An Analysis of Western Pioneer-Era Burials." In *Skeletal Biology and Bioarchaeology of the Northwestern Plains*, ed. G. W. Gill and R. L. Weathermon, 104–27. Salt Lake City: University of Utah Press.

Weddon, William, and Marion Huseas
1984 "Shocking 'Mrs.' Nash." *True West* 31(3):19–21, 59–60.

Welsh, Jack D.
2005 *Medical Histories of Union Generals*. Kent, Ohio: Kent State University Press.

Wengert, James W.
1997 "The Contract Surgeon." *Journal of the West* 36(1):67–76.

Wescott, Daniel J., Lori Baker, D. Clark Wernecke, and Michael B. Collins
2012 "A Mass Grave of Mexican Soldiers from the Resaca de la Palma Battlefield (41CF3): Demography and Battle-Related Injuries." *Bulletin of Texas Archaeological Society* 83:1–21.

White, Samuel S.
1995 *Samuel S. White Catalogue of Dental Instruments and Equipment*. San Francisco, Calif.: Norman Publishing.

Wiche, Sandra
2006 "Battle of the Little Bighorn Campaign Weather." Unpublished MS, National Weather Service, Bismarck, N.Dak.

Wier, James A.
1980 "19th Century Doctors on the Frontier and in Nebraska." *Nebraska History* 61:192–214.

Wilkerson, James A. (ed.)
1985 *Medicine for Mountaineering*. Seattle, Wash.: Mountaineers.

Willey, P.
1997 "Osteological Analysis of Human Skeletons Excavated from the Custer National Cemetery." Technical Report 5. Midwest Archeological Center, National Park Service, Lincoln, Nebr.

Willey, P., Amanda Blanchard, Richard A. Glenner, Thomas D. Holland, and Douglas D. Scott
2003 "A Case of Mistaken Identity" (letter to the editor). *Journal of the American Dental Association* 134:1307.

Willey, P., Amanda Blanchard, Thomas D. Holland, and Douglas D. Scott
2004 "A Case of Mistaken Identity: Skeleton in Custer National Cemetery No Longer Believed to Be Corporal Lell." *Greasy Grass* 20:16–21.

Willey, P., Richard L. Glenner, and Douglas D. Scott
1996 "Oral Health of Seventh Cavalry Troopers: Dentitions from the Custer National Cemetery." *Journal of the History of Dentistry* 44(1):3–14.

Willey, P., Paulette Leach, and Deanna Grimstead
1999 "Analysis of Human Bones Attributed to the Civil War Battle of Wilson's Creek: Kerr-Glidwell and Manion's Auction Collections." Midwest Archeological Center, National Park Service, Lincoln, Nebr.

Willey, P., Daniel Tyree, Nicole Cavales, and Douglas D. Scott
2003 "Analysis of Human Bones from the Civil War Battle of Wilson's Creek: Bray's Collection from the Sinkhole." Midwest Archeological Center, National Park Service, Lincoln, Nebr.

Williams, Guy
1981 *The Age of Miracles: Medicine and Surgery in the Nineteenth Century*. London: Constable and Company.

Wilson, Mary E., and Lin H. Chen
2008 "Travel." In *The Social Ecology of Infectious Diseases*, ed. K. H. Mayer and H. F. Pizer, 17–49. London: Academic Press.

Winkler, Albert
2013 "The Germans in the Seventh U.S. Cavalry at the Battle of the Little Bighorn." *Greasy Grass* 29:10–20.

Wittke, Carl
1967 *We Who Built America: The Saga of the Immigrant*. Cleveland: Press of Case Western Reserve University.

Woodward, J. J.
1867 *Report on Epidemic Cholera in the Army of the United States during the Year 1866*. Surgeon General's Office Circular no. 5. Washington, D.C.: Government Printing Office.
1870 *The Medical and Surgical History of the War of the Rebellion*. Part 1, vol. 1, Medical History. Washington, D.C.: Government Printing Office.

Woodward, Joseph Janvier
2010 *The Hospital Steward's Manual: For the Instruction of Hospi-*

tal Stewards, Ward-Masters, and Attendants in Their Several Duties. Memphis, Tenn.: General Books.

World Health Organization

2012 *International Statistical Classification of Diseases and Related Health Problems* (ISCD; 10th revision, version 2012). http://apps.who.int/classifications/icd10/browse/2010/en.

Young, James Harvey

1961 *The Toadstool Millionaires: A Social History of Patent Medicines in America before Federal Regulation*. Princeton, N.J.: Princeton University Press.

Contributors

COLLEEN CHEVERKO, whose research interests include bioarchaeology and paleoepidemiology, is a doctoral student at Ohio State University.

KATIE COHAN teaches anthropology at Ashford University and assists on disaster relief and recovery projects. Her research interests lie in cultural and physical anthropology and historical studies.

PATRICK J. COLLISON, MD, has been a practicing otolaryngologist for the past thirty-three years and a clinical assistant professor of surgery at the University of South Dakota (USD) since 1995. He also has been involved in research and teaching in the Department of Anthropology and Sociology at USD since 2001.

BILLY MARKLAND is an avocational historian concentrating on the U.S. Army's experiences in the American West. He lives in Kansas City.

COLLEEN MILLIGAN is an assistant professor of anthropology at California State University, Chico. She has studied the Milwaukee County Institutional Grounds Cemetery skeletal collection and U.S. public health in the nineteenth and early twentieth century.

GARY PLANK retired from the Nebraska State Patrol Investigative Services Division and is currently an associate professor of forensic science at Nebraska Wesleyan University in Lincoln.

DOUGLAS D. SCOTT is retired from the National Park Service and is the author of the award-winning book *Uncovering History: Archaeological Investigations of the Little Bighorn*, published by the University of Oklahoma Press. He is currently an adjunct professor at Colorado Mesa University and the University of Nebraska–Lincoln.

P. WILLEY is a professor at Chico State and has studied skeletons from the Little Bighorn Battlefield since 1988.

KRISTINA ZARENKO obtained her master's degree from California State University at Chico and is now working toward her doctorate in anthropology at the University of South Carolina.

Index

References to illustrations appear in italic type; references to tables appear in italic type followed by t.